# The Complete Idiot's Reference Card

## Top-Five Nutrition List

1. Fill up on fresh fruit and veggies. They are loaded with nutrients and are naturally low in fat and calories.
2. Make it a habit to choose low-fat dairy. Low-fat milk, yogurts, and cheese supply protein and calcium—a key player for building and maintaining strong, healthy bones.
3. Stick with the lean sources of protein. Choose chicken breast, turkey breast, lean red meats, seafood and fish, egg whites, tofu, beans, and legumes.
4. Eat plenty of whole grain products. Breads, cereal, pasta, and rice provide B-vitamins and a lot of complex carbohydrates.
5. Take it easy on the fat and sugar. Limit your intake of fried foods, butter, margarine, cream, salad dressings, oils, sugars, soft drinks, rich desserts, candies, cakes, cookies, and so on.

## Top-Five Exercise Tips

1. Set realistic goals. Aim to look and feel your best, not somebody else's best.
2. Pace yourself. It's much better to consistently workout 3 times per week for 30 minutes each session than to come on strong with 2-hour sessions for 7 days straight and then drop out of sight for the next 2 months.
3. Vary your workouts. Don't get caught up in the same exercise routine day in, day out!
4. Keep yourself properly hydrated. Drink plenty of water before, during, and after exercising.
5. Make exercise fun and convenient, not a hassle. Do what works best for you and your schedule, whether it means joining a gym, buying home equipment, or simply walking home from work. If planned exercise is just not your thing, go ahead and break it up into three 10-minute bouts throughout the day; you'll still get the health benefits!

## Calories in Commonly Eaten Foods

| Food | Calories | Food | Calories |
|---|---|---|---|
| Bread (1 slice) | 67 | Low-fat fruit yogurt (1 cup) | 230 |
| Crackers (5) | 60 | Non-fat fruit yogurt (1 cup) | 140 |
| Bagel (1 medium) | 234 | Steak, lean (5 ounces) | 293 |
| Apple (1 medium) | 80 | Chicken breast (5 ounces) | 233 |
| Strawberries (1 cup) | 45 | Hot dog (with bun) | 294 |
| Banana (1 medium) | 105 | Hamburger (with bun) | 393 |
| Orange juice (1 cup) | 110 | Cheeseburger (with bun) | 520 |
| Broccoli (cooked, 1/2 cup) | 25 | Jelly beans (30) | 198 |
| Carrot (1 whole) | 31 | Chocolate chip cookies (3) | 158 |
| Corn (1/2 cup) | 67 | Soda (5 ounces) | 233 |
| 1% low-fat milk (1 cup) | 102 | Hot dog (with bun) | 294 |

## alpha books

tear here

# Calories Burned During Popular Exercises

The following list represents the approximate calories burned during 30 minutes of a particular activity. Notice that the more you weigh, the more you burn—simply because it takes more energy to move a heavier mass. Calculations were based on people weighing 130 pounds and 183 pounds.

|                              | 130 lbs | 183 lbs |                              | 130 lbs | 183 lbs |
|------------------------------|---------|---------|------------------------------|---------|---------|
| Aerobic dance (moderate)     | 183     | 255     | Skiing (moderate speed)      | 210     | 297     |
| Basketball                   | 243     | 345     | Swimming (slow crawl)        | 228     | 318     |
| Bicycling, 9.4 mph           | 177     | 249     | Swimming (breast stroke)     | 288     | 402     |
| Dancing (ballroom)           | 90      | 126     | Tennis, singles (moderate)   | 192     | 270     |
| Horseback riding (trotting)  | 195     | 273     | Volleyball (recreational)    | 90      | 126     |
| Jogging, 9-mile minutes      | 342     | 480     | Walking, 3.5 mph             | 153     | 213     |
| Jumping rope                 | 291     | 408     | Weight lifting, free weights | 150     | 213     |
| Mountain climbing            | 282     | 396     | Weight lifting, machines     | 165     | 231     |

# Nutrition and Fitness Health Directory

For your personal nutrition profile, visit Joy Bauer at www.joyofnutrition.com.

**American Dietetic Association (ADA)**
National Center for Nutrition and Dietetics (NCND)
216 West Jackson Blvd.
Chicago, IL 60606
**Consumer Nutrition Hotline**
800-366-1655
www.eatright.org

**American Heart Association**
National Center
7272 Greenville Ave.
Dallas, TX 75231-4596
800-AHA-USA1 (242-8721)
http://207.211.141.25

**American Cancer Society**
1599 Clifton Rd. NE
Atlanta, GA 30329
800-227-2345

**American Institute for Cancer Research**
1759 R St. NW
Washington, DC 20009
800-843-8114

**American Diabetes Association**
1660 Duke St.
Alexandria, VA 22314
800-DIABETES (342-2383)

**Arthritis Foundation Information Line**
1314 Spring St. NW
Atlanta, GA 30309
800-283-7800

**American College of Sports Medicine (ACSM)**
P.O. Box 1440
Indianapolis, IN 46206-1440
317-637-9200
www.acsm.org/sportsmed

**American Anorexia/Bulimia Association**
165 West 46th St.
Suite 1108
New York, NY 10036
212-575-6200

**Anorexia Nervosa and Associated Disorders (ANAD)**
P.O. Box 7
Highland Park, IL 60035
847-831-3438

**Celiac Disease Foundation**
13251 Ventura Blvd.
Suite 1
Studio City, CA 91604
818-990-2354

**The Food Allergy Network**
10400 Eaton Place
Suite 107
Fairfax, VA 22030
800-929-4040

**National Eating Disorders Organization**
Laureate Eating Disorder Unit
6655 South Yale Ave.
Tulsa, OK 74136
918-481-4044

**Vegetarian Resource Group**
P.O. Box 1463
Baltimore, MD 21203
410-366-VEGE
http://envirolink.org/arrs/VRG/home.html

**Monthly Newsletters**
Consumer Reports on Health
P.O. Box 52148
Boulder, CO 80322
800-234-2188

**Environmental Nutrition**
P.O. Box 420235
Palm Coast, FL 32142-0451
800-829-5384

**Nutrition Action Health Letter**
Center for Science in the Public Interest
1875 Connecticut Ave. NW
Suite 300
Washington, DC 20009
202-332-9110

**Tufts University Diet and Nutrition Letter**
P.O. Box 57857
Boulder, CO 80322-7857
800-274-7581
http://healthletter.tufts.edu

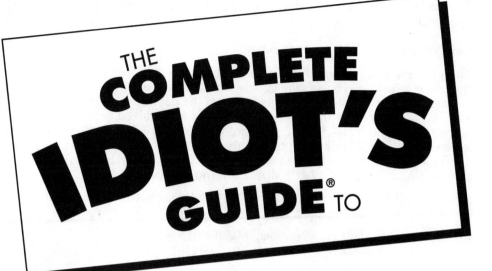

# Total Nutrition

*by Joy Bauer, M.S., R.D.*

## alpha
## books

A Pearson Education Company

*This book is dedicated to my husband, Ian, my daughter, Jesse, and my son, Cole, who are always there to make me smile.*

## Copyright © 1999 by Joy Bauer

International Standard Book Number: 0-02-862956-6
Library of Congress Catalog Card Number: 99-64168

03   02        8   7   6   5   4

Interpretation of the printing code: the rightmost number of the first series of numbers is the year of the book's printing; the rightmost number of the second series of numbers is the number of the book's printing. For example, a printing code of 99-1 shows that the first printing occurred in 1999.

*Printed in the United States of America*

## Alpha Development Team

**Publisher**
*Kathy Nebenhaus*

**Editorial Director**
*Gary M. Krebs*

**Managing Editor**
*Bob Shuman*

**Marketing Brand Manager**
*Felice Primeau*

**Acquisitions Editor**
*Jessica Faust*

**Development Editor**
*Phil Kitchel*
*Amy Zavatto*

**Assistant Editor**
*Georgette Blau*

## Production Team

**Development Editor**
*Phil Kitchel*

**Production Editor**
*Donna Wright*

**Copy Editor**
*Kris Simmons*

**Cover Designer**
*Mike Freeland*

**Photo Editor**
*Richard H. Fox*

**Illustrator**
*Jody P. Schaeffer*

**Book Designers**
*Scott Cook and Amy Adams of DesignLab*

**Indexer**
*Larry Sweazy*

**Layout/Proofreading**
*Angela Calvert*
*Mary Hunt*
*Julie Trippetti*

# Contents at a Glance

# Contents

**xiii**

# Foreword

As a society, we're bombarded with books on how to eat. Well, guess what? In spite of all the texts, we remain undernourished and overfat, and if you look at the latest statistics regarding overweight children, the future doesn't look much brighter. Obviously, we're in dire need of guidance.

As editor-in-chief of *Fit* magazine, I'm probably among the most bombarded with the afore-mentioned nutrition books. Most of them are either driven by an obsessive, unhealthy goal ("Become super-lean tomorrow!"), or suggest ideas like vegetarianism, food-combining, or high-protein-low-carb diets—ways of eating that aren't enjoyable, healthy or realistic for the average Jane.

That's why I'm a huge fan of this book's author, Joy Bauer. Her approach to nutrition is never trendy and is always rock-solid—her advice is consistently backed by the American Dietetic Association and the USDA Food Pyramid.

Yet, what makes Bauer a true treasure is her ability to get you, the reader, excited about nutrition and all it can do for you. Whether she's examining vitamins and minerals, explaining exactly how many carbs you need each day, or guiding you toward permanent weight loss, Bauer makes you *want* to learn about nutrition, which will fuel your desire to improve your own diet. And you won't have to worry about the facts in this book going out of style—as I said before, Bauer isn't trendy. She advocates proper, sensible nutrition, and shuns fads.

This is truly the only nutrition book anyone will ever need, because it is intensely thorough. It tells you exactly how much of what kinds of foods to eat every day, while giving you the facts about sodium, fiber, calcium, iron—Bauer even incorporates an excellent guide to exercise that is realistic and motivating, not overwhelming. I have access to countless nutritionists all over the world, yet I call Bauer whenever I have a question regarding food, diet, or weight loss, because I know I'm going to get the facts explained in an easy-to-understand and interesting way. Now that I have this book at my disposal, however, Bauer is going to hear from me a lot less often.

**—Lisa Klugman**

Lisa Klugman has worked at *Fit* magazine for the past eight years, working her way up from assistant to her present position of editor-in-chief, a position she has held for the past two-and-a-half years. Klugman shapes the magazine around her own personal health and fitness philosophy, which advocates the pursuit of fitness for sake of energy, pleasure, and self-care.

# Introduction

If you're confused by the enormous amount of nutrition information that bombards us on a daily basis—this book is for you! It provides a comprehensive guide to eating smart and becoming fit that's both up-to-date, trustworthy, and, most importantly, reader-friendly. It was written with both my personal and professional experiences in mind for people who want to slim down, bulk up, maintain good health, or just plain look and feel great.

## How to Use This Book

To make the reading easier for you, I've divided these pages into six areas of interest:

**Part 1, "Time for a Nutrition Tune-Up,"** clears up the confusion on the fundamentals of food. This section dissects the dietary guidelines and offers simple strategies to incorporate the five food groups into your life. You'll also get the inside scoop on simple to complex carbohydrates, the power of protein, and the relationship between excessive fat intake and heart disease. In addition, you'll examine the facts on fiber and salt, plus become well versed on the vital vitamins and minerals that your body requires.

**Part 2, "Making Savvy Food Choices,"** shows you that dining healthy does not mean giving up the pleasure of eating. In this section, you'll learn to become Sherlock Holmes in your grocery store—able to decode the nutrition information on product labels and make more informed food purchases. We'll take a trial run through the supermarket and load your cart with healthy food items to stock in your kitchen. You'll also find many easy-to make creative recipes—and personally learn to master the art of low-fat cooking. Further, I provide the best bets in most ethnic cuisines so you'll be ready to tackle any type of restaurant—*plus* you'll learn strategies for trimming down your holiday menus without losing taste or tradition.

**Part 3, "The ABCs of Exercise,"** provides you with the tools and inspiration to get moving and keep moving. That's right—a crash course on becoming physically fit. You'll hear the lowdown on strengthening your heart and lungs through aerobic exercise and tips to buff your bodacious physique through appropriate weight training and conditioning. You'll learn the importance of properly warming up, cooling down, and stretching your body, *plus* get the education you need to enter a gym with confidence. I also take a comprehensive look at sports nutrition and provide the skills you'll need to fuel your body for both casual exercise and competitive sport.

**Part 4, "Beyond the Basics: Nutrition for Special Needs,"** discusses a variety of hot topics within the world of nutrition. First, I discuss how diet can potentially reduce your risk of cancer and zoom in on the common culprits that trigger food allergies and other food sensitivities. I also present the latest scoop on herbal remedies and how they can help to conquer a bunch of bothersome ailments and offer sound information on vegetarian eating plans.

**Part 5, "Pregnancy and Parenting,"** provides essential information that will help you manage your and your growing baby's health. I discuss the importance of sound nutrition and offer specific food guidelines for a healthy pregnancy. You learn how much weight you should gain, the right foods to eat, and which foods to avoid. I also give you surefire tips to help get your kids to eat healthier. This section includes lower-fat after-school snack ideas, strategic ways to disguise vegetables, and tips to encourage more physical activity. I also address the college crowd and map out best bites in the campus dining hall, the real-deal on vending machines, late night munchies, alcohol and partying, and, of course, how to avoid those notorious "freshman 15" pounds of weight that seem to creep up on a lot of college students.

**Part 6, "Weight Management 101,"** provides you with a sensible plan of attack. Whether you want to lose weight, gain weight, or, most importantly, stop obsessing—this final section covers it all. I provide weight-loss programs to help knock off (and keep off) those extra unwanted pounds, along with calorie-cramming strategies to help you skinny folks beef up your bods. I also take a look at life-threatening eating disorders—and where to find help when food and exercise go beyond health and get way out of control.

## Extras

To help you get the most out of this book, I've sprinkled it with the following helpful information boxes.

**Q & A**

The questions we all want to ask and their answers.

**Food for Thought**

Follow these tips on eating and exercising to make everyday nutrition and fitness fun.

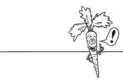

### Nutri-Speak

This box provides definitions of food and exercise jargon.

### Overrated—Undercooked

You should keep in mind these warnings when eating or exercising.

# Acknowledgments

Many thanks to the tremendous number of people who helped to pull this book together. First, let me extend my eternal gratitude to my extraordinary associate Lisa Mandelbaum, who provided her expertise and long hard work!

A special thanks to my great literary agent, Mitch Douglas, for making this book happen. Tremendous thanks to Jessica Faust for wrapping up the entire project and, of course, Phil Kitchel, Kris Simmons, and Donna Wright for their intense dedication on the editing and production end.

Thanks to Tom Gates and Ina for the great cover photo and thank you to Meredith Gunsberg for such delicious vegetarian recipes.

Sincere thanks (as usual) to Geralyn Coopersmith and Evan Spinks, two outstanding fitness consultants who shared their sense of humor and invaluable information. Thanks to Suki Hertz, a talented chef who provided great ideas and creative recipes in the holiday chapter. And a million thanks to Karen Robinowitz, a great writer and an exceptional person.

I am also grateful to many others who contributed to portions of this book, including Frances Aaron, Michael Simon, Elyse Sosin, M.A. R.D., Grace Leder, Meg Fein, Dany Levy, Candy Gulko, Jane Stern, Dr. Catharine Fedeli, and Dr. Susan Wagner.

On a personal note, I would like to extend a sincere thanks to my incredible parents, Ellen and Artie Schloss, who have always taught me that *anything* and *everything* is possible! My Grandma Martha, for sticking around to see my second edition published. "The gang": Debra, Steve, Ben, Glenn, Pam, Dan, Nancy, Jon, Camrin, Harley, Karen, Lisi, Lisa, and Jason. To my saviors on the fourth floor: Vivian, Mary, Cece, and Kiki. To Andrea Mendonca for being the wonderful person she is. My super in-laws, Carol and Vic, along with Grandma Mary and Grandpa Nat for their support and encouragement. And, most of all, my partners in crime, Ian, Jesse, and Cole!

# Part 1

# Time for a Nutrition Tune-Up

*After reading and listening to conflicting food advice from friends, relatives, and hairdressers, it's no wonder people are more confused than ever about what they should be eating.*

*This first part of the book proves that eating healthy does not need to be complicated or restrictive. In fact, it is quite the contrary. This section unravels the colorful Food Guide Pyramid and provides the inside scoop on carbohydrates, protein, fat, fiber, and salt. After grasping these fundamentals of food, you'll be ready to read further into the book and learn the specifics about everything you never understood or realized.*

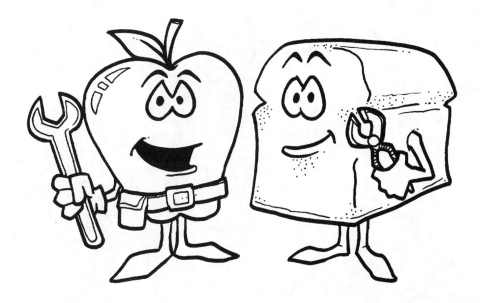

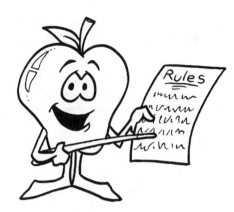

# Chapter 1

# The Dietary Guidelines

## In This Chapter

➤ Unraveling the Food Guide Pyramid

➤ Balancing your food groups

➤ Where do *calories* fit in?

➤ The keys to successful eating

➤ Scheduling time to fuel your body

After thumbing through hundreds of complicated nutrition articles and magazine ads, catching random food advice from friends and relatives, and listening warily to endless infomercials promising an instant bodacious bod, you're probably more confused than ever about what you should be eating.

*So what exactly should you be eating?* Believe it or not, healthy eating doesn't mean driving miles to some obscure health food store in search of organic produce. It also doesn't mean eating bean sprouts sprinkled with wheat germ for dinner (mm, mm). That's a relief, huh? In fact, according to nutrition experts, healthy eating is more basic than you think.

## Solving the Pyramid Puzzle

In 1992, the United States Department of Agriculture (USDA) created the *Food Guide Pyramid*, an updated version of the familiar basic four food groups that have been drilled into your head since the first grade. I'm sure you've seen this colorful Egyptian triangle on the packages of products in the grocery store and on the back of your favorite cereal box. This visual approach to nutrition, a general outline of what you should eat each day, makes healthy eating a lot less complicated. Although individuals vary in their specific requirements, the Food Guide Pyramid provides solid information on dos and don'ts for the general population.

The Food Guide Pyramid emphasizes eating a variety of foods from the five main food groups. (That's right: The USDA separated fruits and vegetables into two different groups.) It also limits the amount of fats, oils, and sweets in your diet. Here's the cast:

**Group 1:** Breads, cereal, rice, and pasta

**Group 2:** Vegetables

**Group 3:** Fruits

**Group 4:** Milk, yogurt, and cheese

**Group 5:** Meat, poultry, fish, dry beans, eggs, and nuts

# Food Guide Pyramid

## A Guide to Daily Food Choices

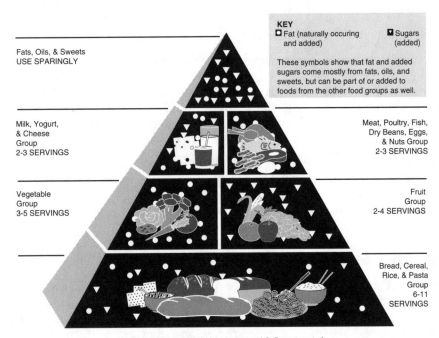

**KEY**
□ Fat (naturally occuring and added)    ◼ Sugars (added)

These symbols show that fat and added sugars come mostly from fats, oils, and sweets, but can be part of or added to foods from the other food groups as well.

Fats, Oils, & Sweets
USE SPARINGLY

Milk, Yogurt,
& Cheese
Group
2-3 SERVINGS

Meat, Poultry, Fish,
Dry Beans, Eggs,
& Nuts Group
2-3 SERVINGS

Vegetable
Group
3-5 SERVINGS

Fruit
Group
2-4 SERVINGS

Bread, Cereal,
Rice, & Pasta
Group
6-11
SERVINGS

Source: U.S. Department of Agriculture - U.S. Department of
Health and Human Services

Let's take a peek at how this model works:

1. **Breads, cereal, rice, and pasta group:** Foods that come from grains sit at the bottom of the pyramid, creating a foundation for building a healthy diet. This foundation provides vitamins and minerals, along with complex carbohydrates (also called carbs or carbos), which serve as an important source of energy. To add some fiber to your diet, eat whole grains whenever possible. USDA guidelines recommend 6–11 servings per day. That might sound like a lot, but serving sizes are deceptively small, so they add up quickly!

   One serving =

   1 slice of bread, or

   $1/2$ English muffin, or

   $1/2$ small bagel, or

   $1/2$ of a large pita bread, or

   1 small roll, or

   1 ounce (approx. $3/4$ cup) ready-to-eat cereal, or $1/2$ cup cooked cereal, rice, or pasta

2. **Vegetable group:** Depending on which ones you choose, veggies are loaded with vitamins and minerals, including vitamins A and C, folate, iron, magnesium, and several others. Vegetables are naturally low in calories and fat, plus packed with fiber (bonus!). USDA guidelines recommend 3–5 servings per day—but certainly you can never get enough.

   One serving = 1 cup of raw, leafy green vegetables, or

   $1/2$ cup cooked or chopped vegetables, or

   $3/4$ cup vegetable juice

3. **Fruit group:** Fruits and fruit juices are terrific sources of vitamins A and C and potassium. Eat whole fruits often: They are higher in fiber than juice. USDA guidelines recommend 2–4 servings per day.

   One serving = 1 medium fruit (apple, banana, orange), or

   $1/2$ mango, or

**Food for Thought**

Look how quickly the grains can add up; bet ya didn't know that...

A common pasta entree = 4–5 grain servings

A large New York bagel = 3–4 servings

A large hot pretzel = 3 servings

**Overrated—Undercooked**

When buying fruit juice, pay close attention to the wording on the juice containers; they might not be as healthy as they sound. For instance, "fruit drinks" and "fruit cocktails" generally contain a lot of added sugar with small amounts of real fruit juice. Instead of falling for these impostors, examine the label and select fruit beverages that contain "100% Fruit Juice."

1 cup of strawberries, blueberries, raspberries, or

³/₄ cup of fruit juice, or

¹/₂ cup chopped, canned, or cooked fruit, or

¹/₄ cup dried fruit, or

1 wedge of melon

4. **Milk, yogurt, and cheese group:** The hands-down winners of the calcium contest, these foods also provide protein and other vitamins and minerals. USDA guidelines recommend 2–3 servings per day—two for most people and three plus for teenagers, young adults under 24, and women who are pregnant or breastfeeding.

   One serving = 1 cup of milk or yogurt, or

   1¹/₂–2 ounces of cheese, or

   ¹/₂ cup ricotta cheese, or

   ³/₄ cup cottage cheese

5. **Meat, poultry, fish, dry beans, eggs, and nuts group:** Along with supplying substantial amounts of protein, this group contains B-vitamins, iron, and zinc. USDA guidelines recommend 2–3 servings per day, the equivalent of 5–7 ounces.

   One serving = 2–3 ounces of cooked lean meat, or

   2–3 ounces of cooked fish or skinless poultry, or

   Count ¹/₂ cup cooked beans, or 1 egg, or 2 tablespoons peanut butter as 1 ounce lean meat.

6. **Fats, oils, and sweets:** The tip of the pyramid is reserved for these "nutrient-free" foods. These spreads, oils, and sugary treats, known as "empty calories," literally offer nothing in the form of nutrition. Every shrewd dieter can tolerate a bit of these foods, but many of us eat far too much fat and sugar, forgetting the important groups that make up 99 percent of the pyramid's foundation. USDA guidelines recommend limiting your intake of salad dressings and oils, cream, butter, margarine, sugars, soft drinks, candies, and rich desserts.

### Food for Thought

Stock your fridge with low-fat dairy products. You'll still get all the good stuff (calcium, protein, and so on), but you'll get a lot less fat. Smart choices include 1% or skim milk, low-fat cheese and yogurts, reduced-fat or fat-free ice cream, or low-fat frozen yogurt.

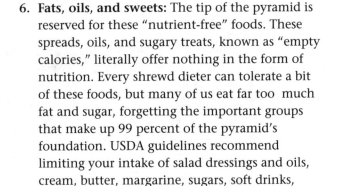

### Food for Thought

Although eggs are a good source of protein, the yolks contain high amounts of cholesterol. Limit your consumption of egg yolks to 3–4 per week. When you do eat eggs, get into the habit of using the egg substitutes (no cholesterol) or mix one whole egg with two or three whites.

# Where Do Calories Fit In?

Practically everyone over the age of 10 has heard the word "calorie"—but few actually understand how calories work in regard to their diets. For some reason, the word calorie gets a bad rap, when a calorie is simply the measurement of food as energy. The more calories you eat, the more energy you supply your body.

All the foods we eat contain calories, some more than others. Here's the ideal situation: *Take in the amount of food energy—calories—that your body needs. No more, no less.*

Although this is easier said than done, this tight-rope walk will help maintain a normal body weight. Unfortunately, it is quite easy to eat more calories than your body actually needs or burns, resulting in weight gain. On the other hand, taking in fewer calories than your body needs can result in weight loss.

**Nutri-Speak**

A **calorie** is the amount of energy food provides. The number of calories is determined by burning it in a device called a **calorimeter** and measuring the amount of heat produced. One calorie is equal to the amount of energy needed to raise the temperature of one liter of water one degree Celsius. Carbohydrates and protein contain 4 calories per gram, fat contains 9 calories per gram, and alcohol has 7 calories per gram.

# How Many Calories Are Right for You?

How can you find the perfect balance between calories in and calories out? Not by nit-picking over calorie counting, that's for sure! You *should* pay attention to what and how much you eat, but not to the point that you carry a calculator and whip it out after each bite of food.

To get a *rough* idea of how many calories you should be taking in, look at the following chart. This chart only offers three general caloric ranges, so keep in mind that your personal daily requirements might fall somewhere between two that are listed. Remember, everyone is different. Caloric intake will vary depending upon your age, sex, size, and level of activity. After you select the caloric amount that seems right for you, simply experiment with the various number of servings in each group (listed underneath your caloric level) until you find what feels most comfortable. You may even keep a food log for a week or so; this way, you can keep track of the groups you need to increase and those you might be overloading.

**Nutri-Speak**

**Sedentary** folks generally have desk jobs, watch a lot of TV, and tend to sit around most of the time. **Active** folks are constantly on the go. They do a lot of walking, taking the stairs, playing sports, or regularly working out.

## General Daily Calorie Requirements

| | |
|---|---|
| 1,600 calories | Number of calories needed for many sedentary women and some older adults. |
| 2,200 calories | Number of calories needed for most children, teenage girls, active women, and many sedentary men. Women who are pregnant and breastfeeding may need some-what more. |
| 2,800 calories | Number of calories needed for teenage boys, many active men, and some very active women. |

*Source: USDA 1992*

Remember that serving sizes are approximations, so a guess is fine. If you have no idea what a serving looks like, you might want to measure it out once or twice for a future comparison. For example, measure a serving of cooked pasta ($^1/_2$ cup) so that you are able to guesstimate that a restaurant entree is probably about 4–5 servings.

Now that you have an idea of how many calories you should be taking in daily, look at the following chart to determine how many servings of each group will be right for you. Keep in mind that these are only the servings for the five food groups—not the fats, oils and sweets.

| | 1,600 calories | 2,200 calories | 2,800 calories |
|---|---|---|---|
| Bread group servings | 6 | 9 | 11 |
| Vegetable group servings | 3 | 4 | 5 |
| Fruit group servings | 2 | 3 | 4 |
| Milk group servings | 2–3* | 2–3* | 2–3* |
| Meat group servings | 2 | 2–3 | 3 |

*With newly increased calcium requirements, all people will benefit from 3 daily servings of low-fat dairy.*

Here are some handy sample menus for each caloric level.

| | 1,600 calories | 2,200 calories | 2,800 calories |
|---|---|---|---|
| **Breakfast** | 1 bowl cereal | 3 pancakes | Bowl of cereal with raisins and low-fat milk |
| | 1 cup low-fat milk | 1 cup berries and some maple syrup | |
| | 1 slice toast with jam | | Large bagel with a smear of cream cheese |
| | | 1 cup low-fat milk | |
| | 1 banana | | Glass of orange juice |

|  | 1,600 calories | 2,200 calories | 2,800 calories |
|---|---|---|---|
| **Lunch** | Turkey breast (approx. 2–3 ounces) | Turkey burger on a roll (about 3 ounces) | Large salad with 1 cup lentils, small amount of oil and vinegar |
|  | 2 slices Swiss cheese | Green salad with vinaigrette | 1 slice of broccoli and cheese pizza |
|  | 2 slices whole wheat bread |  | 1 apple |
|  | Lettuce and tomato Carrot sticks |  |  |
| **Snack** | 1 apple | Medium frozen yogurt Banana | 2 fig bars Strawberry yogurt milkshake |
| **Dinner** | Salad with vinaigrette | Sliced tomato and mozzarella (try low-fat) | 1 dinner roll lightly stir-fried chicken (approx. 5 ounces)—with a lot of vegetables (approx. 2 cups) |
|  | Grilled fish (approx. 3 ounces) | Linguini (approx. 2 cups)—with shrimp (approx. 3 ounces)—and a lot of vegetables in marinara sauce |  |
|  | Rice (approx. 1 cup) |  | Brown rice (approx. 2 cups) |
|  | Broccoli with parmesan cheese | Wedge of melon | 1 orange |

*Adding more tip-of-the-pyramid foods (oil, margarine, dressings, and so on) will increase your daily calories.*

# The Keys to Successful Eating: Variety, Moderation, and Balance

Now that we've covered the daily food requirements, let's find out what kind of an eater you are. Are you one of those people who orders the exact *same* thing, in the *same* restaurant, day after day? Have you packed the same lunch to bring to work for the last 15 years? Or do you skip eating lunch altogether? Do you define the five food groups as McDonald's, Burger King, Pizza Hut, KFC, and Dunkin Donuts? If you answered "yes" to any of these questions, pay close attention to the next few paragraphs.

## Eating a Variety of Healthy Foods

First, understand why variety is important. Varying your food provides a much greater range of nutrients. Eating the same foods day after day supplies your body with the same exact vitamins and minerals over and over again. Although you might be consuming the recommended daily allowance of many beneficial vitamins and minerals, *you miss out on a lot of good stuff that your body needs.*

Furthermore, variety can make your meals much more interesting! Forget about those hum-drum standards; be adventurous!

➤ **Try new cookbooks.** Throw things together that you would have never dreamed of eating.

➤ **Give your palate a worldly kick.** Try a different ethnic restaurant or recipe each week.

➤ **Make a list...**of 20 different fruits, veggies, and grains, and try something new each day. Pick one day a week to create a meal that you've never had before. Your taste buds won't believe what they've been missing.

**Food for Thought**

All calories are not created equal! Although the following foods contain the same amount of calories, notice the difference in nutrition:

Package of licorice: 230 calories; 0 milligrams calcium; 0 protein; 0 IU vitamin D

8-ounce fruit yogurt: 230 calories; 350 milligrams calcium; 8 grams protein; 100 IU vitamin D

Opt for foods rich in nutrients.

## All Foods in Moderation

We need to place greater emphasis on healthy foods and downplay the not-so-healthy stuff. However, there is a place in *every* food plan for *all* kinds of foods (and let's face it—man cannot live on health food alone). Too many of us label high-fat, high-sugar foods as the enemy and, as a result, feel guilty when we allow ourselves to indulge. In fact, imposing too-strict limitations may actually cause people to react by overindulging. Remember, the tip on the pyramid indicates that you should *limit* fat and sugar—not *avoid* it completely.

Take care of your mind as well as your body: If you're absolutely crazy for chocolate cake, then you should have the pleasure of eating it once in a while. Obviously, you shouldn't eat high-fat foods all the time, but there is room for everything—*in moderation.* (People who have specific medical conditions such as heart disease, diabetes, food allergies, gastro-intestinal ailments, and so on might have to completely avoid certain foods altogether. Check with your doctor for more information.)

Eating in moderation also means controlling the *size* of your portions. Once you determine the number of servings that you should be eating from each food group, spread them throughout your daily meals. Proper planning will ensure that you are eating balanced meals in moderation and meeting your daily requirements.

## *Balancing Your Meals with Various Food Groups*

Many people eat excessive amounts of food from one group and completely forget about other groups that offer important vitamins and nutrients. For instance, have you ever watched someone (not *you*, of course) reach for a couple of rolls from the bread basket and then polish off a huge plate of pasta? The meal probably tasted delicious, but that's a lot of grain without much of anything else. What happened to the fruits, vegetables, protein, and dairy?

Once in a while, a meal like that is fine, but as a general rule, incorporate different food groups onto your plate at each meal. For example, choose a house salad, pasta with chicken and broccoli in marinara sauce, and some parmesan cheese. This balanced meal offers a significant amount of nutrition. All you need to do is strategize before throwing something on your plate, and aim for at least three food groups with each meal.

# Scheduling Time for Breakfast, Lunch, and Dinner

What kind of an eating schedule are you on? Do you make time in your day for breakfast, lunch, and dinner; or do you run on empty until dinner and then pig out from starvation? Everyone has his own eating regimen—some better than others. You should be fueling your body *throughout* the day when you need the energy.

## *Breakfast with a Bang*

You've heard it a million times: BREAKFAST IS IMPORTANT!

Think of your body as a car: It needs fuel to run properly. When you wake up from a good night's sleep, your body has been in fasting for about eight hours (if you're lucky enough to get that much sleep). "Break-fast" in the morning helps kick your system into gear by supplying food energy to your body. Without food, you feel tired and sluggish.

Incidentally, breakfast also helps you control your weight: Eating a smart breakfast can help regulate

**Food for Thought**

Eat a variety of foods.

Balance the foods you eat with physical activity to maintain or improve your weight.

Choose a diet low in fat, saturated fat, and cholesterol.

Choose a diet with plenty of grain products, vegetables, and fruits.

Choose a diet moderate in sugars, salt, and sodium.

If you drink alcoholic beverages, do so in moderation.

*\*Developed by the U.S. Departments of Agriculture and Health and Human Services, 1995*

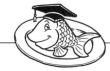

**Food for Thought**

Numerous studies have proven that breakfast eaters are more likely to be productive and attentive in the morning than non-breakfast eaters.

*Source: U.S. Departments of Agriculture and Health and Human Services*

your appetite throughout the day so you eat in moderation during lunch and dinner. Have you ever skipped breakfast to "save calories," only to find yourself so hungry by lunch that you overeat? So much for that diet. Start your day off smart: Schedule time for breakfast.

## Fueling Your Body All Day

Remember, breakfast alone just won't cut it. Your body needs to be constantly energized throughout the day to help keep you going. You don't necessarily have to eat the standard three square meals. In fact, some prefer six mini-meals (or constant snacking) each day. Do whatever works best for your schedule and eating style, but be sure that your daily food totals resemble the guidelines of the Food Guide Pyramid.

---

### The Least You Need to Know

➤ Make sure to eat a variety of foods from the five food groups.

➤ Don't get caught up with counting calories; it can drive you crazy! Simply focus on eating healthy foods in moderation.

➤ Get out of your food rut and be adventurous. Try new and exciting foods, recipes, and restaurants.

➤ Although the food pyramid allows for "some" fat and sugar intake, don't overdo it.

➤ Schedule time to fuel your body *throughout* the day. Food can help keep you alert, energetic, and focused.

---

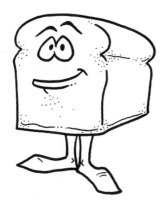

# Chapter 2

# A Close-Up on Carbohydrates

## In This Chapter

➤ What's a carbohydrate?

➤ Simple carbs versus complex carbs

➤ How many carbohydrates should you eat?

➤ Do starchy carbs make you fat?

➤ To artificially sweeten or not

All the foods you eat are composed of three macro-nutrients known as carbohydrate, protein, and fat. Some foods consist primarily of only one macro-nutrient (in other words, bread is mainly carbohydrate, turkey meat is protein, and butter is fat), whereas other foods contain combinations of all three (for example, pizza, sandwiches, and burritos).

Your body needs all three of these macro-nutrients to properly function, but *not* in equal amounts. Most leading health professionals recommend that we eat a daily diet made up of *approximately*

➤ 55 percent carbohydrate

➤ 15 percent protein

➤ No more than 30 percent total fat

By following the general guidelines outlined in the Food Guide Pyramid, you'll automatically meet these proportions.

Fifty-five percent of our daily totals come from carbohydrate; that's more than half your food coming from a single macro-nutrient. Thanks to growing consumer education about nutrition, many people now recognize the benefits of a carbohydrate-rich diet. Remember, carbohydrates provide us with important nutrients, and they are an excellent source of energy—specifically for those of us with active lifestyles. This chapter covers the "real deal" on carbos, from simple to complex.

## What Exactly Is a Carbohydrate?

Technically speaking, a carbohydrate is a compound made up of carbon, hydrogen, and oxygen. Now relax, the technical portion is over. The most basic carbohydrates are called simple sugars and include honey, jams, jellies, syrup, table sugar, candies, soft drinks, fruits, and fruit juices. Glucose (also called dextrose) is a common simple sugar found in fruits, honey, and vegetables. It is also the substance measured in blood. (In other words, blood sugar equals blood glucose.) As you can see from the figure, they are relatively small compounds. When several of these simple sugars are linked together, they form much more complicated molecules known as complex carbohydrates.

Complex carbohydrates that come from plants are called *starch* and are found in quality foods such as grains, vegetables, breads, seeds, legumes, and beans. Whether it's a handful of jelly beans or freshly sliced whole-grain bread, it's all carbohydrate!

### Nutri-Speak

**Legumes** are vegetables in the bean and pea family that are rich in complex carbohydrates, protein, and fiber. They supply iron, zinc, magnesium, phosphorous, potassium, and several B-vitamins, including folic acid. Because these provide both complex carbs and protein, they fit in the meat and beans group *and* the vegetable group. Legumes include black beans, pinto beans, kidney beans, lima beans, navy beans, soybeans (tofu), black-eyed peas, chickpeas (garbonzos), split peas, lentils, and nuts and seeds, which are higher in fat.

*Simple sugar*

## Sweet Satisfaction: the Lowdown on Simple Sugars

So your favorite sugary sweets are classified as carbohydrates—and you're supposed to eat a lot of carbohydrates—*so it's okay to load up on gummy bears and licorice, right?*

Not a chance. Here's why: The *quality* of your carbohydrate matters tremendously. Simple sugars such as candy, sodas, and sugary sweeteners found in cakes and cookies offer little in the form of nutrition except that they provide your body with energy and calories. These foods are literally "empty calories"—calories with no nutritional value. In moderation, simple sugars are perfectly fine (and, I admit, yummy), but people who consistently load up on the sweet stuff often find themselves too full for, or uninterested in, the healthy foods their bodies require. The end result is too much sugar and not enough nutrition.

### Q & A

**Does sugary candy promote dental cavities?**

Actually, all foods that contain carbohydrates (rice, pasta, potato, cakes, cookies, and, yes, candy) can equally mix with the bacteria in plaque and increase your risk for tooth decay. But don't panic: By brushing a few times each day, flossing daily, and swishing water around in your mouth after eating, you can fight off the drill.

## Where Do Fruits and Fruit Juices Fit In?

There are some exceptions to the "no sugar" rule. For example, fruits and fruit juices contain fructose (a natural simple sugar) and provide several vitamins and minerals. Eating fresh fruit or drinking 100 percent fruit juice is far from pumping "empty calories" into your system. When you can, choose whole fruit over fruit juice: You get the same nutrients, as well as more complex carbohydrates and fiber. You'll read more about this in Chapter 6, "In and Out with Fiber."

As you can see in the following table, juice and cola both contain simple sugars, but juice provides a lot more nutrition.

| 8 ounces of orange juice | 8 ounces of cola |
| --- | --- |
| 110 calories | 100 calories |
| 26 grams carbohydrate | 26 grams carbohydrate |
| 25 grams sugar | 26 grams sugar |
| 120% daily vitamin C | 0% daily vitamin C |
| 12% daily potassium | 0% daily potassium |
| 20% daily folic acid | 0% daily folic acid |

# All About Complex Carbohydrates

Now that you know what you shouldn't load up on, let's take a look at the foods you should eat. By now, you should be clued-in to which foods are rich in complex carbohydrates (pasta, rice, grains, breads, cereal, legumes, and vegetables). Although they're actually made from hundreds—or even thousands—of simple sugars linked together, they react quite differently inside your body. After you ingest a complex carbohydrate (or starch), several enzymes break it down into its simplest form, called glucose. Glucose is the simple sugar that your body recognizes and absorbs. All types of carbohydrate (simple and complex) must be broken down and converted into glucose before your body can absorb and use it for energy.

If all carbs wind up as glucose, why can't we just eat simple sugars? I've already touched on the first reason: Many simple sugars are nutrition zeroes, whereas complex carbs often provide vitamins, minerals, and even fiber, depending on the food.

Check out this comparison: a small baked potato (complex carbo) versus an 8-ounce glass of cola (simple carbo). Although both provide about 100 calories, that's where the similarity ends. The potato supplies vitamin C, potassium, and fiber, along with several other vitamins and minerals. And the cola—you probably guessed—*provides zilch*. As you can see, eating complex carbs certainly does make a difference, even though it all ends up as glucose.

Another reason to choose complex carbohydrates is that the glucose created during digestion gets released into your blood more slowly. Simple carbohydrates are already broken down—they go straight into the blood, resulting in what is unofficially known as the "sugar rush"—whereas complex carbohydrates are larger molecules that must be broken down. As your body processes complex carbs, small glucose molecules are released into the blood over an extended period of time. This helps to regulate blood-sugar levels, especially in people who may have problems with their blood sugars (for example, people with hyperglycemia, hypoglycemia, or diabetes mellitus).

### Nutri-Speak

**Simple carbohydrates (simple sugars)** are molecules of single sugar units or pairs of small sugar units bonded together. **Complex carbohydrates (complex sugars)** are compounds of long strands of many simple sugars linked together.

### Nutri-Speak

**Hyperglycemia** is a condition resulting in abnormally high blood-glucose (blood-sugar) concentration. *Hyper* means "too much," *glyce* means "glucose," and *emia* means "in the blood." **Hypoglycemia** is characterized by abnormally low blood-sugar. Here, *hypo* means "too little." **Diabetes mellitus** is a disorder of blood-sugar regulation usually caused by the body's inability to either produce enough insulin or use it effectively.

# How Much Carbohydrate Should You Eat?

As mentioned earlier, 55 percent of your total food for the day should consist of carbohydrates, specifically complex carbohydrates. In fact, 80 percent or more of your total carbohydrate intake should come from complex carbs and naturally occurring sugars in fruits and vegetables.

What exactly does this mean in terms of food? You'll need to fill more than half of your plate at each meal with carbohydrate-rich foods. Instead of the typical bacon and eggs for breakfast, boost your carbohydrate intake with cereals, waffles, pancakes, oatmeal, or bagels. For lunch, eat vegetable soups, salads with beans, whole-grain breads, pasta salads, and fresh fruit. With dinner, include plenty of rice, couscous, pasta, vegetables, legumes, and all types of potatoes. (Go easy on the fried potatoes, though.) The idea is to have *larger* amounts of carbohydrates and much *smaller* amounts of protein and fat.

Note: In extremely rare instances, due to medical conditions such as diabetes, some people cannot tolerate these recommended carbohydrate amounts and should be under a doctor's supervision for dietary guidance.

Wanna get more specific? Calculate the amount of carbohydrate you need:

1. Take your total calories for the day.

2. Multiply by .55 (or 55 percent).

3. Divide by 4 (which will convert your carbohydrate calories into grams because 1 gram carbohydrate = 4 carbohydrate calories).

| Daily Calories | Cals from Carbs | Grams of Carbs |
|---|---|---|
| 1,600 cals = | 880 | 220 |
| 1,800 cals = | 990 | 248 |
| 2,200 cals = | 1,210 | 303 |
| 2,800 cals = | 1,540 | 385 |

The amount of carbohydrate grams remains proportional to your caloric requirements. The more calories you require, the more carbohydrates you need to eat.

# Do Pasta and Other Carbohydrates Make You Fat?

One day, you hear you should load up on carbs, and the next day, an article claims that pasta will make you fat. Ever feel like a nutrition yo-yo? What gives?

The story is that bread, pasta, and all other complex carbohydrates supply primo quality calories and should be included in every healthful food plan. Why all the confusion? Well for starters, some people confuse weight-gain from fat with

**Food for Thought**

Some excellent sources of carbohydrates include fruits, vegetables, legumes, pasta, rice, barley, couscous, oatmeal, pita bread, pretzels, tortillas, unsweetened cereal, potatoes, air-popped popcorn, fig bars, rice cakes, and low-fat muffins.

weight-gain from carbohydrates. One gram of fat has more than double the amount of calories as one gram of carbohydrate. What some people don't realize is that fat usually accompanies carbohydrates at a meal. For instance, people remember that they had pasta for dinner but forget that the pasta was swimming in oil, butter, cheese, or Alfredo sauce. Clearly, the culprit for weight gain was the fat (butter, oil, and so on), not the carbohydrate (pasta).

Another example is many a New Yorker's favorite staple—the bagel. Alone, a bagel is a wonderful complex carbohydrate. Add all that butter or cream cheese, and you'll wind up with a lot more calories and fat than you bargained for. The next time you question whether pasta or other carbos make you fat, re-evaluate. It's more likely the fat that is making you fat.

Expand your grain vocabulary:

➤ **Couscous**—A staple in Mediterranean countries, it is one of the easiest grains to cook and can be found in many grocery stores.

➤ **Quinoa** (pronounced "keen-wah")—It is high in protein, calcium, and iron. Quinoa is a native South American grain that is good in puddings, soup, and stir-fry.

➤ **Barley**—Good in soups, stews, side dishes, puddings, and cereals, barley is found in grocery stores and available as "pot" or "scotch barley."

➤ **Millet**—Millet is available in health-food stores. It is good as a side dish or stuffing for poultry and is high in phosphorus and B-vitamins.

➤ **Wild rice**—This pseudo-grain is really a grass seed. It is high in protein and a good source of B-vitamins.

➤ **Amaranath**—High in protein, iron, and calcium, amaranath is from South America and available in health-food stores and some upscale grocery stores. It serves as a good side dish or cereal.

➤ **Wheat berries**—Found in most grocery stores and health food stores, it serves as a good high-fiber cereal or substitute for rice.

## Carbo-Addicts Beware

There are, of course, some exceptions to the rule that it's fat and not carbohydrates making people fat. We call them the "carbo-addicts." These people go overboard on the starchy carbs and can, in fact, gain weight. Do you eat two large bagels for breakfast, a jumbo muffin for lunch, and a family-sized bag of pretzels for snack, and then polish off a big bowl of pasta at dinner? Note that *watching* "Monday Night Football" doesn't require carbo-loading! Unless you're actually playing the game, you're eating too many carbs, specifically those denser in calories, unlike fruits and vegetables. With this daily food intake, you've probably taken in more carbohydrates and calories than your body requires.

Remember, to maintain an ideal weight, you need that balance of "calories in, calories out." It doesn't matter if those extra calories come from carbohydrates, protein, or fat: *Excessive calories will be stored by your body as fat.* I'm not saying that carbohydrates are fattening. I'm saying almost *anything* you eat too much of can put on the pounds.

## To Artificially Sweeten or Not

People often have to use artificial sweeteners because of a medical condition. For example, sugar substitutes can be a great for diabetics, who can't tolerate *real* sugar because their bodies can't produce the hormone insulin. Insulin delivers the sugar from our blood to our cells, where we utilize it as energy. When your body doesn't have enough insulin, sugar builds up in the blood and doesn't get into the cells. This condition is known as high blood-sugar and can be extremely dangerous for people with diabetes. Because sugar substitutes do not contain any glucose (and therefore do not require insulin), they can be effective sweeteners for people with diabetes.

A more popular reason for using artificial sweeteners is saving calories. However, this notion might not be as effective as you think. Although it is true that diet soft drinks and other artificially sweetened foods can save you a lot of sugar calories, several studies have shown that people who "save calories" with these diet foods usually wind up eating those saved calories somewhere else. Pretty ironic, huh? Other studies suggest that artificial sweeteners might, in fact, make you hungrier. Did you know that a real sugar packet (that's 1 teaspoon) has only 16 calories. You can easily burn that off walking an extra flight of stairs. It's certainly something to think about the next time you grab artificial sweetener.

Artificial sweeteners are the subject of much controversy. Before you tear open your gazillionth non-sugar packet, read the following and learn the facts.

One of the first sugar substitutes to receive U.S. Food and Drug Administration (FDA) approval was saccharin (Sweet & Low), and it continues to be popular. Although several studies suggest that saccharin in large quantities can cause cancer (specifically bladder tumors) in laboratory rats, no harmful effects have been shown in humans.

Another popular artificial sweetener is aspartame, better known as Nutrasweet or Equal. Aspartame consists of two protein fragments (phenylalanine and aspartic acid) and has had FDA approval since 1981. It is presently found in more than 5,000 different products, and there is no evidence of any harmful effects from its use. However, because aspartame does contain phenylalanine, individuals with the metabolic disorder PKU (an inherited disease in which the body cannot dispose of excess phenylalanine) should consult their physicians before using this sweetener.

The most recent artificial sweetener to come into the market is called acesulfame K. This FDA-approved sweetener is sold under the brand name Sunett, and to date, studies have shown it perfectly safe for human consumption.

The bottom line is that artificial sweeteners can safely be part of a well-balanced diet. Just don't get so carried away that you view sugar as the enemy. Remember, the dietary guidelines suggest eating real sugar *in moderation*, not avoiding it altogether.

---

### The Least You Need to Know

➤ Approximately 55 percent of your total food for the day should come from carbohydrates (mostly complex carbohydrates). Carbohydrate-rich foods include fruit, vegetables, legumes, bread, cereal, rice, pasta, and all other grain products.

➤ Limit your intake of candy, cola, and other sugary sweets. Although they are carbohydrates, simple sugars provide you with nothing more than "simply sugar."

➤ Fruit and fruit juices are the exception to the "simple sugar" rule. Although considered simple carbohydrates, they provide a variety of important nutrients.

➤ Carbs aren't fattening; however, almost anything you consistently overeat will put on the pounds—including carbohydrates.

➤ In moderation, artificial sweeteners can be an effective sugar substitute for people with diabetes mellitus and part of a well-balanced diet for the general population. The choice between sugar and substitutes is yours.

---

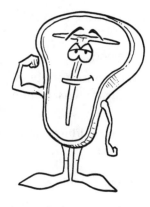

# Chapter 3

# The Profile on Protein

---

**In This Chapter**

➤ The importance of protein

➤ Amino acids—the building blocks

➤ Animal protein versus vegetable protein

➤ Combining incomplete proteins

➤ Your personal requirements

➤ The facts, the fallacies

---

It's time to learn the many powers of protein—one incredibly versatile molecule. Almost everyone seems to have a basic idea of which foods are rich in protein, but do you actually know your personal requirements or understand why protein is important and how it works? Stay tuned: This chapter presents the facts.

## What's So Important About Protein?

First, protein is not just in food; it's floating around *all over* your body. Did you know that your bones, organs, tendons, ligaments, muscle, cartilage, hair, nails, teeth, and skin are all made up of protein? That's just the beginning. *Working proteins* are busy performing specific tasks in your body. These include:

➤ **Enzymes**—Proteins that facilitate and accelerate chemical reactions. They are also known as protein catalysts. Each enzyme has a specific function to perform in the body.

➤ **Antibodies**—Proteins that help fight illness and disease. They are found in red blood cells.

➤ **Hemoglobin**—Proteins that transport oxygen all over the body.

➤ **Hormones (most)**—Proteins that regulate many body functions. Hormones signal enzymes to do their job, such as equalizing blood-sugar levels, insulin levels, and growth.

➤ **Growth and maintenance proteins**—Proteins that serve as building materials for the growth and repair of body tissues.

The list is endless. But I promise not to take you back to high school biology.

**Food for Thought**

Protein was named over 150 years ago after the Greek word *proteios,* meaning "of prime importance."

**Nutri-Speak**

**Proteins** are compounds composed of carbon, hydrogen, oxygen, and nitrogen and arranged as strands of amino acids.

# A Brief Return to Chemistry 101

Protein consists of carbon, hydrogen, oxygen, and nitrogen. The addition of nitrogen gives protein its unique distinction from carbohydrate and fat, along with establishing the signature name, amino acid. Much like simple sugars, which link together to form a *complex* carbohydrate (Chapter 2, "A Close-Up on Carbohydrates"), amino acids are the building blocks for the more complicated protein molecule.

## Amino Acids: the Building Blocks of Protein

There are a total of 20 different amino acids, and depending upon the sequence in which they appear, a specific job or function is carried out in your body. Think of amino acids as similar to the alphabet—26 letters that can be arranged in a million different ways. These arranged letters create words, which then translate into an entire language. The arrangement of amino acids is your body's "protein language," which dictates the exact tasks that need to be carried out. Therefore, proteins that make up your enzymes will have one sequence, whereas those that form your muscles will have a completely different one.

## Your Bod: the Amino Acid Recycling Bin

Your body continually gets the amino acids it needs from its own amino-acid pool and from a diet that meets your daily protein requirements. After you eat a food that contains protein, your body goes to work, breaking it down into various amino acids. (Different foods yield different amino acids.) When the protein is completely dissected, your body absorbs the amino acids (resulting from your digested food) and rebuilds them into the sequence that you need for a specific body task. Your body is sort of like a recycling bin.

Let's take this amino acid talk a bit further. Out of 20 amino acids, 11 can actually be manufactured within your body. However, that means nine cannot be manufactured. You cannot function without each and every amino acid. It is "essential" that you get these nine from outside food sources. Therefore, they are appropriately called *essential amino acids*.

**Nutri-Speak**

**Amino (a–MEEN-o) acids** are the building blocks for protein that are necessary for every bodily function.

| Essential Amino Acids | Nonessential Amino Acids |
| --- | --- |
| Histidine | Glycine |
| Isoleucine | Glutamic acid |
| Leucine | Arginine |
| Lysine | Aspartic acid |
| Methionine | Proline |
| Phenylalanine | Alanine |
| Threonine | Serine |
| Tryptophan | Tyrosine |
| Valine | Cysteine |
| | Asparagine |
| | Glutamine |

# Animal Protein Versus Vegetable Protein

In general, animal proteins (meat, fish, poultry, milk, cheese, and eggs) are considered good sources of *complete proteins*. Complete proteins contain ample amounts of all essential amino acids.

On the other hand, vegetable proteins (grains, legumes, nuts, seeds, and other vegetables) are *incomplete proteins* because they are missing, or do not have enough of, one or more of the essential amino acids. That's not such a big deal. You already know that grains and legumes are rich in complex carbohydrate and fiber. Now you learn that they can be an excellent source of protein as well; it just takes a little bit of work and know-how. By combining foods from two or more of the following

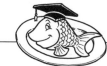

**Food for Thought**

Gelatin is the only animal protein that is not considered a complete protein.

columns—voilà—you create a self-made complete protein. You see, the foods in one column may be missing amino acids that are present in the foods listed in another column. When eaten in combination at the same meal (or separately throughout the day), your body receives all nine essential amino acids.

You can combine the following vegetable proteins to make complete proteins.

## Sources of Complementary Proteins

| Grains | Legumes | Nuts/Seeds |
| --- | --- | --- |
| Barley | Beans | Sesame seeds |
| Bulgur | Lentils | Sunflower seeds |
| Cornmeal | Dried peas | Walnuts |
| Oats | Peanuts | Cashews |
| Buckwheat | Chickpeas | Pumpkin seeds |
| Rice | Soy products | Other nuts |
| Pasta | | |
| Rye | | |
| Wheat | | |

## Combinations to Create Complete Proteins

| Combine Grains and Legumes | Combine Grains and Nuts/Seeds | Combine Legumes and Nuts/Seeds |
| --- | --- | --- |
| Peanut butter on whole-wheat bread | Whole-wheat bun with sesame seeds | Humus (chickpeas and sesame paste) |
| Rice and beans | Breadsticks rolled with sesame seeds | Trail mix (peanuts and sunflower seeds) |
| Bean soup and a roll | Rice cakes with peanut butter | |
| Salad with chickpeas and cornbread | | |
| Tofu-vegetable stir-fry over rice or pasta | | |
| Vegetarian chili with bread | | |

Also, by adding small amounts of animal protein (meat, eggs, milk, or cheese) to any of the groups, you create a complete protein. Here are some examples:

➤ Oatmeal with milk

➤ Macaroni and cheese

➤ Casserole with a small amount of meat

➤ Salad with beans and a hard cooked egg

➤ Yogurt with granola

➤ Bean and cheese burrito

# Your Personal Protein Requirements

This chart presents the Recommended Dietary Allowances (RDAs) of protein for a variety of age categories:

| Infants | Up to 5 mos | 13 grams |
| | 5 mos–1 year | 14 grams |
| Children | 1–3 years | 16 grams |
| | 4–6 years | 24 grams |
| | 7–10 years | 28 grams |
| Males | 11–14 years | 45 grams |
| | 15–18 years | 59 grams |
| | 19–24 years | 58 grams |
| | 25+ years | 63 grams |
| Females | 11–14 years | 46 grams |
| | 15–18 years | 44 grams |
| | 19–24 years | 46 grams |
| | 25+ years | 50 grams |
| Pregnant | | 60 grams |
| Lactating | 1st six months | 65 grams |
| | 2nd six months | 62 grams |

## *Protein for the Day in a Blink of an Eye*

The previous chart gave you a number; let's see how quickly 63 grams can translate into food. The following chart lists the protein content of commonly eaten foods.

**Nutri-Speak**

**Complementary proteins** are two incomplete proteins in a food that compensate for one another's shortfalls when combined.

**Food for Thought**

Hey, did you know that the mineral iron is best absorbed from the following animal proteins: liver, beef, pork, lamb, chicken, turkey, shellfish, and other fish?

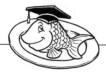

**Food for Thought**

Keep in mind that pregnant or lactating women have increased protein requirements. Pregnant women need an additional 10 grams of protein a day, whereas breast-feeding women need 12–15 extra grams a day for the first 6 months.

## Protein Content of Common Foods

| Animal Proteins | Grams of Protein | Vegetable Proteins | Grams of Protein |
|---|---|---|---|
| Steak, sirloin | 26 | Peanuts (1 oz) | 7 |
| Ground meat | 20 | Walnuts (1 oz) | 4 |
| Hamburger | 14 | Peanut butter (2 Tbs) | 8 |
| Bologna | 10 | Sesame seeds (1 oz) | 5 |
| Hot dog | 10 | Sunflower seeds (1 oz) | 6 |
| Bacon (1 slice) | 2 | Kidney beans ($1/2$ cup) | 8 |
| Ham | 21 | Lentils ($1/2$ cup) | 9 |
| Turkey breast | 26 | Chickpeas ($1/2$ cup) | 10 |
| Roast beef | 21 | Split peas ($1/2$ cup) | 8 |
| Chicken, light without skin | 26 | Tofu (5 oz) | 10 |
| Swordfish | 17 | Oatmeal (1 cup) | 6 |
| Tuna, white, in water | 25 | Pasta (1 cup) | 7 |
| Flounder | 19 | Brown rice (1 cup) | 5 |
| Shrimp | 17 | White rice (1 cup) | 3 |
| Cottage cheese ($1/2$ cup) | 14 | Whole-wheat bread (2 slices) | 5 |
| Cheddar cheese (1 oz) | 7 | Potato, baked (small) | 3 |
| American cheese (1 oz) | 6 | Broccoli ($1/2$ cup) | 2 |
| Whole milk (1 cup) | 8 | Corn ($1/2$ cup) | 2 |
| Skim milk (1 cup) | 8 | Spinach ($1/2$ cup) | 3 |
| Low-fat plain yogurt (1 cup) | 10 | Green peas ($1/2$ cup) | 4 |
| Low-fat fruit yogurt (1 cup) | 10 | | |
| Egg (1) | 6 | | |

*All are 3-ounce servings (approximately the size of a deck of cards) unless otherwise indicated.*

*Source: 1996 First Databank*

You can imagine how quickly these numbers add up, especially because most people tend to eat much more than a 3-ounce serving in one shot.

Let's take a look at a typical day:

**Breakfast:**

2 scrambled eggs

3 strips of bacon

2 slices of toast with margarine

Glass of milk

**Lunch:**

A big fat tuna-salad sandwich (6 oz)

2 slices of bread

Apple

**Dinner:**

Steak (6 oz)

Some veggies and rice

**Total protein = 137 grams** (yikes!)

**Food for Thought**

Your leanest protein sources include turkey breasts, skinless chicken breasts, egg whites, lean red meats, low-fat yogurt, skim or 1% milk, low-fat cheese, beans and lentils, all seafood and fish, split peas, chickpeas, and tofu.

As mentioned earlier, people in industrialized countries don't have a problem meeting their protein requirements. In fact, as you can see, it's easy to *exceed* the amount you need because our society tends to focus on meat, fish, eggs, seafood, or dairy with most every meal.

## Should You Worry About Overeating Protein?

Well, maybe. The problem is that your body only uses what it needs. And the rest? Well, some protein may be used for energy, but most is just a lot of extra calories and usually not just protein calories. Many of these high-protein foods are also packaged with fat; therefore, excess calories, which can translate into weight gain, can be a major concern. Furthermore, filling up on enormous portions of animal protein might crowd out grains, fruits, and veggies, which would create "macro-nutrient chaos."

Go ahead and determine your personal protein needs—and then adjust your meals accordingly. You might want to prepare smaller pieces of animal protein (about 3 ounces) and load a variety of veggies and grains onto your plate.

Also, watch out for "high-protein" diets, which promise quick weight loss by encouraging large amounts of protein while severely limiting carbohydrate intake (no bread, potatoes, rice, pasta, cereal, and so on). You might lose weight, but not from any magical combination of "high protein/low carbohydrates." One reason may be loss of water because the breakdown of excessive protein causes frequent urination. Another explanation may be that your total calories usually decrease when you're limited to high-protein foods. How much plain protein can you really eat?

Furthermore, these high protein/low carb eating plans can be unhealthy (unless you are clinically diagnosed with hyperinsulinemia by your physician). Your body cannot burn fat efficiently without adequate carbohydrates. As a result, you produce compounds called *ketones*, which can accumulate in the blood and leave you feeling dizzy, nauseous, fatigued, and headachy—and give you incredibly bad breath. What's more, excessive protein can also put an added strain on your kidneys. It's pretty ironic when the goal of losing weight should be to improve your health, not make it worse.

## Does Excessive Protein Build Larger Muscles?

Okay, let's set the record straight. It's true that protein is needed for the development of muscle, but it's not true that "extra" protein will build bigger biceps. Body builders and other athletes do need more protein than the RDA; however, this increase is already accounted for in the typical American diet. As mentioned earlier, we cannot store excess protein. Therefore, all those extra protein calories (and the fat that came along with them) will most likely wind up on your...well, let's just say I'm not talking about your quads!

In addition, anyone eating excessive protein will urinate more frequently because the breakdown of protein produces an increase in *urea*, a waste product in urine. You can imagine the inconvenience of running to the bathroom every 10 minutes, let alone your risk of becoming dehydrated. Furthermore, body builders who take tremendous amounts of protein tend to skimp on carbohydrates—the key energy-providing ingredient for an optimal workout.

## The Scoop on Amino-Acid Supplements

Amino-acid supplements are unnecessary. Your body only needs a certain amount of each amino acid, and most of us receive far more than this amount from the food we eat (both animal and vegetable protein). Although the amount that you need is vital, there is nothing miraculous about megadosing. In fact, overkill can be expensive and inefficient. Think about it: For next to nothing, you can prepare a piece of grilled chicken with a meal instead of spending more than double that for one of those "amino-acid" shakes.

## The Least You Need to Know

➤ A total of 20 different amino acids act as building blocks for the more complicated protein molecules. Nine of these amino acids must be obtained from outside food sources and are called "essential amino acids."

➤ Animal proteins are considered "complete proteins" because they contain ample amounts of all nine essential amino acids. Vegetable proteins are "incomplete proteins" because they are missing one or more of the essential amino acids. By combining two or more incomplete vegetable proteins during the day, you can create a complete protein with all nine essential amino acids.

➤ Some people have a tendency to go *protein overboard*, which can also mean more fat and calories because foods high in protein may also be high in fat.

➤ Excessive protein and amino acid supplements do not build larger muscles. In fact, these myths can lead to a host of problems, including dehydration and increased fat intake.

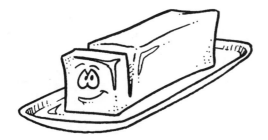

# Chapter 4

# Chewing the Fat

---

## In This Chapter

➤ Various types of fat

➤ The heart disease connection

➤ Your cholesterol numbers and what they mean

➤ Gaining weight from excessive fat

➤ Living a low-fat lifestyle

---

Unless you've been living on another planet, you've heard that too much fat can create a lot of problems. Ironically, despite the "fat warnings" that bombard us every day, we remain an overweight society that eats far too much. It's one thing to *know* what to eat (and I'm sure we would all do pretty well in the "Fat" category on *Jeopardy*), but it's a whole different ball game to actually commit to eating healthy and follow through with it.

Let's not forget the flip side: Low-fat does not mean no-fat. Some people take this new "low-fat religion" to radical extremes. "I'll have a broiled fish, dry, no oil; salad with mustard on the side, no dressing; steamed veggies, nothing on them; and a baked potato, plain." You might as well remove your taste buds before digging into that meal! Come on, food is supposed to be enjoyable, right?

This chapter shows that excessive fat can lead to a host of problems, including weight gain and disease. However, it will also emphasize to all the "fat-phobics" out there that *some* fat is perfectly okay, and with some hard work and realistic planning, everyone can find his or her happy medium.

# Why Fat Is Fabulous

Before we begin a fat-bashing session, let's look at all the positives about fat. You heard right; there are actually good things about the three-letter macro-nutrient:

➤ Fat provides you with a ready source of energy.

➤ Children need fat to grow properly.

➤ Fat supports the cell walls within your body.

➤ Fat enables your body to circulate, store, and absorb the fat-soluble vitamins A, D, E, and K. Without any fat, you would become deficient.

➤ Fat supplies essential fatty acid that your body can't make and must therefore get from foods.

➤ Fat helps promote healthy skin and hair.

➤ Fat makes food taste better by adding flavor, texture, and aroma.

➤ Fat provides a layer of insulation just beneath the skin. People who are extremely thin are often cold because they lack this layer of subcutaneous fat. Overweight people tend to have too much of this insulation and become uncomfortably warm in hot weather.

➤ Fat surrounds your vital organs for protection and support.

**Nutri-Speak**

**Fat-soluble** nutrients dissolve in fat. Some essential nutrients such as the vitamins A, D, E, and K require fat for circulation and absorption.

# Are All Fats Created Equal?

Fat comes in a variety of packages; some are more harmful than others. In addition to watching your total fat intake, you must also pay attention to the *type* of fat you take in. Let's start from the beginning and figure out what's what in the world of fat.

First, here's all of the "fat vocabulary" you will ever need to speak like an expert at your next social function:

➤ **Triglyceride**—The general term used for the main form of fat found in food. The structure of a TG (that's fat slang for triglyceride) is a *glycerol* (carbon atoms linked together) plus three fatty acids. There are several triglyceride categories, and depending upon the fatty acid composition, a TG is classified as saturated, monounsaturated, or polyunsaturated.

You may also hear about your "triglyceride level" when the doctor takes your blood. That's because TGs, like cholesterol, are a storage form of fat in your body—circulating in the bloodstream and deposited in adipose tissue (better known as flub).

➤ **Monounsaturated fats**—As mentioned earlier, the molecular composition of a triglyceride can vary. When one double carbon bond is present in the fatty acid molecule (c=c) the fat is grouped as "monounsaturated" (one spot that is *not* saturated). Olive oils, peanut oils, sesame seed oils, canola oils, and avocados are high in monounsaturated fat. According to studies, these fats may help to lower blood cholesterol. But go easy with that olive oil if your weight is an issue. This "good" fat is still loaded with fat calories.

➤ **Polyunsaturated fats**—Another type of unsaturated fat is polyunsaturated. Where a "mono" has one double carbon bond, the "poly" fat has several (c=c=c, several spots that are *not* saturated). Corn oils, cotton seed oils, safflower oils, sunflower oils, soybean oils, and mayonnaise are all predominant in polyunsaturated fat. The fat in fish is also polyunsaturated (a type called omega-3 fatty acids). Didn't think fish had any fat? Well, it does (especially mackerel, salmon, albacore tuna, and sardines), but much less than most meats. What's more, the poly-fats have also been shown to help reduce the risk of heart disease. So fish away—just don't fry it.

**Nutri-Speak**

**Fish-oil supplements** can be a useful tool for helping to lower triglyceride levels and reducing the symptoms of arthritis. Speak with your physician if you think you may benefit.

**Overrated—Undercooked**

*All* types of fat when eaten in excess can cause weight gain, but overloading on saturated fat, specifically, can also put you at risk for serious health problems, including heart disease.

➤ **Saturated fats**—When triglyceride molecules contain only single carbon bonds (c-c-c, unlike the double bonds you saw in mono and polyunsaturated), the fat is grouped as "saturated." Saturated fats are the demons of all fats because they can raise your blood cholesterol, which, in turn, can lead to heart disease. Hard to believe a simple molecular change can make such a difference, but it can, and these guys are destructive. Animal fats found in meat, poultry, and whole-milk dairy products are all high in saturated fats. Although most vegetable oils are unsaturated, some "saturated" exceptions include coconut, palm, and palm kernel oils (found in cookies, crackers, nondairy creamers, and other baked products). Do your body a favor: Make a concerted effort to cut back on these fats. You'll help protect yourself from heart disease, certain cancers, and other potential health problems.

➤ **Trans-fatty acids**—This type of fat is *not* naturally occurring but is created when innocent unsaturated fats undergo a manufacturing process called hydrogenation.

**33**

Hydrogenation is when a liquid or semisoft fat is transformed into a more solid state. Trans-fatty acids can be harmful because they act like saturated fats inside the body and raise blood cholesterol. What's more, these fats do not appear on a nutrition label since the government does not regulate them to date.

Why mess with a good thing and "hydrogenate?" The process can help preserve food or enable a food company to change the texture of a product. For example, margarine in the liquid form is unsaturated, but with some hydrogenation, it becomes semisoft (tub margarine). With further hydrogenation, it becomes hard (stick margarine). Unfortunately, most people prefer tub and stick over liquid margarines and end up paying the "trans-fatty" penalty. Other trans-fatty culprits include partially hydrogenated vegetable oils, commonly found in cakes, crackers, cookies, and other baked goods. If you ever read the ingredients on food products, you'll know that trans-fats are everywhere.

What can you do? It would be almost impossible to avoid trans-fat completely. Reducing your total fat and limiting the processed products that contain partially hydrogenated oils can significantly reduce the intake of trans-fatty acids.

### Q & A

**Is it better to use butter or margarine?**

Butter is loaded with saturated fat; margarine is packed with trans-fatty acids. Which one do you choose? Although both contain artery-clogging fat, a serving of butter contains *more* artery-clogging fat than most margarines. Give your blood vessels a break and spread on the margarine (specifically soft tub over stick). Better still, go all the way and buy reduced-fat tub spreads. You will save yourself both fat and calories.

## Most Fats Contain Combinations of All Three Types of Fat but Are Predominantly One Type

| Saturated | Monounsaturated | Polyunsaturated |
| --- | --- | --- |
| Beef fat | Canola oil | Corn oil |
| Butter | Olive oil | Cottonseed oil |
| Whole milk | Peanut oil | Safflower oil |
| Cheese | Sesame oil | Soybean oil |

| Saturated | Monounsaturated | Polyunsaturated |
|-----------|-----------------|-----------------|
| Coconut oil | Most nuts | Sunflower oil |
| Palm oil | Avocados | Margarine (soft) |
| Palm kernel oil | | Mayonnaise |
| | | Fish oils |
| | | Sesame oil |

# The Cholesterol Connection and Heart Disease

If you have ever read a nutrition label, you know that dietary fat and cholesterol make up two very different categories. In fact, they are even measured in different units; fat is shown in grams, whereas cholesterol is shown in milligrams. We've already explored the facts on fat, now it's time for cholesterol.

Cholesterol is a waxy substance that contributes to the formation of many essential compounds, including vitamin D, bile acid, estrogen, and testosterone. At this point, you might be thinking, "Hey, if this stuff does so many great things, why can't I eat as much as I want?" The problem is that your liver makes all the cholesterol you'll ever need, and the unused portion all too often gets stored as plaque in your arteries.

All animal-related foods and beverages contain cholesterol because all animals have livers. Eggs, meats, fish, cheese, milk, and poultry are all sources of cholesterol. Needless to say, a slab of liver is loaded with the stuff. What's more, plant foods do not contain cholesterol, simply because they never had a liver.

## Q & A

**How do you lower triglycerides?**

Reduce your fat intake, specifically saturated fat; cut down on simple sugars such as candy, fruit juice, and so on; avoid alcoholic beverages; and engage in regular aerobic exercise.

## Don't Be Fooled by Misleading Labels

When a label reads "no cholesterol," the food in question is not necessarily low in calories and fat. Here is a perfect example. I walked into a famous cookie store and noticed these incredibly decadent peanut butter cookies. Next to them was a sign proclaiming "No-Cholesterol Cookies." Well, as far as I know, a peanut has never had a liver, and therefore, peanut butter doesn't have any cholesterol. But WOW, those cookies were packed with fat; the ingredients included peanut butter, margarine, and vegetable oil. Unfortunately, the majority of people mistook these cookies for low calorie/low-fat just because of the no-cholesterol label. The next time you grab something that reads "no cholesterol," check out the fat content; it might not be all it's cracked up to be.

How does saturated fat work its way into the cholesterol picture? This artery-clogging culprit can also raise blood cholesterol levels. Just imagine how harmful the high-fat animal foods such as marbled red meats and whole-milk dairy products can be; they contain *both* saturated fat and cholesterol.

## Total Fat, Saturated Fat, and the Cholesterol Content of Common Foods

| Food Name | Portion | Total Fat (g) | Saturated Fat (g) | Cholesterol (mg) |
|---|---|---|---|---|
| Ground beef, med. fat | 3 oz | 17.7 | 6.9 | 76 |
| Ground beef, lean | 3 oz | 15.7 | 6.2 | 74 |
| Frankfurter | 3 oz | 24.8 | 9.1 | 43 |
| Chicken breast, no skin | 3 oz | 3.0 | 0.9 | 72 |
| Turkey breast, no skin | 3 oz | 1.0 | 0.2 | 71 |
| Liver, braised | 3 oz | 4.2 | 1.6 | 331 |
| Sole/flounder | 3 oz | 1.3 | 0.3 | 58 |
| Swordfish | 3 oz | 4.4 | 1.2 | 43 |
| Salmon, Atlantic | 3 oz | 6.9 | 1 | 60 |
| Whole egg | 1 | 5.0 | 1.6 | 213 |
| Egg yolk | 1 | 5.0 | 1.6 | 213 |
| Egg white | 1 | 0.0 | 0.0 | 0 |
| Whole milk | 1 cup | 8.1 | 5.1 | 33 |
| Skim milk | 1 cup | 0.4 | 0.3 | 4 |
| Cheddar cheese | 1 oz | 9.4 | 6.0 | 30 |
| American cheese | 1 oz | 8.8 | 5.6 | 27 |
| Mozzarella/skim milk | 1 oz | 4.5 | 2.9 | 16 |
| Nuts | 1 oz | 14.1 | 2.0 | 0 |
| Butter | 1 Tbs | 11.4 | 7.1 | 31 |
| Margarine | 1 Tbs | 11.4 | 2.1 | 0 |
| Margarine, red. fat | 1 Tbs | 5.7 | 1.0 | 0 |
| Olive oil | 1 Tbs | 13.5 | 1.8 | 0 |

*Source: First Databank*

## *Your Cholesterol Report Card*

Yikes! The doctor just sent you a report indicating that your blood cholesterol level is high. Are you now at risk for heart disease?

Although it's certainly not in your favor to have clogged arteries, don't give away your prized possessions yet. In fact, most people have tremendous control over lowering their numbers by limiting the fats and oils in their diet, increasing foods rich in soluble fiber, losing weight if it's warranted, and becoming more physically active.

What do those numbers on the report card mean anyway?

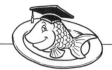

**Food for Thought**

Although shellfish contains a considerable amount of cholesterol, it has substantially less total fat and saturated fat than red meat and is clearly a leaner choice.

➤ **Total blood cholesterol**—This number refers to the amount of cholesterol circulating in the bloodstream and provides a direct correlation to the amount of plaque deposited in your arteries. It is a combination of both types of cholesterol—HDL (good) and LDL (bad). Total cholesterol levels less than 200mg/dL are considered desirable. To help remember which "DL" is which, just remember this: "L" in LDL stands for "lousy," and "H" in HDL stands for "helpful."

➤ **HDL**—The "good guys" actually help your body get rid of the cholesterol in your blood (sort of like garbage men clearing out the garbage). Thus, the higher your HDL-cholesterol number, the better off you are. An HDL-cholesterol less than 35mg/dL is considered low and increases your risk for heart disease.

**Food for Thought**

Some people are born with a genetic predisposition to high cholesterol and therefore might need the assistance of cholesterol-lowering medication.

➤ **LDL**—The "bad guys" cause the cholesterol to build up in the walls of your arteries. Thus, the higher your LDL-cholesterol number, the greater your risk for heart disease. Desirable LDL-cholesterol is less than 130mg/dL.

# Getting Fat from Eating Fat

The consequence from eating excessive fat is one that most of us know all too well: *weight gain*. Gram for gram, fat delivers more than twice as many calories as carbohydrates and protein. In other words, high-fat foods (such as chips, cakes, and whole-milk dairy products) are more calorically dense than low-fat foods (grains, fruits, and veggies), and boy, those fat calories can add up quickly. A measly chocolate bar contains 240 calories; by contrast, so does an entire plateful of low-fat foods such as an

Moo!

apple, a banana, and a handful of pretzels. There is no comparison; you get a lot more quantity for the same amount of calories when you go low-fat. Sure, the candy bar might sound more appealing, but consider the other fats you may have consumed that same day: salad dressings, fried foods, whole-milk dairy, and fatty meats. That's a lot of fat, which means a tremendous amount of calories.

Don't get me wrong: No one should deprive himself of the things he loves; however, as with money, you must budget your fat so you don't go overboard by the end of the day. In this case, consistently going over budget won't leave you broke; it will leave you fat.

Filling up on fatty foods might also crowd out the healthy stuff that keeps us fit. Great—chubby and malnourished! Believe me, I sympathize. It's tough limiting all those delicious donuts, cakes, and gooey, chocolate treats. I'm certainly not one of those "genetic lean machines" who can eat whatever he wants and not gain an ounce. (I hate every one of them.) For most people, maintaining an ideal weight means watching total fat intake.

## How Much Fat and Cholesterol Should We Eat?

The American Heart Association recommends the following:

➤ Less than 30 percent of the day's total calories should come from fat.

➤ Less than 10 percent of the day's total calories should come from saturated fat.

➤ Less than 300 milligrams of dietary cholesterol is the total you should consume in a day.

### A Guide to Recommended Daily Fat Intake

| Daily Calories | Fat Calories | Total Fat Grams | Saturated Fat Grams |
| --- | --- | --- | --- |
| 1,200 | <360 | <40 | <13 |
| 1,500 | <450 | <50 | <17 |
| 1,800 | <540 | <60 | <20 |
| 2,000 | <600 | <67 | <22 |
| 2,500 | <750 | <83 | <28 |
| 2,800 | <840 | <93 | <31 |
| 3,000 | <900 | <100 | <33 |

## Some Fats Are Easier to Spot Than Others

Although some fats and oils are rather obvious, others are hidden deep within our food. Take a look:

➤ **Visible fats**—butter*, cream cheese*, lard*, sour cream*, mayonnaise, oil-based salad dressings, cream-* or cheese-based salad dressings, animal shortenings*, guacamole, cooking oils, peanut butter, and margarine.

➤ **Invisible fats**—whole-milk dairy*, high-fat meats* (including bologna, pepperoni, sausage, bacon, pastrami, spare-ribs, and hot dogs), doughnuts*, cakes*, cookies*, nuts, candy bars*, chocolate chips*, avocado, ice cream*, fried foods, pizza*, cole slaw, macaroni salad, and potato salad.

*Contains saturated fat*

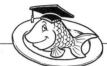

**Food for Thought**

Forty to sixty percent of all cancers may be diet-related. Evidence strongly suggests that people who eat low-fat diets have substantially less risk for certain types of cancer.

## Slicing Off the Fat Without a Knife

These are tips to help you reduce the fat in your diet. Read through them and learn how to painlessly develop a low-fat lifestyle:

➤ Choose low-fat dairy products whenever possible: skim or 1% milk, low-fat cheese and yogurts, low-fat sour creams, and reduced-fat ice cream.

➤ Prepare foods by roasting, baking, broiling, boiling, steaming, lightly stir-frying, or grilling.

➤ Use non-fat cooking sprays or non-stick pans when frying.

➤ Remove all skin from poultry and trim all visible fat from meats.

➤ Limit your intake of red meats and try to completely avoid the higher-fat selections, including salami, bologna, sausage, pepperoni, bacon, and hot dogs.

➤ Buy reduced-fat versions of margarine, butter, mayonnaise, and cream cheese.

➤ Buy low-fat salad dressings, or make your own by mixing balsamic vinegar, a lot of spices, and a drop of olive oil.

➤ Instead of using butter and oily sauces, flavor your vegetables with herbs and seasonings. Also try lemon juice, spicy mustard, salsa, and flavored vinegars.

➤ Watch out for pastas swimming in oil and cream sauce. Instead, substitute marinara or other tomato-based sauces.

➤ Opt for egg-white omelets (or egg substitutes) rather than whole eggs with yolk. If you can't live without eating whole eggs, limit yourself to three to four yolks per week.

➤ Pass on the ice cream, chips, and cookies. Instead, snack on pretzels, fig bars, fresh fruit, and frozen yogurt.

➤ Use extra-lean ground turkey breast instead of ground beef in your favorite recipes.

# The "Fat-Phobic" Generation

Sure, a low-fat lifestyle is the way to go, but some misinterpret this message and become utterly neurotic. Are you afraid to even touch anything that might have once possibly come in contact with fat? When ordering in a restaurant, do you create such chaos that your waiter is off and running to his or her shrink?

It might sound funny, but it's no laughing matter to be completely preoccupied with fat. Certainly, a low-fat diet is an essential part of being healthy; however, taking this concept to radical extremes can place serious restraints on social eating, let alone set you up for a serious eating disorder. If your reason is weight control, think again. Some fat is fine, and I promise you can maintain your ideal body weight (within reason, of course) and still allow yourself to enjoy foods with fat every once in a while.

In fact, joining a "fat-free cult" doesn't necessarily mean that you automatically lose weight. Quite frequently, I meet clients who cannot seem to drop an aggravating 5 or 10 pounds—even while following a strictly fat-free regimen. How can that be?

The answer is rather obvious: They simply overcompensate with the fat-free products. For the most part, the explosion of lower-fat foods on the market has been a wonderful tool, enabling people to painlessly lower their cholesterol and total fat intakes. Unfortunately for some people, the expression "low-fat" means carte-blanche to eating huge amounts. Just because a product is fat-free doesn't mean it's calorie-free. As a matter of fact, many lower-fat foods can pack in just as many calories as their original fat-containing counterparts.

Do you have a friend who will not go near a "real" chocolate-chip cookie but doesn't hesitate to inhale half a box of the fat-free version? Which is worse: the cookie with fat at 75 calories or 15 no-fat cookies at a whopping 750 calories? Remember, no matter where they come from, calories still count in the battle of the bulge.

## The Least You Need to Know

➤ Fats perform vital roles in the body, including providing stored energy, storing and circulating fat-soluble vitamins, and providing a layer of insulation underneath the skin.

➤ All types of fat, when eaten in excess, can cause a variety of health problems, including weight gain.

➤ Saturated fat has the destructive capability to increase blood cholesterol and therefore promote heart disease.

➤ Live a "low-fat lifestyle" by limiting your intake of red meat, whole-milk dairy, fried foods, high-fat spreads, and oily sauces. Switch to low-fat milk, yogurts, and cheese while jazzing up foods with herbs, spices, lemon juice, and Dijon mustard.

➤ Although low-fat and fat-free foods are great for your diet, every diet must have some sort of fat in it. A totally "fat-free diet" is dangerous because fat is responsible for vital body functions.

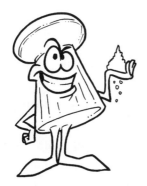

# Chapter 5

# Don't As-*salt* Your Body

---

### In This Chapter

➤ All about salt

➤ Sodium and water retention

➤ The high blood pressure connection

➤ How much is recommended

➤ Decreasing your intake

---

True story: I had a friend in college who would buy a large bucket of salted popcorn at the movie theater. Once in her seat, she'd whip out a salt shaker hidden in her jacket and heavily salt each handful before popping it in her mouth. The sign of a true salt addict!

A lot of your salt habit has to do with the way you grew up and your cultural background. (Some ethnic cuisines are loaded with salty condiments and seasonings.) Were your parents into the salt shaker? Were the first three ingredients in grandma's secret recipes salt, salt, and salt? If so, you were clearly "salt corrupted" as a kid. What about our convenience-food generation? Nowadays, people are so happy to buy prepared, prepackaged, frozen, and microwaveable meals, they don't realize the colossal amounts of salt they're putting in their bodies.

So what's the problem? Well, using excessive amounts might lead to uncomfortable water retention and the more serious problem of high blood pressure. Although it has been proven that *not* everyone is "salt sensitive," there is no way to tell who is—and it is certainly better to be safe than sorry when your health is at stake. Read on and learn how to give up the shakes without giving up taste.

# All About Salt

Salt is composed of 40 percent sodium and 60 percent chloride. When most people speak of the problems associated with salt, they are usually referring to the part of salt called sodium. What exactly is sodium and what does it do?

Sodium is a mineral that is essential for many important functions, such as

➤ Controlling the fluid balance within your body

➤ Transmitting electrical nerve impulses

➤ Contracting muscles (including your heart)

➤ Absorbing nutrients across cell membranes

➤ Maintaining your body's acid/base balance

With such a wonderful résumé for sodium, why worry about your sodium intake? Although sodium is essential for good health, your body requires less than $^1/_{10}$ teaspoon of salt each day. Would you believe the average American consumes 5 to 18 times more than that every day? This is one salty society we live in. In fact, most people could stand to substantially cut back.

**Nutri-Speak**

**Hyponatremia** is the excessive loss of sodium and water due to persistent vomiting, diarrhea, or profuse sweating. In this case, both water and salt must be replenished to maintain the correct balance for your body.

# Feeling a Bit Waterlogged?

Have your fingers ever been so swollen that it's literally impossible to get your rings on or off? Oh, the uncomfortable effects of excess salt.

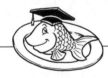

**Food for Thought**

Although your salt intake might vary from day to day, the amount of sodium in your body doesn't generally vary by more than two percent. Your body is efficient at conserving sodium if you need it or excreting it if you have a surplus.

It's common to experience a temporary bloating or swelling after eating highly salted foods. You see, your body requires a certain balance of sodium and water at all times. Extra salt requires extra water, resulting in water retention. Where does this extra water or fluid come from? Usually your glass. Salt triggers your thirst response to balance out the sodium-water concentration. Ever wonder why you're so thirsty after munching on salty pretzels or nuts? It's no coincidence that the snacks offered in drinking establishments are covered with salt. What a strategy: The more you eat, the more you drink!

Try performing this test: Record your weight one morning. Then, before going to bed that night, eat a large serving of heavily salted popcorn or other food (drink a lot of water). Weigh yourself again the next morning. It is amazing how much water that salt can retain. All you dieters out there, remember that this is water weight—not fat weight. Don't panic; it will be gone in a couple of hours.

Note: Do not, under any circumstances, try the preceding test if you have any medical condition.

# Can't Take the Pressure!

For reasons that are not completely understood, salt can play an active role in raising the blood pressure in people who are salt-sensitive.

## *What Exactly Is High Blood Pressure?*

When your heart beats, it pumps blood into your arteries and creates a pressure within them. High blood pressure (also known as hypertension) occurs when too much pressure is placed on the walls of the arteries. This can occur if there is an increase in blood volume or the blood vessels themselves constrict or narrow.

People who are genetically sensitive to salt can't efficiently get rid of extra sodium through their urine. Therefore, that extra sodium hangs around, drawing in extra water, which means an increase in blood volume. This increased blood volume can then stimulate the vessels to constrict, creating increased pressure.

Imagine a garden hose with a normal flow of water running through it. No problem. Now, think about the increased pressure on the hose when you drastically turn up the amount of water rushing out. What if you were to pinch off spots of this hose, like a constricted blood vessel? A garden hose might endure the wear and tear, but your arteries can become extremely damaged by such constant pressure—so damaged that the end result might include a heart attack, stroke (a brain attack), or kidney disease.

**Nutri-Speak**

**Hypertension** is the medical term for sustained high blood pressure. It has nothing to do with being tense, nervous, or hyperactive.

**Food for Thought**

1.5 million Americans suffer a heart attack every year.

500,000 Americans suffer a stroke every year.

*Source: American Heart Association, 1996*

## *What Causes High Blood Pressure?*

According to recent statistics, one out of every four American adults—nearly 60 million people—has high blood pressure. In a small percentage of people, this increased

**45**

pressure is from an underlying problem such as kidney disease or a tumor of the adrenal gland. However, in 90–95 percent of all cases, the cause is unclear. That's why it is known as the *silent killer*; it just creeps up without any warning. Whereas some of the contributing factors are *not* controllable, others can be quite controllable.

Risk factors that cannot be controlled are

➤ **Age:** The older you get, the more likely you are to develop high blood pressure.

➤ **Race:** African-Americans tend to have high blood pressure more often than whites. They also tend to develop it earlier and more severely.

➤ **Heredity:** High blood pressure can run in families. If you have a family history, you're twice as likely to develop it than others.

### Q & A

**What's a normal blood pressure reading?**

Normal blood pressure readings fall within a range. It is not one set of numbers; however, it should be less than 140/90 if you are an adult.

**How do you know if you have high blood pressure?**

You don't! High blood pressure is known as the "silent killer" because it has no symptoms. In fact, many people can have hypertension for years without knowing it; by that time, their body organs may have already been damaged. Stay on top of your health and have your blood pressure checked regularly by a qualified health professional.

Risk factors that can be controlled are

➤ **Obesity:** Being extremely overweight is clearly related to high blood pressure. In fact, nearly 60 percent of all high blood pressure cases concern overweight patients. By losing weight—even a small amount—obese individuals can significantly reduce their blood pressure.

➤ **Sodium consumption:** Reducing the intake of salt can lower blood pressure in people who are salt sensitive.

➤ **Alcohol consumption:** Regular use of alcohol can dramatically increase blood pressure in some people. Fortunately, alcohol's effect on blood pressure is completely reversible. Limit yourself to a maximum of two drinks a day.

➤ **Smoking**: Although the long-term effect of smoking on blood pressure is still unclear, the short term effect is that it can raise blood pressure briefly. However, given that both smoking and high blood pressure have been linked to heart disease, smoking compounds the risk.

➤ **Oral contraceptives:** Women who take birth control pills may develop high blood pressure.

➤ **Physical inactivity:** Lack of exercise can contribute to high blood pressure. By becoming more active with moderate exercise, an inactive person can get into better shape, feel terrific, and help keep his or her blood pressure in check.

## Investigating Your Blood Pressure Numbers

Your doctor measures two numbers when checking your blood pressure, systolic and diastolic. *Systolic pressure* is the top, larger number. This represents the amount of pressure that is in your arteries while your heart contracts (or beats). During this contraction, blood is ejected from the heart and into the blood vessels that travel throughout your body.

*Diastolic pressure* is the bottom, smaller number. This represents the pressure in your arteries while your heart is relaxing between beats. During this relaxation period, your heart is filling up with blood for the next squeeze. Although both numbers are critically important, your doctor might be more concerned with an elevated diastolic number because this indicates that there is increased pressure on the artery walls even when your heart is resting.

## How to Lower High Blood Pressure

If your blood pressure is high, don't panic. Most people can significantly lower their numbers with know-how and determination. A diagnosis of high blood pressure often requires reducing salt intake, losing excess weight, increasing exercise, and in some instances, taking medication:

➤ **Diet:** Lose weight if you are overweight by cutting back on calories and fat. Reduce your consumption of sodium by avoiding salty foods, and limit the amount of alcohol you drink. Better yet, avoid alcohol completely.

➤ **Exercise:** Become physically active and get some type of exercise at least four times a week. Check with your doctor before beginning any diet or exercise program.

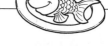

**Food for Thought**

Studies suggest that calcium, potassium, and magnesium may also play a beneficial role in the regulation of blood pressure. Consult with your doctor for further information.

➤ **Medication:** For some people, diet and exercise are just not enough. In this case, your doctor might give you medication to help lower your blood pressure.

➤ **If you smoke—QUIT!**

# How Much Sodium Is Recommended?

Many question the "one size fits all" recommendation because not everyone is salt-sensitive. However, there is no test for salt sensitivity; therefore, it makes sense for *everyone* to play it safe and follow a prudent approach. Most health professionals recommend limiting your intake of sodium to no more than 2,400 milligrams per day. This includes both the salt you add and the sodium that is already present in foods you eat. Become familiar with the following list of high-sodium foods, and learn to balance your diet so you don't go sodium overboard. Note, if you have high blood pressure, your doctor might prescribe a more severe sodium restriction.

## Common Foods That Are High in Sodium

| Seasonings and Cooking Aids | Portion Size | Sodium (mg) |
| --- | --- | --- |
| Baking powder | 1 tsp | 426 |
| Baking soda | 1 tsp | 1,259 |
| Table salt | 1 tsp | 2,300 |
| Garlic salt | 1 tsp | 2,050 |
| Bouillon cube, chicken | 1 item | 1,152 |
| Bouillon cube, beef | 1 item | 864 |
| Monosodium glutamate (MSG) | 1 Tbs | 1,914 |
| Salad dressing, Italian | 1 Tbs | 116 |
| Soy sauce | 1 Tbs | 1,029 |
| Low-sodium soy sauce | 1 Tbs | 660 |
| Butter buds | 1 Tbs | 177 |

| Canned Food Items | Portion Size | Sodium (mg) |
| --- | --- | --- |
| Tuna, canned | 3 oz | 303 |
| Sardines, canned | 3 oz | 261 |
| Caviar, black and red | 1 Tbs | 240 |
| Chicken noodle soup | 1 cup | 1,106 |
| Vegetable soup | 1 cup | 795 |
| Veg. beef soup (low-sodium) | 1 cup | 57 |
| Corn, canned | ½ cup | 266 |
| Asparagus, canned | ½ cup | 472 |
| Sauerkraut, canned | ½ cup | 780 |

| Processed/Cured and Smoked Meats | Portion Size | Sodium (mg) |
|---|---|---|
| Bologna | 3 oz | 832 |
| Salami | 3 oz | 1,922 |
| Hot dog | 1 item | 639 |
| Smoked turkey | 3 oz | 916 |
| Smoked fish | 3 oz | 619 |
| Smoked sausage | 3 oz | 853 |

| Snack Foods | Portion Size | Sodium (mg) |
|---|---|---|
| Salted nuts | 1 oz | 230 |
| Pretzels | 1 oz | 476 |
| Corn chips | 1 oz | 164 |
| Potato chips | 1 oz | 133 |
| Popcorn | 1 oz | 179 |
| Saltines | 5 crackers | 180 |
| Peanut butter | 1 Tbs. | 76 |

| Dairy Products | Portion Size | Sodium (mg) |
|---|---|---|
| American cheese | 1 oz | 336 |
| Cheddar cheese | 1 oz | 176 |
| Parmesan cheese | 1 oz | 527 |
| Cottage cheese | $1/2$ cup | 459 |
| Butter | 1 Tbs | 116 |
| Margarine | 1 Tbs | 132 |

| Common Breakfast Cereals | Portion Size | Sodium (mg) |
|---|---|---|
| Rice Krispies | 1 oz | 294 |
| Corn Flakes | 1 oz | 351 |
| All-Bran | 1 oz | 320 |
| Cheerios | 1 oz | 307 |
| Special K | 1 oz | 306 |
| Raisin Bran | 1 oz | 155 |

*Source: First Databank, 1996 and Bowes & Church's Food Values of Portions Commonly Used, 15th ed., 1989*

# Salt-Less Solutions

Giving up salt doesn't mean giving up the pleasure of eating. However, you'll need to be a bit more selective with certain food products and much more creative in the seasoning department. The following guidelines can show you how to drastically cut the amount of salt in your food and body:

➤ Enhance the flavor of your foods with spices and herbs. Try allspice, basil, bay leaves, chives, cinnamon, curry powder, dill, garlic (not garlic salt), onion (not onion salt), rosemary, nutmeg, thyme, sage, turmeric, mace, and salt substitutes.

➤ Avoid putting a salt shaker on your breakfast, lunch, or dinner table.

➤ Choose fresh and frozen vegetables when possible. (The canned versions generally contain a lot of salt.) When canned is the only option, reduce the salt by draining the liquid and rinsing the vegetables in water before eating.

➤ Here I go with another plug for fresh fruit: It's naturally low in sodium.

➤ Go easy on condiments that contain considerable amounts of salt, including catsup, mustard, monosodium glutamate (MSG), salad dressings, sauces, bouillon cubes, olives, sauerkraut, and pickles. Stock your kitchen with low-sodium versions of soy sauce, teriyaki sauce, steak sauce, and anything else you might find in your travels.

➤ Select unsalted (or reduced salt) nuts, seeds, crackers, popcorn, and pretzels.

➤ Take it easy with cheese. Unfortunately, it not only has a lot of fat, but sodium as well. If you're feeling extra motivated, stock your fridge with low-salt/low-fat brands.

➤ Read labels carefully and choose foods lower in sodium, especially when choosing frozen dinners, canned soups, packaged mixes, and combination dishes.

➤ Beware of processed luncheon cold cuts, as well as cured and smoked meats, because they are saturated with sodium. This includes bacon, bologna, salami, sausages, hot dogs, smoked turkey, fish, and beef. Also be aware that most varieties of canned fish (tuna, salmon, and sardines) are extremely high in sodium.

➤ When dining in Chinese or Japanese restaurants, ask for meals without MSG or added salt. Nowadays, you can also request low-sodium soy sauce for your table. If they don't have any, dilute the regular by adding a tablespoon of water.

### Overrated—Undercooked

Be aware that some over-the-counter medicines contain a lot of sodium. For example, two tablets of dissolvable Alka-Seltzer (plop plop fizz fizz) have a whopping 1,134 milligrams of sodium. (Each single tablet provides 567 milligrams.) Instead, opt for the caplets that you swallow; they contain *only* 1.8 milligrams. Quite a drastic difference.

## The Least You Need to Know

➤ Salt consists of 40 percent sodium and 60 percent chloride. The mineral sodium is essential for many important functions. It maintains body fluids and the contraction of muscles and transmits nerve impulses.

➤ Eating a high-sodium diet can increase blood pressure in people who are "salt-sensitive."

➤ People diagnosed with high blood pressure often need to reduce their salt intake, lose excess weight, increase exercise, and in some instances, take blood pressure-lowering medication.

➤ Because salt sensitivity is *not* something we are tested for, everyone should limit her sodium intake to less than 2,400 milligrams per day.

➤ Reduce your sodium intake by using herbs, spices, and seasonings instead of salt. Limit canned food items, salty snack foods, luncheon cold cuts, and meats that have been smoked or cured. Go easy on high-sodium condiments such as soy sauce, teriyaki sauce, mustard, catsup, olives, pickles, and sauerkraut. Also read labels carefully and opt for the lower sodium foods.

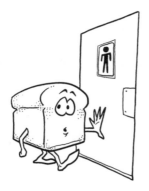

# Chapter 6

# In and Out with Fiber

> ### In This Chapter
>
> ➤ What is fiber?
>
> ➤ The different kinds of fiber
>
> ➤ Benefits from a fiber-rich diet
>
> ➤ How much do you need?
>
> ➤ Increasing your daily fiber intake

Say you're a little constipated? Got high cholesterol? Want to reduce your risk of colon cancer? Have I got a food for you! What is this magical food? Where can you get some? Well, the nice part is that you don't have to buy any special potions or formulas or seek the advice of your local medicine man. This incredible healer is conveniently found in some of your favorite carbohydrate-rich foods.

## Fiber Facts: What Is Fiber Anyway?

Fiber is a mix of many different substances found in plant cell walls and is not digestible by the human body. *In it comes and out it goes.* How can a substance we cannot even digest (and, by the way, has no nutritional value) be so beneficial? Might sound crazy, but once inside your body, fiber does some pretty amazing things. The term *dietary fiber,* when listed on a nutrition label, simply refers to the amount of these indigestible substances in a specific food product. This way, you can identify a food rich in fiber.

Fiber fits in two categories, insoluble and soluble, depending upon its ability to dissolve (or not dissolve) in water. Some foods contain *both* soluble and insoluble fiber, whereas others are predominant in only one. The key is to eat a variety of fiber-rich foods each day and receive the beneficial effects from both types.

# Soluble Fiber

*Water-soluble* fiber readily dissolves in water. Technically speaking, soluble fibers include pectins, gums, and mucilages. It's obvious, however, that these terms won't be of any help to you in your grocery store. Translated into "real-food" terminology, you'll find soluble fiber in the following:

➤ Oats

➤ Brown rice

➤ Barley

➤ Oat bran

➤ Dried beans and peas

➤ Rye

➤ Seeds

➤ Vegetables (especially carrots, corn, cauliflower, and sweet potatoes)

➤ Fruits (especially apples, strawberries, oranges, bananas, nectarines, and pears)

Why all the hoopla? Well for starters, foods rich in soluble fiber have been shown to help decrease blood cholesterol, therefore reducing the risk of heart disease. Another benefit comes from its ability to slow the absorption of glucose (sugar in the blood), which might in turn help control blood-sugar levels in diabetics.

# Insoluble Fiber

The type of fiber that does not readily dissolve in water is called *water-insoluble*. Insoluble fiber includes lignin, cellulose, and hemicellulose. Once again, converted into understandable food terms, we are talking about the following:

➤ Wheat bran

➤ Corn bran

➤ Whole-wheat breads and cereals

➤ Fruits

➤ Vegetables (especially potatoes with skin, parsnips, green beans, and broccoli)

As you can see, some foods are mentioned on both lists, indicating that they provide both soluble *and* insoluble fiber.

Insoluble fiber is primarily responsible for accelerating intestinal transit time, along with increasing and softening stools. In other words, insoluble fiber is responsible for "moving things along," if you know what I mean. In addition to promoting regularity, insoluble fiber has been shown to decrease your risk for colon cancer and diverticulosis.

## Reducing Your Risk of Colon Cancer

Can a diet rich in fiber actually lower your chance of developing colon cancer? Several studies say yes, and it makes perfect sense. Think about it. *Insoluble fiber* helps move waste material through your intestines more quickly. Therefore, there is less time for suspicious substances to lurk around and possibly damage your colon and rectal area. In addition, fiber may bind with possibly harmful bacteria, transporting it through the intestines and out of your body. While we're down there, it's a perfect time to point out that softer more regular bowel movements can also prevent constipation and reduce your chance of getting hemorrhoids.

## Lowering Your Cholesterol Level

If your cholesterol tends to be a bit high, or you'd just like to maintain an already low number, you might want to increase your *soluble fiber*. Soluble fibers have been shown to bind with cholesterol and pull it out of the body. Fruits, vegetables, legumes, oats, and all foods made with oat bran can therefore reduce your risk for heart and artery disease by lowering blood cholesterol. Another thought is that high-fiber foods can displace some of the high-fat, artery-clogging foods in your diet—a double impact!

## Feeling Fuller with Less Food

Did you ever feel as though a plate of vegetables expanded in your stomach after you ate it? Well, it did! Eating fiber-rich foods can make you feel full because they absorb water and swell inside you. You might also feel full longer if you choose a meal with some soluble fiber. Unlike insoluble fiber, which quickly moves food through your body, soluble fiber tends to stick around a while, keeping you full and satisfied.

Does this mean you'll lose weight from eating a lot of fiber? It does if you eat these foods *instead* of the high-fat, high-calorie stuff. If you eat them in addition to all the junky food, your chance of becoming slim is slim.

**Nutri-Speak**

**Diverticulosis** is an illness or condition where tiny pouches (called diverticula) form in the wall of the colon. The condition is often without symptoms, but when the pouches become infected or inflamed, it can be painful. When this happens, the condition is known as diverticulitus, which can cause fever, abdominal pain, and diarrhea.

**Overrated—Undercooked**

Just because a food sounds healthy doesn't necessarily mean that it is. Some bran muffins are loaded with fat and sugar—certainly not worth the small amount of fiber they provide.

# How Much Fiber Do You Need?

Although there's no Recommended Daily Amount (RDA) for fiber, most health experts agree that we should aim for 20–35 grams of dietary fiber each day (a mix of both soluble and insoluble). On the following page are a few ideas to help you raise your intake of fiber.

**Ready-Made Menu**

This sample day provides about 31 grams of fiber:

| | |
|---|---|
| Breakfast | Bowl of **bran cereal** with milk |
| | Banana |
| | Glass of juice |
| Lunch | Roast beef sandwich on wheat bread |
| | Cup of **vegetable barley soup** |
| | Apple with skin |
| | A lot of water |
| Snack | **Chewy fruit bar** |
| | Low-fat yogurt |
| Dinner | **Mixed green salad** |
| | Grilled fish with **sautéed carrots** |
| | Baked sweet potato |
| | Fresh strawberries |
| | Club soda with lemon |

## Tips to Increase the Fiber in Your Diet

As you read the following tips, keep these points in mind. It's important to increase your fiber *gradually* (sometimes over several weeks) because your body needs time to adjust. For example, if you are a newcomer to the world of fiber, start with 20 grams each day for the first week. Increase to 25 grams per day the second week, and—if your stomach can handle it—graduate to 30+ grams per day by week three. Also, drink plenty of fluids. Fiber acts as a bulking agent by absorbing some of the fluid in your body. Extra fluids will prevent you from becoming dehydrated, and most importantly, help that bulk to move merrily on its way.

➤ Read nutrition labels. Generally, a good source of fiber should have at least 2.5 grams per serving.

➤ Start your day with a high-fiber breakfast cereal. Supermarkets are flooded with them. Read the nutrition label and select a cereal that offers more than 2 grams per serving.

➤ Add a few tablespoons of wheat bran to your cereal, cottage cheese, yogurts, and salads.

➤ Include plenty of fresh or frozen vegetables in your day. Add them to soups, pizza, sandwiches, stir-frys, pastas, omelets, rice, and anything else you can think of.

➤ Eat breads and pasta made from wheat, rye, and oat products, along with brown rice, barley, and bulgur.

➤ Add fruit to your cereal (hot or cold), top off your pancakes and waffles with fruits, mix fruits into yogurts and salads, or simply enjoy them plain. Remember, whole fruit, with seeds and peels intact, provides more fiber than most fruit juice.

➤ Cook with beans and lentils. They are loaded with fiber. Enjoy them in soups, stews, salads, burritos, and a million other creative entrees.

➤ Get your fiber from food sources, not supplements. Food is a natural provider not only of fiber, but other essential nutrients as well.

### Q & A

**How much fiber do kids need?**

Just tack on an extra 5 grams to their age; this works for healthy kids from age 3–18. Your child's age plus five equals the grams of dietary fiber they require each day.

The following table lists foods rich in fiber:

## Foods Rich in Fiber

| Fruits | Grams of Fiber |
| --- | --- |
| Raspberries (1 cup) | 5.50 |
| Pear (1) | 4.65 |
| Blueberries (1 cup) | 4.00 |
| Prunes (5) | 3.00 |
| Apple (1) | 3.00 |
| Orange (1) | 3.00 |
| Strawberries (1 cup) | 2.70 |
| Grapes (1$^1$/$_2$ cups) | 2.30 |
| Banana (1) | 2.00 |
| Peach (1) | 2.00 |
| Grapefruit ($^1$/$_2$) | 1.70 |
| Nectarine (1) | 1.60 |

*continues*

*continued*

| Vegetables (All Servings ¹/₂ Cup Cooked) | Grams of Fiber |
|---|---|
| Green Peas | 4.00 |
| Broccoli | 3.60 |
| Brussels sprouts | 3.00 |
| Sweet potato (small) | 3.00 |
| Baked potato with skin (small) | 2.50 |
| Carrots | 2.50 |
| Spinach | 2.20 |
| Corn | 1.70 |

| Breads and Grains | Grams of Fiber |
|---|---|
| Barley (1 cup cooked) | 8.80 |
| Whole wheat bread (2 slices) | 3.20 |
| Brown rice (³/₄ cup cooked) | 2.50 |
| Bran muffin (1) | 2.50 |

| Cereals (Measured by Weight; Serving Sizes Will Vary) | Grams of Fiber |
|---|---|
| Fiber One (¹/₂ cup) | 12.90 |
| 100% Bran (¹/₂ cup) | 9.75 |
| All Bran (¹/₃ cup) | 8.40 |
| Bran Buds (¹/₃ cup) | 7.70 |
| Bran Flakes (³/₄ cup) | 5.00 |
| Raisin Bran (³/₄ cup) | 4.50 |
| Shredded Wheat (³/₄ cup) | 4.00 |
| Oatmeal (¹/₂ cup cooked) | 2.20 |
| Wheat bran (4 Tbs.) | 2.00 |
| Wheat germ (2 Tbs.) | 1.50 |

| Beans (All Servings Equal; ¹/₂ Cup Cooked) | Grams of Fiber |
|---|---|
| Pinto | 6.40 |
| Navy | 4.70 |
| White | 4.40 |
| Kidney | 4.30 |
| Black | 3.60 |

*Sources: First Databank, 1996 and Bowes & Church's Food Values of Portions Commonly Used, 15th Ed., 1989*

## Don't Overdo It!

Can you ever eat too much fiber? You sure can, especially if your body is not used to it. I remember a client who ate half of a large box of high-fiber cereal and spent the entire day doubled over in his bathroom. Overloading on fiber can cause severe bloating, cramping, gas, diarrhea, and other abdominal discomforts. Furthermore, excessive amounts of fiber (generally 50 grams or more per day) can decrease the absorption of important vitamins and minerals—specifically calcium, zinc, magnesium, and iron. With all this in mind, once again, be sure to increase your fiber *gradually*, over a period of several weeks, and drink plenty of extra fluids to help the fiber pass through your system. The key is to pay attention to your body's response so you can figure out the amount you can handle at one time.

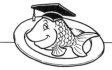

### Food for Thought

Watch how the amount of fiber can decrease as food changes form:

Apple with peel = 3.0 grams

Apple without peel = 2.4 grams

$\frac{1}{2}$ cup apple juice = 0 grams

---

### The Least You Need to Know

➤ Fiber is the indigestible substance found in plants and is classified in two categories: water-soluble and water-insoluble.

➤ Most foods contain combinations of both fibers. Foods particularly rich in soluble-fiber include oats, oat bran, legumes, rye, fruits, and vegetables. Foods rich in insoluble-fiber include wheat bran, whole wheat breads and cereals, fruits, and vegetables.

➤ Evidence suggests that soluble fiber can help lower blood cholesterol and improve the control of blood sugar in diabetics. Insoluble fiber has been reported to decrease the risk for colon cancer and diverticulosis, along with preventing hemorrhoids and constipation.

➤ The recommended fiber intake is 20–35 grams a day and is an important part of every well-structured food-plan for the average adult.

➤ Increase your fiber gradually to give your body time to adjust. Also, be sure to drink plenty of extra fluids.

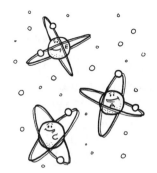

# Vitamins and Minerals: The "Micro" Guys

A woman walked into my office for an initial consult. After introducing herself, she pulled open a large duffel bag filled to the rim with vitamin and mineral bottles. "I take one of each, every day," she claimed. "Why?" I asked. "Well, a neighbor told me about extra Bs, and my hairdresser recommended extra iron, and the others I can't seem to remember."

Unfortunately, this story is not uncommon. Popping pills has certainly become a popular morning ritual throughout this country. And why not? We've all heard the dramatic tales of vitamins and minerals. From health-food stores to infomercials, everyone seems to be buzzing about megadosing on one thing or another. Needless to say, the vitamin industry is big business, with annual sales reaching the *multi-billion dollar* level.

Do you really need all of the pills? Chances are you don't. With so much misinformation floating around, it's no wonder some people swallow exorbitant amounts of supplements they don't need. By the way, those extra supplements are literally money down the toilet because your body usually filters out the extra stuff. What's worse, some vitamins do not get flushed out and can potentially become toxic.

Don't get me wrong, vitamins and minerals are essential for normal functioning, and without them, you could not survive. However, your body requires only minute amounts of these "micro-guys," and most nutrition experts agree that the best way to get all the vitamins and minerals you need is to eat a balanced, varied diet. Although some groups of people *can* benefit from supplements, it is important to check with a competent health professional before running out to your nearest drugstore.

Get ready to buckle in and find out whether you are getting what your body needs. This chapter will help to clear up the facts on vitamins and minerals.

# What Are Vitamins and Minerals?

In previous chapters, you became familiar with the macro-nutrients carbohydrate, protein, and fat. Now it's time to understand the micro-nutrients (in other words, vitamins and minerals), which exist *within* the macro-nutrients. Although the macro-nutrients receive top billing, these micro-guys are equally important in our diets because they perform specific jobs that enable your body to operate efficiently.

Think about carbohydrate, protein, and fat as the rock stars on stage. Now, imagine the vitamins and minerals as the backup singers, the band, and all the people who help produce the concert. The big guys and little guys work together to get the job done, and the result is one dynamite show.

That's how your body works. You eat the carbohydrate, protein, and fat, which in turn supply your body with the 13 vitamins and at least 22 minerals you need. Although tiny in size and quantity, these nutrients accomplish the mighty tasks that keep your body going. Furthermore, a lack of any one will cause a unique deficiency that can only be corrected by supplying that particular nutrient.

## The RDAs: Recommended Dietary Allowances

The Recommended Dietary Allowances (RDAs) are standards set by an expert committee known as the Food and Nutrition Board of the National Academy of Sciences/National Research Council. These recommendations list the average daily requirements for a variety of nutrients (in other words, vitamins and minerals) and are intended for healthy people.

Note: People with certain illnesses might require more or less of specific nutrients. The RDA guidelines are set slightly higher than the level your body actually needs, building in a precautionary safety net.

**Food for Thought**

For your personal nutrition profile, visit my Web site at www.joyofnutrition.com. Simply fill out your food for a typical day (plus list your height, weight, and age), and I'll show how you measure up to your daily requirements for vitamins, minerals, calories, carbohydrate, protein, fat, sugar, fiber, and much more.

## The DRIs: Dietary Reference Intakes

Because scientific knowledge regarding diet and health has increased, the Food and Nutrition Board has recently expanded its framework and developed the Dietary Reference Intakes (DRI's) for several vital nutrients. It is forecasted that over the next 3–4 years additional groups of nutrients including phtyoestrogens, antioxidants and phytochemicals will also be slated for review toward DRI development. These new DRI standards include the RDAs as goals for intakes, plus three new reference values; the estimated average requirement (EAR), the tolerable upper limit (UL), and the adequate intake (AI). On the two reference charts provided here, you'll notice that some nutrients are listed as DRIs, some as RDAs, and some as AIs—a bit confusing—but all you'll need to understand is the actual recommended amount.

FOOD AND NUTRITION BOARD, NATIONAL ACADEMY OF SCIENCES–NATIONAL RESEARCH COUNCIL
RECOMMENDED DIETARY ALLOWANCES,[a] Revised 1989 (Abridged)
*Designed for the maintenance of good nutrition of practically all healthy people in the United States*

| Category | Age (years) or Condition | Weight[b] (kg) | (lb) | Height[b] (cm) | (in) | Protein (g) | Vitamin A (µg RE)[c] | Vitamin E (mg α-TE)[d] | Vitamin K (µg) | Vitamin C (mg) | Iron (mg) | Zinc (mg) | Iodine (µg) | Selenium (µg) |
|---|---|---|---|---|---|---|---|---|---|---|---|---|---|---|
| Infants | 0.0–0.5 | 6 | 13 | 60 | 24 | 13 | 375 | 3 | 5 | 30 | 6 | 5 | 40 | 10 |
| | 0.5–1.0 | 9 | 20 | 71 | 28 | 14 | 375 | 4 | 10 | 35 | 10 | 5 | 50 | 15 |
| Children | 1–3 | 13 | 29 | 90 | 35 | 16 | 400 | 6 | 15 | 40 | 10 | 10 | 70 | 20 |
| | 4–6 | 20 | 44 | 112 | 44 | 24 | 500 | 7 | 20 | 45 | 10 | 10 | 90 | 20 |
| | 7–10 | 28 | 62 | 132 | 52 | 28 | 700 | 7 | 30 | 45 | 10 | 10 | 120 | 30 |
| Males | 11–14 | 45 | 99 | 157 | 62 | 45 | 1,000 | 10 | 45 | 50 | 12 | 15 | 150 | 40 |
| | 15–18 | 66 | 145 | 176 | 69 | 59 | 1,000 | 10 | 65 | 60 | 12 | 15 | 150 | 50 |
| | 19–24 | 72 | 160 | 177 | 70 | 58 | 1,000 | 10 | 70 | 60 | 10 | 15 | 150 | 70 |
| | 25–50 | 79 | 174 | 176 | 70 | 63 | 1,000 | 10 | 80 | 60 | 10 | 15 | 150 | 70 |
| | 51+ | 77 | 170 | 173 | 68 | 63 | 1,000 | 10 | 80 | 60 | 10 | 15 | 150 | 70 |
| Females | 11–14 | 46 | 101 | 157 | 62 | 46 | 800 | 8 | 45 | 50 | 15 | 12 | 150 | 45 |
| | 15–18 | 55 | 120 | 163 | 64 | 44 | 800 | 8 | 55 | 60 | 15 | 12 | 150 | 50 |
| | 19–24 | 58 | 128 | 164 | 65 | 46 | 800 | 8 | 60 | 60 | 15 | 12 | 150 | 55 |
| | 25–50 | 63 | 138 | 163 | 64 | 50 | 800 | 8 | 65 | 60 | 15 | 12 | 150 | 55 |
| | 51+ | 65 | 143 | 160 | 63 | 50 | 800 | 8 | 65 | 60 | 10 | 12 | 150 | 55 |
| Pregnant | | | | | | 60 | 800 | 10 | 65 | 70 | 30 | 15 | 175 | 65 |
| Lactating | 1st 6 months | | | | | 65 | 1,300 | 12 | 65 | 95 | 15 | 19 | 200 | 65 |
| | 2nd 6 months | | | | | 62 | 1,200 | 11 | 65 | 90 | 15 | 16 | 200 | 75 |

**NOTE:** This table does not include nutrients for which Dietary Reference Intakes have recently been established (see *Dietary Reference Intakes for Calcium, Phosphorus, Magnesium, Vitamin D, and Fluoride* [1997] and *Dietary Reference Intakes for Thiamin, Riboflavin, Niacin, Vitamin B6, Folate, Vitamin B12, Pantothenic Acid, Biotin, and Choline* [1998]).

[a] The allowances, expressed as average daily intakes over time, are intended to provide for individual variations among most normal persons as they live in the United States under usual environmental stresses. Diets should be based on a variety of common foods in order to provide other nutrients for which human requirements have been less well defined.
[b] Weights and heights of Reference Adults are actual medians for the U.S. population of the designated age, as reported by NHANES II. The median weights and heights of those under 19 years of age were taken from Hamill et al. (1979). The use of these figures does not imply that the height-to-weight ratios are ideal.
[c] Retinol equivalents. 1 retinol equivalent = 1 µg retinol or 6 µg β-carotene.
[d] α-Tocopherol equivalents. 1 mg d-α tocopherol = 1 α-TE.

FOOD AND NUTRITION BOARD, INSTITUTE OF MEDICINE–NATIONAL ACADEMY OF SCIENCES
DIETARY REFERENCE INTAKES: RECOMMENDED INTAKES FOR INDIVIDUALS

| Life-Stage Group | Calcium (mg/d) | Phosphorus (mg/d) | Magnesium (mg/d) | Vitamin D (μg/d)[a,b] | Fluoride (mg/d) | Thiamin (mg/d) | Riboflavin (mg/d) | Niacin (mg/d)[c] | Vitamin B$_6$ (mg/d) | Folate (μg/d)[d] | Vitamin B$_{12}$ (μg/d) | Pantothenic Acid (mg/d) | Biotin (μg/d) | Choline[e] (mg/d) |
|---|---|---|---|---|---|---|---|---|---|---|---|---|---|---|
| Infants | | | | | | | | | | | | | | |
| 0–6 mo | 210* | 100* | 30* | 5* | 0.01* | 0.2* | 0.3* | 2* | 0.1* | 65* | 0.4* | 1.7* | 5* | 125* |
| 7–12 mo | 270* | 275* | 75* | 5* | 0.5* | 0.3* | 0.4* | 4* | 0.3* | 80* | 0.5* | 1.8* | 6* | 150* |
| Children | | | | | | | | | | | | | | |
| 1–3 yr | 500* | 460 | 80 | 5* | 0.7* | 0.5 | 0.5 | 6 | 0.5 | 150 | 0.9 | 2* | 8* | 200* |
| 4–8 yr | 800* | 500 | 130 | 5* | 1* | 0.6 | 0.6 | 8 | 0.6 | 200 | 1.2 | 3* | 12* | 250* |
| Males | | | | | | | | | | | | | | |
| 9–13 yr | 1,300* | 1,250 | 240 | 5* | 2* | 0.9 | 0.9 | 12 | 1.0 | 300 | 1.8 | 4* | 20* | 375* |
| 14–18 yr | 1,300* | 1,250 | 410 | 5* | 3* | 1.2 | 1.3 | 16 | 1.3 | 400 | 2.4 | 5* | 25* | 550* |
| 19–30 yr | 1,000* | 700 | 400 | 5* | 4* | 1.2 | 1.3 | 16 | 1.3 | 400 | 2.4 | 5* | 30* | 550* |
| 31–50 yr | 1,000* | 700 | 420 | 5* | 4* | 1.2 | 1.3 | 16 | 1.3 | 400 | 2.4 | 5* | 30* | 550* |
| 51–70 yr | 1,200* | 700 | 420 | 10* | 4* | 1.2 | 1.3 | 16 | 1.7 | 400 | 2.4[f] | 5* | 30* | 550* |
| >70 yr | 1,200* | 700 | 420 | 15* | 4* | 1.2 | 1.3 | 16 | 1.7 | 400 | 2.4[f] | 5* | 30* | 550* |
| Females | | | | | | | | | | | | | | |
| 9–13 yr | 1,300* | 1,250 | 240 | 5* | 2* | 0.9 | 0.9 | 12 | 1.0 | 300 | 1.8 | 4* | 20* | 375* |
| 14–18 yr | 1,300* | 1,250 | 360 | 5* | 3* | 1.0 | 1.0 | 14 | 1.2 | 400[g] | 2.4 | 5* | 25* | 400* |
| 19–30 yr | 1,000* | 700 | 310 | 5* | 3* | 1.1 | 1.1 | 14 | 1.3 | 400[g] | 2.4 | 5* | 30* | 425* |
| 31–50 yr | 1,000* | 700 | 320 | 5* | 3* | 1.1 | 1.1 | 14 | 1.3 | 400[g] | 2.4 | 5* | 30* | 425* |
| 51–70 yr | 1,200* | 700 | 320 | 10* | 3* | 1.1 | 1.1 | 14 | 1.5 | 400 | 2.4[f] | 5* | 30* | 425* |
| >70 yr | 1,200* | 700 | 320 | 15* | 3* | 1.1 | 1.1 | 14 | 1.5 | 400 | 2.4[f] | 5* | 30* | 425* |
| Pregnancy | | | | | | | | | | | | | | |
| ≤18 yr | 1,300* | 1,250 | 400 | 5* | 3* | 1.4 | 1.4 | 18 | 1.9 | 600[h] | 2.6 | 6* | 30* | 450* |
| 19–30 yr | 1,000* | 700 | 350 | 5* | 3* | 1.4 | 1.4 | 18 | 1.9 | 600[h] | 2.6 | 6* | 30* | 450* |
| 31–50 yr | 1,000* | 700 | 360 | 5* | 3* | 1.4 | 1.4 | 18 | 1.9 | 600[h] | 2.6 | 6* | 30* | 450* |
| Lactation | | | | | | | | | | | | | | |
| ≤18 yr | 1,300* | 1,250 | 360 | 5* | 3* | 1.5 | 1.6 | 17 | 2.0 | 500 | 2.8 | 7* | 35* | 550* |
| 19–30 yr | 1,000* | 700 | 310 | 5* | 3* | 1.5 | 1.6 | 17 | 2.0 | 500 | 2.8 | 7* | 35* | 550* |
| 31–50 yr | 1,000* | 700 | 320 | 5* | 3* | 1.5 | 1.6 | 17 | 2.0 | 500 | 2.8 | 7* | 35* | 550* |

NOTE: This table presents Recommended Dietary Allowances (RDAs) in **bold type** and Adequate Intakes (AIs) in ordinary type followed by an asterisk (*). RDAs and AIs may both be used as goals for individual intake. RDAs are set to meet the needs of almost all (97 to 98 percent) individuals in a group. For healthy breastfed infants, the AI is the mean intake. The AI for other life-stage and gender groups is believed to cover needs of all individuals in the group, but lack of data or uncertainty in the data prevent being able to specify with confidence the percentage of individuals covered by this intake.

a As cholecalciferol. 1 μg cholecalciferol = 40 IU vitamin D.
b In the absence of adequate exposure to sunlight.
c As niacin equivalents (NE). 1 mg of niacin = 60 mg of tryptophan; 0–6 months = preformed niacin (not NE).
d As dietary folate equivalents (DFE). 1 DFE = 1 μg food folate = 0.6 μg of folic acid (from fortified food or supplement) consumed with food = 0.5 μg of synthetic (supplemental) folic acid taken on an empty stomach.
e Although AIs have been set for choline, there are few data to assess whether a dietary supply of choline is needed at all stages of the life cycle, and it may be that the choline requirement can be met by endogenous synthesis at some of these stages.
f Because 10 to 30 percent of older people may malabsorb food-bound B$_{12}$, it is advisable for those older than 50 years to meet their RDA mainly by consuming foods fortified with B$_{12}$ or a supplement containing B$_{12}$.
g In view of evidence linking folate intake with neural tube defects in the fetus, it is recommended that all women capable of becoming pregnant consume 400 μg of synthetic folic acid from fortified foods and/or supplements in addition to intake of food folate from a varied diet.
h It is assumed that women will continue consuming 400 μg of folic acid until their pregnancy is confirmed and they enter prenatal care, which ordinarily occurs after the end of the periconceptional period—the critical time for formation of the neural tube.

# Fat-Soluble Vitamins

Vitamins are organic compounds (compounds that contain carbon), and of the 13 that your body needs, 4 are called fat-soluble (A, D, E, and K). Fat-soluble vitamins do not dissolve in water and are stored in your body's fat and liver. As a result, these vitamins can build up in the tissues and become toxic (specifically vitamins A and D).

Vitamins fall into two classes: fat-soluble and water-soluble.

| Fat-Soluble Vitamins | Water-Soluble Vitamins |
| --- | --- |
| Vitamin A | B-vitamins |
| Vitamin D | Thiamin |
| Vitamin E | Riboflavin |
| Vitamin K | Niacin |
| | Vitamin B-6 |
| | Folate |
| | Vitamin B-12 |
| | Pantothenic acid |
| | Biotin |
| | Vitamin C |

## *Vitamin A (Retinol)*

Like Mom always said, eat plenty of carrots and you'll see in the dark. That's because carrots contain beta-carotene, a substance that is converted into vitamin A by your body. Vitamin A promotes good vision, as well as healthy skin and the normal growth and maintenance of your bones, teeth, and mucous membranes. What Mom didn't tell you was that beta-carotene is also found in most orange-yellow fruits and vegetables, along with dark-green vegetables.

Your body converts beta-carotene into vitamin A only when you need it, so eating foods rich in beta-carotene cannot cause vitamin A toxicity. However, eating huge amounts might turn your skin slightly orange. Not to worry, this condition isn't serious. Simply lay off the orange veggies for a few days and the color will disappear.

Although your body controls the creation of vitamin A from beta-carotene, it has no control when you ingest straight vitamin A, which can be found in vitamin tablets. Over-supplementation can be extremely toxic, resulting in general fatigue and weakness, severe headaches, blurred vision, insomnia, hair loss, menstrual irregularities, skin rashes, and joint pain. In extreme cases, there can be liver and brain damage. Huge doses taken in the prenatal period can cause birth defects.

What happens if you don't get enough? Vitamin-A deficiency can cause night blindness, total blindness, and lowered resistance to infection because vitamin A plays a key role in the structural integrity of your cells. Here come the germs!

Foods rich in vitamin A:

> Liver
>
> Eggs
>
> Milk
>
> Butter
>
> Margarine
>
> Cheese

Foods rich in beta-carotene:

> Cantaloupe
>
> Carrots
>
> Sweet potato
>
> Winter squash
>
> Spinach
>
> Broccoli

# Vitamin D: the Sunshine Vitamin

Vitamin D plays an indispensable role in building and maintaining strong bones and teeth. In fact, vitamin D is responsible for the body's absorption and utilization of the mineral calcium. Insufficient amounts of this key vitamin can lead to serious bone abnormalities, including rickets in children (bones that are soft and malformed) and osteoporosis or osteomalacia (softening of the bone) in adults.

On the other hand, vitamin D is fat-soluble, so taking large supplemental doses can be dangerous. Some of the toxic effects involve drowsiness, diarrhea, loss of appetite, headaches, high blood pressure, high cholesterol, fragile bones, and calcium deposits throughout your body (including your heart, kidneys, and blood vessels). If you are taking supplements, make sure you're not getting much more than the recommended amount for your age category; you'll notice that folks over 50 need more. Also, note that the adequate intake (AI) for vitamin D is given in micrograms on the chart; the vitamin D in food and supplements is usually measured in international units (IU). The conversion is one microgram = 40 international units (IU).

Foods rich in vitamin D:

| | |
|---|---|
| Fortified milk | Margarine |
| Egg yolk | Tuna |
| Salmon | Canned sardines |
| Cod-liver oil | Shrimp |
| Mackerel | |

Your body can also synthesize it's own Vitamin D when your skin is exposed to sunlight for 10–20 minutes. In fact, three sunny days per week can provide you with all the vitamin D you need.

## Vitamin E (Tocopherols)

Talk about a hot nutrient! Later, I explain vitamin E's tremendous role as an antioxidant, but for now, let's investigate its traditional side.

Vitamin E aids the formation and functioning of your red blood cells, muscle, and other tissues and protects essential fatty acids (special fats that are needed by your body). Because vitamin E is found in a variety of foods, deficiency is rare. However, an extreme case of vitamin-E deficiency involves wasting of the muscles and neurological disorders. To date, there have been no shown toxic effects from taking doses well over the RDA.

Foods rich in vitamin E:

| | |
|---|---|
| Vegetable oils | Margarine |
| Salad dressings | Whole-grain cereals |
| Green leafy vegetables | Nuts and seeds |
| Peanut butter | Wheat germ |

## Vitamin K

Thanks to vitamin K, you won't bleed to death after an injury. That's because vitamin K is essential for normal blood clotting. Current research also suggests that this vitamin might play a role in maintaining strong bones in the elderly. Where do you get this vitamin? Interestingly enough, bacteria that live in your intestines help to make 80 percent of the vitamin K that you need, and the rest can be found in a variety of foods listed here.

A vitamin K deficiency can cause hemorrhaging (uncontrollable bleeding), mainly in newborn infants because their immature intestinal tracts might not have enough bacteria to make this vitamin. In addition, people taking antibiotics might temporarily lose the ability to make vitamin K because the medication destroys all bacteria, good and bad.

Foods rich in vitamin K:

| | |
|---|---|
| Turnip greens | Cauliflower |
| Spinach | Beef liver |
| Broccoli | Kale |
| Cabbage | |

# Water-Soluble Vitamins

Unlike fat-soluble vitamins, water-soluble vitamins can easily dissolve in the watery fluids of your body. Because excessive amounts are generally excreted in the urine, there is less chance for toxic side effects but more chance for deficiencies. Therefore, it is important to regularly replenish these vitamins by eating healthy foods that supply ample amounts. Be extra careful during food preparation. Because some of these vitamins are easily washed away or destroyed by light, air, and heat, use small amounts of water, avoid overcooking, and only cut your fruits and vegetables right before you eat them. The following provides a quick rundown on each of the nine water-soluble vitamins, eight B-vitamins, and vitamin C.

## Thiamin (B-1)

Thiamin is needed for the conversion of carbohydrate-rich foods into energy. B-1 also plays a role in keeping your brain, nerve, and heart cells healthy. A deficiency will lead to loss of energy, nausea, depression, muscle cramps, nerve damage, and muscular weakness. Although uncommon in the United States, a severe depletion of thiamin can result in the disease beriberi, causing potential muscle wasting and paralysis.

Foods rich in thiamin (B-1 ):

| | |
|---|---|
| Pork | Beef |
| Liver | Peas |
| Seeds | Legumes |
| Whole-grain products | Oatmeal |
| Lamb | |

## Riboflavin (B-2)

Like its buddy thiamin, riboflavin plays a key role in the metabolism of energy. Furthermore, this vitamin is involved in the formation of red blood cells and is necessary for healthy skin and normal vision.

A riboflavin deficiency will cause dry, scaly skin, accompanied by cracks on your lips and in the corners of your mouth. If that's not enough, getting insufficient amounts can also make your eyes extremely sensitive to light.

Foods rich in riboflavin (B-2):

| | |
|---|---|
| Milk | Yogurt |
| Cheese | Whole-grain breads and cereals |
| Green leafy vegetables | Meat |
| Eggs | Beef liver |

Note: This vitamin is easily destroyed with exposure to sunlight; therefore, store these foods in the fridge, cabinet, or pantry.

# Niacin (B-3)

This B-vitamin is also involved in energy-producing reactions in the cells that convert food to energy. In addition, niacin helps maintain healthy skin, nerves, and your digestive system. In some instances, you can use large doses of niacin as a cholesterol-lowering medication. However, you should only do this under the supervision of your doctor. Megadoses can cause hot flashes, itching, ulcers, high blood-sugar, and liver damage.

In the rare case of a niacin deficiency, symptoms include diarrhea, mouth sores, changes in the skin, nervous disorders, and pellagra disease known to cause the "four Ds": diarrhea, dermatitis, dementia (mental confusion), and death.

Foods rich in niacin (B-3):

| | |
|---|---|
| Meat | Poultry |
| Liver | Eggs |
| Nuts | Enriched breads and cereals |
| Brown rice | Baked potato |
| Fish | Peanut butter |
| Milk | Whole grains |

# Pyridoxine (B-6)

Vitamin B-6 is a vital component for chemical reactions involving proteins and amino acids. (Remember those protein-building blocks?) It also participates in the formation of red blood cells, antibodies, and insulin, in addition to maintaining normal brain function. Deficiency causes skin changes, convulsions in infants, dementia, nervous disorders, and anemia.

Foods rich in pyridoxine (B-6):

| | |
|---|---|
| Lean meats | Fish |
| Legumes | Green leafy vegetables |
| Raisins | Corn |
| Whole-grain cereals | Pork |
| Bananas | Lentils |
| Mangos | Poultry |

# Cobalamin (B-12)

Vitamin B-12 assists in the formation of red blood cells and the normal functioning of your nervous system and is required for the synthesis of DNA (your genetic résumé). Because B-12 is only found in foods of animal origin, strict vegetarians might need to take a supplement to avoid a deficiency. Furthermore, this unique vitamin needs the help of another substance called *intrinsic factor* to be absorbed. Because intrinsic factor is made by the lining of the stomach, people with gastrointestinal disorders (especially in the elderly) might need to get B-12 shots directly into the bloodstream. Symptoms of B-12 deficiency include nervous disorders and pernicious anemia.

Because a good amount of vitamin B-12 can be stored in the liver, it might take years for a deficiency to be recognized. As a result, people should have their B-12 levels checked starting at age 60 and every decade thereafter.

Foods rich in cobalamin (B-12):

| | |
|---|---|
| Meat | Fish |
| Poultry | Eggs |
| Milk products | Clams |

## Folic Acid (Folacin, Folate)

Folic acid appropriately gets its name from the word *foliage* because it's primarily found in leafy, dark-green vegetables. In addition to playing a vital role in cell division and red blood cell formation, this vitamin is needed to make the genetic material DNA.

In recent years, folic acid has gained a lot of attention for its ability to reduce neural-tube birth defects in newborn babies. Needless to say, it is imperative that pregnant mothers and women of childbearing years (because some women do not even know they are pregnant until after the fact) get appropriate amounts of folic acid by both foods and supplementation. For this reason, folic acid is a key ingredient in most prenatal vitamins. Because this nutrient is involved in cell division, a deficiency will leave you vulnerable to anemia and an abnormal digestive function because your blood cells and cells of the intestinal tract divide most rapidly.

**Food for Thought**

Folic acid has recently been shown to decrease your risk for colon cancer. If you have ulcerative colitis or feel that you are at a high risk for colon cancer—speak to your if possible physician about supplementation.

Folic Acid can also reduce the risk of heart disease by lowering the levels of a harmful substance called homocysteine in the blood.

Foods rich in folic acid:

| | |
|---|---|
| Spinach | Liver |
| Beans (all types) | Peas |
| Asparagus | Lima beans |
| Oranges | Brussel sprouts |
| Collard greens | Avocado |

## Pantothenic Acid and Biotin

Pantothenic acid and biotin are both part of the "B-vitamin gang" that participates in the metabolism of energy. In addition, pantothenic acid also plays a role in the formation of certain hormones and neurotransmitters. Although both vitamins are vital for normal functioning, as of today there isn't a set RDA for either one. This is because deficiencies are so rare, and they are both found in a wide variety of plant and animal foods.

# Vitamin C (Ascorbic Acid)

Now for the million dollar question, "Can vitamin C ward off the common cold?" The scientists say no. To date, there is no documented evidence supporting this notion. Interestingly enough, this vitamin might lessen the severity of those lousy symptoms experienced *during* a cold because vitamin C has a mild antihistaminic effect.

What else can vitamin C do? Let's just say if all the vitamins and minerals were on a pay scale according to the jobs they perform, vitamin C would be rolling. Vitamin C wears many hats, from helping to keep your bones, teeth, and blood vessels healthy to healing wounds, boosting your resistance to infection, and participating in the formation of collagen (a protein that helps support body structures). Another benefit from eating vitamin-C–rich foods is that you increase the absorption of the mineral iron—good news for people with greater iron requirements or deficiencies.

Although vitamin C deficiency is uncommon, it can cause a lowered resistance to infection, sore gums, hemorrhages, and in severe cases, the disease scurvy.

On the flip side, some studies have shown that megadosing on vitamin C might help reduce the risk of certain diseases. (This is further discussed in the section on antioxidants.) However, large doses might also lead to uncomfortable side effects, including diarrhea and nausea.

Foods rich in vitamin C:

| | |
|---|---|
| Melons | Berries |
| Tomatoes | Potatoes |
| Broccoli | Fortified juices |
| Guava | Kiwi |
| Mango | Papaya |

Citrus fruits (oranges, grapefruits, etc.)
Yellow peppers

**Nutri-Speak**

**Scurvy** is a disease resulting from a deficiency of vitamin C, characterized by bleeding and swollen gums, joint pain, muscle wasting, and bruises. Scurvy is now very rare, except among alcoholics, and can be cured by as little as five to seven milligrams of vitamin C.

**Overrated—Undercooked**

For reasons that are unclear, cigarette smokers seem to require 50 percent more of vitamin C than non-smokers. Instead of popping more vitamin C, why not just quit smoking?

# A Day in the Life of an Antioxidant

We've all heard the news: Antioxidants reduce your risk for heart disease and certain cancers and boost your immune system. So what exactly are antioxidants and how do they work?

**Nutri-Speak**

**Free radicals** can be described as unstable, hyperactive atoms that literally trek around your body damaging healthy cells and tissue.

**Overrated—Undercooked**

Although beta-carotene is still considered a powerful antioxidant, it is no longer recommended in supplemental form. Several years ago, a study found that smokers who took beta-carotene supplements showed an increased risk of lung cancer. However, these findings certainly do not mean that beta-carotene has lost any importance among the antioxidant world. It does mean that until we have further information, people should solely focus on getting beta-carotene from food sources rather than supplemental megadoses.

As you know, every cell in your body needs oxygen to function normally. Unfortunately, the utilization of this oxygen produces harmful by-products called *free radicals*. Free radicals are also created from environmental pollution, certain industrial chemicals, and smoking.

Outside the body, the process of oxidation is responsible for a sliced apple turning brown and the rusting of metal. Inside the body, oxidation contributes to heart disease, cancer, cataracts, aging, and a slew of other degenerative diseases. In other words, free radicals are the enemy.

So why isn't everyone falling apart? Your cells have their own special defense technique to fight off these radical monsters. What's more, scientists have unfolded compelling evidence suggesting that certain vitamins (specifically C, E, and beta-carotene) can actually enhance your body's ability to ward off these free radicals and therefore prevent oxidation. Appropriately, we call these vitamins antioxidants.

## What Can Antioxidants Do?

To date, numerous studies have shown that antioxidants may protect against the following:

➤ **Cardiovascular disease:** Findings from studies suggest that vitamins C and E might play a role in future strategies for heart disease prevention by reducing the amount of LDL-cholesterol lodged in the arteries. (Remember these bad guys from an earlier chapter?)

➤ **Cancer:** Studies suggest that vitamins E and C and beta-carotene might have a protective effect against several types of cancers. Keep in mind that many factors appear to influence the development of cancer, including heredity, smoking, nutritional excesses and deficiencies, and the environment.

➤ **Cataracts:** Scientists suspect that cataracts develop from the oxidation of the proteins in the lens of the eye. Antioxidants might help to reduce the risk of developing this disease.

➤ **Immunity:** Researchers theorize that antioxidants might help to strengthen the immune system by preventing the action of free radicals.

➤ **Exercise-induced free radical damage:** Recent studies have shown increased free radical activity following strenuous exercise. Therefore, vitamin E might play a role in reducing muscle inflammation and soreness after bouts of vigorous workouts.

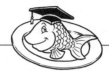

**Food for Thought**

Popeye was sure on to something. With just one can of spinach (2 cups), he swallowed down about 29,000 IUs of beta-carotene, 50 milligrams of vitamin C, and 12 milligrams of vitamin E. That's one heck of a healthy sailor!

## How Much Should You Take?

Your primary (and secondary) focus should be on eating *foods* rich in antioxidant vitamins. Contrary to what people might think, there are no magic bullets (or pills) to good health. Another plug for food is that scientists are constantly discovering new food substances that might help with the quest for well-being. Furthermore, future findings may even reveal that it's not just one isolated vitamin but interactions between several food ingredients that enhance disease prevention.

To date, no harmful side effects have been reported from supplemental doses well above the RDA for vitamins E and C. However, the science of nutrition is constantly being challenged with new discoveries—something to think about before popping the next pill. We know that getting your nutrients from food sources is safe and effective, but we don't know everything about supplemental megadosing.

The bottom line: If you decide to take antioxidant supplements, stay on top of the current research and speak with a competent health professional.

## The Scoop on Minerals

Together with vitamins, at least 22 minerals are needed by your body to make things happen. Major minerals such as calcium and potassium are needed in large amounts, whereas trace minerals such as iron and zinc are only required in minute amounts. Just because a mineral is classified as trace doesn't mean it is any less important. The small

**Food for Thought**

What most people *do* know is that in large quantities, arsenic becomes a lethal poison. What most people *don't* know is that in very small amounts, arsenic is an essential mineral that your body needs to function properly.

RDA for iron is just as important to your body as the large RDA for calcium. Sort of like bread—a lot of flour with a drop of yeast...both are equally important for that perfect baked loaf.

Here's the master list of minerals. The following chapter focuses on two powerhouse players: calcium and iron.

| Major Minerals | Trace Minerals |
| --- | --- |
| Calcium | Iron |
| Chloride | Zinc |
| Magnesium | Iodine |
| Phosphorus | Selenium |
| Potassium | Copper |
| Sodium | Manganese |
| Sulfur | Fluoride |
| | Chromium |
| | Molybdenum |
| | Arsenic |
| | Nickel |
| | Silicon |
| | Boron |
| | Cobalt |

## The Least You Need to Know

➤ More than 13 vitamins and 22 minerals are essential for normal body function. Eating a well-balanced, varied diet will supply your body with the all the right ingredients.

➤ Water-soluble vitamins (eight B-complex vitamins and vitamin C) can easily dissolve in the watery body fluids, and excessive amounts are generally excreted through the urine.

➤ Fat-soluble vitamins (A, D, E, and K) do not dissolve in water and are stored in the body's fat. As a result, these vitamins have the potential to build up in tissues and become toxic with large supplemental doses (specifically A and D).

➤ Antioxidants can help to prevent certain cancers, heart disease, cataracts, exercise-induced soreness, and other degenerative diseases by protecting against free radical damage. Eat plenty of foods rich in vitamins C and E and beta carotene to reap the benefits.

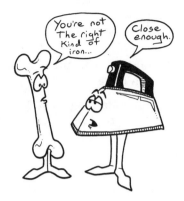

# Chapter 8

# Mighty Minerals: Calcium and Iron

> **In This Chapter**
>
> ➤ All about calcium and iron
>
> ➤ How much do you need
>
> ➤ Where to find the best food sources
>
> ➤ Are you a candidate for a vitamin or mineral supplement?

As you've learned from the preceding chapter, at least 22 minerals are essential for a number of vital functions and body processes. Because not a day goes by without a client or friend asking for some sort of information regarding calcium or iron, I've dedicated this entire chapter to these powerhouse minerals.

## Calcium and Healthy Bones

Calcium is by far the most abundant mineral in your body, with about 99 percent of the stuff stored in your bones. The other 1 percent is located in your body fluids, where it helps to regulate functions such as blood pressure, nerve transmission, muscle contraction (including the heart beat), clotting of blood, and the secretion of hormones and digestive enzymes. Make no bones about it: Calcium, along with vitamin D, fluoride, and phosphorus, is best known for its ability to promote strong, healthy bones. Calcium serves a vital role in bone structure, providing integrity and density to your skeleton. In turn, your bones act as a "calcium bank," releasing calcium into your blood when your diet might be deficient (which we hope is not too often).

Many people think that once you're past a certain age, you don't have to worry about getting enough calcium. Wrong! Adequate calcium is important *throughout* your life: first and foremost for optimal bone building, and later on for bone maintenance.

Generally, the first 24 years are important because your body is laying down the foundation for strong skeletal bones and teeth. In the first three decades of life, your bones reach their *peak adult bone mass*. (Bones are done growing in size and density.) Children who drink plenty of milk and eat other dairy products will enter adulthood with stronger bones than those who skimp on calcium-rich foods.

Calcium intake in the later years is equally important for maintaining healthy bones. (I hope you already did all the right things in your first 30 years.) With age, your bones gradually lose their density (that is, calcium), which is especially true in menopausal women. People who take in adequate amounts of calcium can help slow down this process and defy those brittle bones of old age.

## Q & A

**Why bother with calcium?**

Imagine your bones as your calcium bank. Over the years, you can develop quite an extensive savings account by taking in plenty of calcium-rich foods and supplementing your diet with calcium pills. Keep up the good work as an adult and your bones stay calcium-rich!

On the other hand, regularly skimp on this mineral, and you'll wind up calcium-broke! Your body fluids still need calcium to regulate normal body functions. What these fluids don't get from food must be borrowed from the calcium-bone bank. Borrowing day after day, year after year, will deplete the savings account and leave you with osteoporosis (brittle bones that break easily).

# How Much Calcium Is Recommended?

The DRIs (Dietary Reference Intake) for calcium are laid out for various age categories; here are the recommendations:

| Group | DRI (mg/d) |
|---|---|
| *Infants* | |
| Birth–6 months | 210 |
| 6 months–1 year | 270 |
| *Children* | |
| 1–3 years | 500 |
| 4–8 years | 800 |

| Group | DRI (mg/d) |
|---|---|
| *Male* | |
| 9–13 years | 1,300 |
| 14–18 years | 1,300 |
| 19–30 years | 1,000 |
| 31–50 years | 1,000 |
| 51–70 years | 1,200 |
| >70 years | 1,200 |
| *Females* | |
| 9–13 years | 1,300 |
| 14–18 years | 1,300 |
| 19–30 years | 1,000 |
| 31–50 years | 1,000 |
| 51–70 years | 1,200 |
| >70 years | 1,200 |
| *Pregnancy/Lactation* | |
| 18 years or less | 1,300 |
| 19–30 years | 1,000 |
| 31–50 years | 1,000 |

# Are You Getting Enough Calcium? The Foods to Choose

Browse through the following chart and notice that dairy foods, along with fortified juice and sardines, provide the most calcium hands down. One more thing: Don't be put off by the high amounts of fat in cheese. Simply shop for the low-fat brands in your local store. They have less fat but still retain ample amounts of calcium.

## The Best Sources of Calcium in Various Foods

| Milk Group | Amount | Calcium in mg |
|---|---|---|
| Yogurt, plain (low-fat) | 1 cup | 415 |
| Yogurt, fruit-flavored (low-fat) | 1 cup | 345 |
| Milk, nonfat (dry) | $1/4$ cup | 377 |
| Milk, skim | 1 cup | 302 |
| Milk, 1%–2% | 1 cup | 300 |
| Milk, whole* | 1 cup | 291 |
| Buttermilk | 1 cup | 285 |
| Milk, chocolate (low-fat) | 1 cup | 284 |
| Cheese, Parmesan (grated) | $1/4$ cup | 338 |

*continues*

*continued*

| Milk Group | Amount | Calcium in mg |
|---|---|---|
| Cheese, Swiss* | 1 oz | 272 |
| Cheese, Monterey Jack* | 1 oz | 212 |
| Cheese, mozzarella low moisture, part skim | 1 oz | 207 |
| Cheese, cheddar* | 1 oz | 204 |
| Cheese, colby* | 1 oz | 194 |
| Cheese, American* | 1 oz | 174 |
| Ice cream* | $1/2$ cup | 88 |
| Cottage cheese, creamed 1% | $1/2$ cup | 63 |

| Fruit and Vegetable Group | Amount | Calcium in mg |
|---|---|---|
| Collards, cooked | $1/2$ cup | 168 |
| Turnip greens, cooked | $1/2$ cup | 134 |
| Kale, cooked | $1/2$ cup | 103 |
| Spinach, cooked | $1/2$ cup | 84 |
| Broccoli, cooked | $1/2$ cup | 68 |

| Fruit and Vegetable Group | Amount | Calcium in mg |
|---|---|---|
| Chard, cooked | $1/2$ cup | 64 |
| Carrot, raw | 1 med. | 27 |
| Orange | 1 med. | 60 |
| Dates, chopped | $1/2$ cup | 26 |
| Raisins | $1/2$ cup | 22 |

| Protein Group (Meat, Beans, Eggs) | Amount | Calcium in mg |
|---|---|---|
| Sardines (canned, w/bones) | 3 oz | 372 |
| Salmon, pink (canned, w/bones) | 3 oz | 165 |
| Tofu (processed, w/calcium) | 4 oz | 145 |
| Almonds, shelled* | 1 oz | 66 |
| Soybeans, cooked | $1/2$ cup | 66 |
| Dried beans, cooked (lima, navy, kidney) | $1/2$ cup | 35–60 |
| Egg | 1 large | 27 |
| Peanut Butter* | 2 Tbsp. | 18 |
| Beef patty, cooked* | 3 oz | 9 |

| Grain Group | Amount | Calcium in mg |
|---|---|---|
| Calcium fortified cereals (Total) with $1/2$ cup milk | 1 oz | 350 |

| Grain Group | Amount | Calcium in mg |
| --- | --- | --- |
| Farina, enriched (instant, cooked) | 1 cup | 189 |
| Tortilla, corn | 1 medium | 60 |
| Bread, whole wheat | 1 slice | 25 |

| Calcium-Fortified Foods | Amount | Calcium in mg |
| --- | --- | --- |
| Orange juice and grapefruit juice (Citrus Hill, Minute Maid) | 8 oz | 300 |
| Calcium fortified cereals (Total) | 1 cup | 300 |

*Denotes foods that are also high in fat*

*Source: Calcium Information Center*

**Q & A**

**Should I take calcium supplements?**

If you are having a problem consistently getting enough calcium from food sources, you might want to speak with your doctor about supplementation. Stick with a calcium supplement in the form of calcium carbonate or calcium citrate, and do not take more 500–600 milligrams in one dose. (Anything more than 500–600 mg will not be absorbed.) Also be aware that some calcium supplements need to be taken with food or juice for proper absorption.

If you're over 50, you might want to pick up a calcium supplement with added vitamin D. Just remember that your daily totals of vitamin D (from your multivitamin/mineral and calcium supps) should not exceed 600 I.U.

# Iron Out Your Body

Iron deficiency is the most widespread type of vitamin or mineral deficiency in the world. Do you constantly experience sluggishness, irritability, and headaches? Perhaps you suffer from this condition. Let's take a closer look and find out.

About 70 percent of the iron in your body is located in a portion of your red blood cells known as *hemoglobin*. Hemoglobin is your oxygen delivery service, supplying every cell with the oxygen it needs to perform essential metabolic functions. Iron is also a component of *myoglobin*. Like the hemoglobin in red blood cells, myoglobin ensures adequate oxygen delivery to all your muscles. At this point, you're probably starting to understand the importance of iron in this equation: too little iron, too little oxygen. The result is fatigue, irritability, weakness, headaches, tendency to feel cold, and in the case of severe depletion, iron-deficiency anemia.

Fortunately, iron is found in a variety of animal and plant foods, making it easy to get your daily requirement. *Heme* iron, the type found in animal products (red meats, liver, poultry, and eggs), is more readily absorbed than *nonheme* iron, which can be found in vegetables and other plant foods (beans, nuts, seeds, dried fruits, and fortified breads and cereals). Interestingly enough, the body adjusts the amount it absorbs according to the body's need. In other words, a person with iron-deficient anemia will absorb about two to three times more iron after eating exactly the same meal than a person with normal iron status.

Certain groups of people are at increased risk for developing an iron deficiency. If you think you might fall into one of the following categories, ask your doctor to check your iron status before self-prescribing supplementation. (A simple blood test can tell if you are deficient.)

Groups at risk for iron deficiency include

➤ Infants and children: Their rapid growth and finicky eating habits demand that they get iron in a variety of ways.

➤ Women who bleed heavily during menstruation: They lose iron-rich blood each month.

➤ Pregnant women with increased blood volume: They are supporting their growing babies' needs as well as their own.

➤ Strict vegetarians who take in only nonheme sources of iron: Remember, nonheme plant foods are *much* less absorbent than iron-rich animal foods.

➤ People who lose a lot of blood during surgery or other bleeding injuries.

➤ "Chronic dieters" who bounce from one crash diet to another: People suffering from eating disorders might not eat enough iron-rich foods to meet their requirements.

# Tips to Boost Your Dietary Iron Intake

Here's information that will help you increase your iron intake and its absorption within your body.

➤ Make a point of eating iron-rich foods, both animal (heme) and non-animal (nonheme) sources each day.

➤ When eating nonheme foods, couple them with some vitamin C. (See the list of vitamin-C–containing foods.) Vitamin C can increase the absorption of iron.

➤ Avoid drinking coffee or tea with an iron-rich meal; they inhibit the absorption of iron.

➤ Calcium interferes with the absorption of iron, so if you take calcium supplements do not take them with an iron-rich meal. Try them with a snack or some juice because you usually do need some food for your calcium pills.

➤ Cook casseroles, stews, and sauces in cast iron cookware. Believe it or not, some of the iron will seep into the food.

➤ The presence of heme iron (even very small amounts) at a meal with nonheme iron will enhance the absorption of the nonheme iron.

Best sources of iron (heme) are

> Lean red meats
> Turkey
> Chicken
> Pork
> Lamb
> Veal
> Egg yolk
> Liver (although it's very high in cholesterol)

Good iron sources (nonheme) are

> Beans
> Lentils
> Whole grains
> Dried fruit
> Broccoli
> Spinach
> Collard greens
> Nuts and seeds
> Chickpeas
> Fortified cereals
> Blackstrap molasses
> Barley
> Wheat germ

**Nutri-Speak**

Although not very common, **iron toxicity** is a serious problem that occurs from either a genetic abnormality causing the body to store excessive amounts or the unnecessary over-supplementation of iron. The result can be liver and other organ damage.

# Are You a Candidate for a Vitamin or Mineral Supplement?

Ideally, you should be getting your daily supply of vitamins and minerals from your diet, not from pill-popping. There are exceptions to this rule, but don't abandon good eating habits for a little brown bottle; it just doesn't work that way. Generally speaking, nutrients from food are absorbed more readily by your body, the way nature intended. And food provides you with energy in the form of calories—something you don't get from pills.

Although pill-popping is not the most desired method of getting your nutrients, some people do need assistance to receive the required daily allowances. Check out the following list to see if you fall into one of the categories that require a little help. If you do, speak with your doctor or a registered dietitian (a registered dietitian, or R.D., is a board-certified nutritionist with the proper education and credentials) about appropriate supplementation.

Groups at nutritional risk include people with these qualities:

➤ Do you constantly skip meals, grabbing only snack foods throughout the day? Do you eat fewer than five fruits and vegetables each day? You might benefit from a multivitamin/mineral supplement (supplying up to 100 percent of the RDAs) to fill in the nutrition gaps.

➤ Are you a vegan, a strict vegetarian who consumes absolutely no meat, dairy, or other animal products? You might benefit from a supplement that supplies the RDA for vitamins D and B-12 and the mineral calcium.

➤ Are you over 60 years old? People in this category might have a decline in the absorption of the following vitamins: B-6, B-12, C, D, E, folic acid, and the mineral calcium. A one-a-day multivitamin/mineral might provide some extra backup. Also think about some extra calcium if you are not eating enough calcium-rich food.

➤ Do you regularly drink alcohol or smoke? Excessive amounts of alcohol and smoking interfere with the body's ability to absorb and utilize certain vitamins and minerals. In this case, a supplement recommendation is not the advice. You get the picture!

➤ Are you a professional dieter—on/off every wacky fad diet out there? Chances are you're cheating your body of important nutrients and would probably benefit from the backup of a one-a-day multivitamin/mineral supplement.

➤ Do you completely avoid specific types of foods? Some people stay away from certain foods for reasons including food allergies, intolerances, or just plain dislikes. In these cases, supplements of specific nutrients might be needed.

For women only, ask yourself these:

➤ Do you experience heavy bleeding during monthly menstruation? If so, you might lose iron-rich blood. Check with your doctor whether you will benefit from taking a supplement with iron. Note; iron supplements tend to cause constipation.

➤ Are you currently pregnant or breastfeeding? Women in this category have greater needs for the vitamins A, C, B-1, B-6, B-12, and folic acid, as well as the minerals iron and calcium. These extra amounts are usually included in prenatal vitamins—although, you might need more calcium than the prenatal supps supply, so speak with your doctor if you aren't eating enough calcium-rich food.

# Are Your Vitamin and Mineral Supplements Absorbable?

Most people automatically assume that their supplements will absorb after they swallow them. It's a fair assumption. Unfortunately, it doesn't always work that way. Here are two ways to know whether your vitamin and mineral supplements are doing you any good.

## Home Testing

You can always test your own supplements at home by immersing the individual pill in enough household vinegar to cover it—and letting it stand for one hour. (You can stir it a bit.) The vinegar should cloud up and the pill should at least disintegrate (fall into pieces), if not completely dissolve. If it remains intact, there's a chance that it won't disintegrate in your stomach but will pass right through you undigested.

This type of home testing might tell you something, but it's only a rough approximation of what happens in the stomach. No guarantee.

## Look for the USP Stamp

The USP (U.S. Pharmacopeia) is an independent, nonprofit testing organization that tests vitamin and mineral supplements under controlled laboratory conditions—operating since 1820. This company sets legally enforceable standards for the identity, strength, quality, purity, packaging, and labeling of drug products. USP also develops and publishes authoritative drug information for healthcare professionals, patients, and consumers. (Visit the USP Web site at www.usp.org/did/mgraphs.)

It means that the product has met USP standards, including one for disintegration, dissolution, quality, strength, and purity to name a few, and has been tested in a controlled environment. These USP tests don't 100 percent guarantee absorption of all nutrients; absorbability is very difficult to test or predict. However, if a pill does disintegrate in the digestive tract, it certainly improves the chance of the nutrients within the pill being absorbed by the body.

Unfortunately, vitamins and minerals do not have to conform to USP standards to be marketed in this country. Most brand-name vitamins are not labeled USP because the manufacturer either doesn't want to perform the tests or prefers to guarantee the vitamin through the brand name. My recommendation is to buy products with USP on the label. These tend to be generic or store brands; sometimes, they're cheaper. There is no guarantee, but your chances for absorption will be *greatly* improved.

---

### The Least You Need to Know

➤ Adequate calcium intake is required throughout the life cycle: the early years for bone building and the later years for bone maintenance. Make it a habit to load up on low-fat dairy products and other calcium-rich foods.

➤ The mineral iron is responsible for delivering oxygen to every cell in your body and is found in a variety of foods.

➤ *Heme* iron, the most absorbable type, is found in animal products such as meat, liver, and poultry. *Nonheme* iron, found in plants, is less absorbable and is found in dried fruits, nuts, beans, seeds, and fortified grains.

➤ Boost the absorption rate of nonheme iron by combining foods high in vitamin C with an iron-rich meal (such as iron-fortified cereal with a glass of orange juice).

➤ Although certain groups of people can benefit from vitamin and mineral supplementation, most nutrition experts agree that a well-balanced diet should be your primary focus for optimal nutrition.

➤ If you think you might be a candidate for supplementation, speak with your doctor or a Registered Dietitian (a nutritionist with proper education).

---

# Part 2
# Making Savvy Food Choices

*Decisions, decisions! With all the gazillions of foods offered in grocery stores, restaurants, delis, and even your own kitchen, it's a nightmare trying to decide what to eat— let alone choose something nutritious to eat. But it shouldn't be that way. In fact, thanks to the growing number of health-conscience consumers, most grocery stores and restaurants are now well-equipped to cater to your special food concerns. You simply need to know what to look for.*

*This part covers every angle. You'll learn how to decode the information on nutrition labels so you can make informed food choices in your local grocery store. Then, we'll put your know-how into action by scouting out the supermarket, aisle by aisle, introducing you to the smart food items to load into your shopping cart. You'll also master low-fat cooking techniques so you're ready to wow your friends, family, and taste buds with some knockout meals at home. You certainly won't need to give up dining out. This section fills you in on the best bets for most all ethnic cuisine. Bon appétit!*

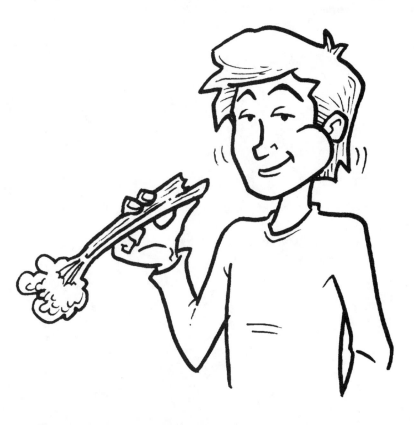

# Chapter 9

# Decoding a Nutrition Label

---

**In This Chapter**

➤ How to read a nutrition label

➤ Understanding the Daily Percent Values

➤ Testing your label savvy

---

Now that you have some solid nutrition know-how, let's put this knowledge to work and decode all that mumbo-jumbo written on prepackaged food products. Once you can interpret the information on nutrition labels, you'll become quite a detective in your local grocery store, further enhancing your skills as a healthy eater. You'll be able to make more informed food choices, as well as compare similar food products to see which brand is nutritionally superior. Best of all, the government has set up strict food label laws and regulations to prevent companies from printing misleading or falsified claims on food items so you can actually believe what you read. This section will provide the whole truth on the foods you love to gobble down.

## Serving Size

First, figure out how much food was analyzed by the folks who prepared the nutrition label. *Serving size* clearly describes this set amount of food. Of course, most packages contain more than one serving, and Servings Per Container refers to the number of single servings in the entire package. For example, the label shown on the next page reports that a serving size is $1/2$ cup and there are four servings per container. Therefore, there must be 2 full cups in the entire package because $1/2$ cup $\times$ 4 = 2 cups.

**Nutrition Facts**

Serving Size ¹/₂ cup (114g)
Servings Per Container 4

**Amount Per Serving**

**Calories** 90          Calories from Fat 30

|  | % Daily Value* |
|---|---|
| **Total Fat** 3g | **5%** |
| Saturated Fat 0g | **0%** |
| **Cholesterol** 0mg | **0%** |
| **Sodium** 300mg | **13%** |
| **Total Carbohydrate** 13g | **4%** |
| Dietary Fiber 3g | **12%** |
| Sugars 3g | |
| **Protein** 3g | |

| Vitamin A | 80% | • | Vitamin C | 60% |
|---|---|---|---|---|
| Calcium | 4% | • | Iron | 4% |

* Percent Daily Values are based on a 2,000 calorie diet. Your daily values may be higher or lower depending on your calorie needs:

| | Calories | 2,000 | 2,500 |
|---|---|---|---|
| Total Fat | Less than | 65g | 80g |
| Sat Fat | Less than | 20g | 25g |
| Cholesterol | Less than | 300mg | 300mg |
| Sodium | Less than | 2,400mg | 2,400mg |
| Total Carbohydrate | | 300g | 375g |
| Fiber | | 25g | 30g |

Calories per gram:
Fat 9    •    Carbohydrate  4    •    Protein 4

Do you eat the amount of food defined as one serving? Remember, fat and calorie measurements on the label are for a single serving size only. And we know it's easy to eat more than one measly serving. Here's a perfect example of the difference between serving size and the actual servings eaten: One serving of ice cream (¹/₂ cup) has approximately 12 grams of fat. Most of the people I know can easily eat 1 cup in a sitting—and you know what that means. When you double the serving size, you double everything: the calories, protein grams, carbohydrate grams, and, of course, the fat grams. Pay close attention to the amount per serving. If you go over (or under) on servings, keep that in mind when reading the remaining information.

# Calories

When calories are listed on a label, they refer to the amount of calories in a single serving. Plain and simple. The sample label shows 90 calories per serving. What about those "lo-cal" claims frequently displayed on the packaging? Luckily, the following key words are now defined by the Government and must mean what they say:

➤ **Calorie-free**—Less than 5 calories per serving.

➤ **Low-calorie**—40 calories or less for most foods items; 120 calories or less for main dish products (lentil soup, turkey burger, chicken breast, and so on).

➤ **Reduced-calorie**—Must be at least 25 percent fewer calories than the regular version of that food item.

# Total Fat

This section lists the total number of fat grams from all types of fat—saturated, monounsaturated, and polyunsaturated. As you can see, the label reveals that there are 3 grams of fat per serving. Another listing titled "Calories from Fat" converts the total fat grams into fat calories (# of fat grams × 9 = calories coming from fat). Again, the sample label reports 30 calories from fat per serving. This is valuable information because it allows you to identify the percentage of fat in a particular food. Ideally, you should choose foods with a big difference between the total number of calories and calories coming from fat. The bigger the gap, the less the percentage of total calories coming from fat.

Here are some of the common "fat" phrases that appear on packaged food products and how they are defined by the Government:

➤ **Fat-free**—Less than 0.5 grams of fat per serving.

➤ **Low-fat**—3 grams of fat (or less) per serving.

➤ **Reduced-fat**—At least 25 percent less fat per serving than the original version of a food product.

## Saturated Fat

This number reveals the amount of "artery-clogging" fat in a food product. Even though saturated fat is part of the total fat in food, it gets listed by itself because it can be extremely bad for you. As you can see, the sample label shows no saturated fat—good deal! In general, avoid foods that are high in saturated fat. This type of fat is responsible for increasing your risk of heart disease and other illnesses.

Here are some of the common "saturated fat" phrases that appear on packaged food products and how they are defined by the Government:

➤ **Saturated fat-free**—Less than 0.5 grams per serving.

➤ **Low in saturated fat**—1 gram or less in a serving size or no more than 10 percent of calories coming from saturated fat.

➤ **Reduced saturated fat**—At least 25 percent less saturated fat than the original version.

# Cholesterol

Remember this waxy guy? Together with its partner in crime—fat—dietary cholesterol is a key player in raising blood cholesterol and therefore increasing your risk for heart disease. You'll notice that the cholesterol content of a food product is measured in milligrams. Budget your foods and eat less than 300 milligrams of dietary cholesterol per day.

Understand the following claims when they appear on food labels:

➤ **Cholesterol-free**—Less than 2 milligrams of cholesterol and 2 grams (or less) of saturated fat per serving.

➤ **Low-cholesterol**—20 milligrams (or less) of cholesterol and 2 grams (or less) of saturated fat per serving.

These cholesterol claims are only allowed when a food product contains 2 grams (or less) of saturated fat as well.

# Sodium

Don't let the terminology confuse you. The label calls it sodium (300 mg reported on the sample label), but most people know it as salt. Remember, sodium is only a component of salt. However, that one component is responsible for water retention and high blood pressure in salt-sensitive people. Limit the amount of high-sodium foods in your diet, and aim for a daily intake of 2,400 milligrams or less.

Here's some sodium lingo and what it means:

➤ **Sodium-free**—Less than 5 milligrams of sodium per serving.

➤ **Low-sodium**—140 milligrams (or less) of sodium per serving.

➤ **Reduced sodium**—At least 25 percent less sodium than the original food version.

# Total Carbohydrate

In Chapter 2, "A Close-Up on Carbohydrates," you became well versed on the various types of carbohydrates. Now, you can use the label information to identify whether a food contains a lot of simple sugar or complex carbohydrate.

First, look for the listing titled "Total Carbohydrate." This will reveal the amount of *all types* of carbs (simple and complex) in a single serving of a food. Next, look for the smaller listing located underneath total carbohydrate titled "Sugars." This indicates how much simple sugar is in a serving of that particular food. Obviously, the less simple sugar, the better. Now, you're ready to determine the amount of complex carbohydrate in a food by simply subtracting the total carbs from the sugars.

Let's look at the previous label for an example:

| Total Carbohydrate | 13 grams |
|---|---|
| Sugars | 3 grams |

These numbers indicate that the majority of carbohydrates are coming from more complex sources, 10 grams to be exact.

Located under Total Carbohydrates is Dietary Fiber. Dietary fiber is predominantly found in carbohydrate-rich foods and includes both soluble and insoluble fiber sources. Because fiber promotes regularity, along with reducing the risk of heart disease and certain cancers, choose foods with at least 3 grams of dietary fiber per serving, and aim for a total intake of 20–35 grams each day.

# Protein

As you know from Chapter 3, "The Profile on Protein," most Americans eat far more protein than they actually need (0.36 grams per pound of body weight). Although some of the best protein sources, unfortunately, do not carry a nutrition label (such as beef, poultry, eggs, and fish), nutrifacts posters are required in meat and produce departments, so ask your grocer and take a look. On the other hand, most dairy products and prepackaged food items do list the grams of protein in a single serving. It's interesting to see that there are even small amounts of protein in foods you might not expect.

# Percent Daily Values

Now for the confusing part: What are those "%" signs floating all over the label? They're called Percent Daily Values (DV) and are based on a 2,000-calorie reference diet. In other words, these percentages indicate how much of the RDA for each nutrient is present in a single serving. Of course, your job is to ultimately eat a variety of foods that supply 100 percent of all nutrients needed. For example, one serving of yogurt provides 35 percent daily calcium and 0 percent iron. It's clearly a great source of calcium, but lousy for iron.

What happens if you eat more or less than 2,000 calories? You can slightly adjust the percentages up or down if you're good with numbers (and extremely motivated). In general, the 2,000-calorie reference diet provides appropriate guidelines for almost everyone (adults and children over 4) to follow.

For total fat, saturated fat, cholesterol, and sodium, choose foods with low percent daily values. On the other hand, you want to choose foods with higher percent DVs for total carbohydrate, dietary fiber, and all vitamins and minerals.

The following are the set daily values. They are specifically used for food labels and are based on a 2,000 calorie reference diet.

## Daily Values for Nutritional Items

| Food Component | Daily Value |
| --- | --- |
| Total Fat | 65 grams |
| Saturated Fat | 20 grams |
| Cholesterol | 300 mg |
| Sodium | 2,400 mg |
| Potassium | 3,500 mg |
| Total Carbohydrate | 300 grams |
| Dietary Fiber | 25 grams |

*continues*

**91**

*continued*

| Food Component | Daily Value |
| --- | --- |
| Protein | 50 grams |
| Vitamin A | 5,000 IU |
| Vitamin C | 60 mg |
| Calcium | 1,000 mg |

| Food Component | Daily Value |
| --- | --- |
| Iron | 18 mg |
| Vitamin D | 400 IU |
| Vitamin E | 30 IU |
| Vitamin K | 80 mcg |
| Thiamin | 1.5 mg |
| Riboflavin | 1.7 mg |
| Niacin | 20 mg |
| Vitamin B-6 | 2.0 mg |
| Folate | 400 mcg |
| Vitamin B-12 | 6.0 mcg |
| Biotin | 0.3 mg |
| Pantothenic Acid | 10 mg |
| Phosphorus | 1,000 mg |
| Iodine | 150 mcg |
| Magnesium | 400 mg |
| Zinc | 15 mg |
| Copper | 2.0 mg |
| Selenium | 70 mcg |
| Manganese | 2.0 mg |
| Chromium | 120 mcg |
| Molybdenum | 75 mcg |
| Chloride | 3,400 mg |

*mg = milligrams; mcg = micrograms; IU = International Units*

*Source: Title 21 "Code of Federal Regulations" Parts 100–169, April 1, 1995, Section 101.9*

# Take the Nutrition Label Challenge

Put your know-how to the test and answer the following questions according to the nutrition label on the following page:

1. How many servings are there in the entire package?

2. How many calories are there in two servings of this food product?

3. How much of your daily percent of iron does one serving of this food provide?

4. Knowing the daily percent of iron in one serving, calculate the amount of iron in milligrams that this product supplies.

**Nutrition Facts**
Serving Size 2 Tbsp (32g)
Servings Per Container about 16

Amount Per Serving

**Calories** 190  Calories from Fat 130

% Daily Value*

| | |
|---|---|
| **Total Fat** 16g | 25% |
| Saturated Fat 3g | 15% |
| **Cholesterol** 0mg | 0% |
| **Sodium** 150mg | 6% |
| **Total Carbohydrate** 7g | 2% |
| Dietary Fiber 2g | 8% |
| Sugars 3g | |
| **Protein** 8g | |

| | | |
|---|---|---|
| Vitamin A 0% | • | Vitamin C 0% |
| Calcium 0% | • | Iron 4% |

*Percent Daily Values are based on a 2,000 calorie diet

5. How much more dietary fiber must you get from other food sources after eating one serving of this food item?

6. How many grams of unsaturated fat are in one serving of this product?

7. Would you consider this food a good source of calcium?

8. Do you think this is an artery-clogging food?

9. How many grams of protein are there in one serving?

10. Any idea what this food may be?

**Answers to Quiz:**

1. 16 servings in the entire package.

2. $190 \times 2$ servings = 380 calories.

3. 4% daily iron.

4. 4% of 18 milligrams = 0.72 milligrams.

5. This product only provides 2 grams of dietary fiber per serving. You'll still need about 20 more grams from other food sources.

6. Because this product supplies 16 grams of total fat, and 3 grams of saturated fat per serving, the remaining 13 grams of fat are unsaturated.

7. This product is not a good source of the mineral calcium. At the bottom of the label, notice "Calcium 0%." To be considered a good source of a nutrient, a food must provide at least 10 percent of the DV for that nutrient.

8. This food is *not* artery clogging because it does not contain any cholesterol and the majority of fat is unsaturated.

9. 8 grams of protein in one serving.

10. Did you guess peanut butter?

---

### The Least You Need to Know

➤ The nutrition information provided on prepackaged food labels can help you make more informed food choices and compare similar food items for the healthier buy.

➤ All the nutrition information provided is based on one serving size. Check to see how much of a particular food is considered one serving, and if you eat more or less, adjust the nutrition information accordingly.

➤ Choose foods that have a big difference between the number of total calories and the number of fat calories. This indicates that a food is not primarily made of fat.

➤ Daily Percent Value refers to how much of a day's recommended amount for certain nutrients is supplied in one serving of a food product. Read carefully and generally stick with foods that have a low daily percentage for fat, cholesterol, and sodium while choosing foods that have a high daily percentage for total carbohydrate, dietary fiber, and all other vitamins and minerals.

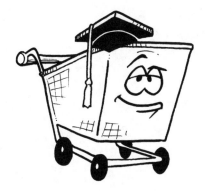

# Shopping Smart

How many times have you eaten unhealthy food just because you didn't have any nutritious food in the house? Are cookies, cakes, and chips constantly on display on your shelves, or do you fill your pantry with fresh fruit and whole grains? Let's face it: When you get those midday munchies, the last thing you want to do is drive to a supermarket to buy an apple. You're going to grab whatever's closest to the couch—and who knows what that might be.

Half the battle of healthy eating is having a variety of nutritious foods on hand so when the "food mood" strikes, you've got the supplies to satisfy that growling belly with some savvy food choices. Grab a cart and read on; you're about to go grocery shopping.

## The Shopping List

The nice part about food shopping today is that supermarkets are responding to nutrition-conscience consumers and shelving healthier foods than ever before. So set up a shopping list by different food categories—and get organized.

➤ Vegetables

➤ Fruits

➤ Dairy

➤ Grains (bread, cereal, pasta, and others)

➤ Protein foods (meats, poultry, fish, eggs, and legumes)

➤ Frozen meals and canned items

➤ Snack foods

➤ Condiments

➤ Fats, oils, dressings, and other spreads

# Aisle One: Starting with the Produce Section

The produce aisle will provide you with a lot of nutritional bang for your buck. Spend a lot of time walking through, and load up your wagon.

## Voluptuous Veggies

Vegetables are naturally low in calories and fat, and they provide an array of vitamins, minerals, and fiber. Unfortunately, bundles of fresh produce don't carry nutrition labels, but you might see posters in the produce area revealing the benefits of specific items. Rest assured: Label or no label, you can never eat too many of these guys!

Most fresh veggies can be judged for freshness and quality by their appearance; closely examine your produce and avoid any decaying or bruising. Another piece of advice is to buy only what you need for the next few days. Fresh veggies will go bad if they sit around for a long time. If you don't shop often, or you don't have the time to wash and chop your vegetables, your best bet is to stuff your freezer. Frozen vegetables come in a variety of combinations (cut, whole, chopped, and pureed, along with medleys of premixed veggie concoctions), and all you have to do is pop them in a pot to cook. Even lazy people have no excuse. What's more, the freezer keeps the nutrients locked in, so there's no rush to eat them before they go bad. Also, frozen (and canned) vegetables have labels telling all the facts, so take advantage and read the impressive profile.

Here are some general shopping tips for buying produce:

➤ Buy fresh fruits and vegetables that are in season to keep the prices reasonable.

➤ Examine your fruits and vegetables for freshness; avoid bruises and other deformities.

➤ Because fresh produce is perishable, buy only what you need. If you're shopping for an extended period of time, load up on the frozen varieties.

➤ Read the labels on frozen and canned vegetables to make sure there isn't a lot of added fat or salt. Read labels on frozen and canned fruits to make sure there isn't a lot of added sugar or heavy syrup.

➤ If you're into "super-convenience," buy the prewashed, precut bags of salad, carrots, celery, and anything else offered at your supermarket. Look for premade fruit salads in either the fresh or frozen sections of your grocery store.

➤ Check out the salad bar in your grocery store. This way you can get the exact amount of anything you need, and it's already precut and prewashed for you.

➤ Speak with the person in charge of produce at your local supermarket, ask about unfamiliar fruits and vegetables, and then try something new!

## Getting to Know 'Em

Here is a quick rundown on some common vegetables and what to look for when buying fresh selections:

➤ **Artichokes** provide potassium and folic acid. Look for artichokes that are plump and heavy in relation to size. The many leaf-like parts are called "scales" and should be thick, green, and fresh-looking. Avoid artichokes with any brownish discoloration or moldy growth on the scales.

➤ **Asparagus** provides vitamins A and C, niacin, folic acid, potassium, and iron. Look for closed, dense tips with smooth, deep green spears. Avoid tips that are spread open or seem to have any mold or decay.

➤ **Broccoli** provides calcium, potassium, iron, fiber, vitamins A and C, folic acid, and niacin. Look for stalks that are not too tough with compact, firm, bud clusters and that are dark green or sage green in color. Avoid broccoli with a wilted appearance, yellowish-green discoloration, or bud clusters that are spread open. These are all signs of over-maturity.

➤ **Brussels sprouts** provide vitamins A and C, folic acid, potassium, iron, and fiber. Look for Brussels sprouts with a bright-green color and tight-fitting outer leaves. Avoid Brussels sprouts that appear to be wilting or have blemishes.

➤ **Cabbage** provides vitamin C, potassium, folic acid, and fiber. Whether it's green or red, cabbage can be used in coleslaw, salads, and a variety of cooked dishes. Look for a dense, heavy head of cabbage relative to its size, with outer leaves that display a green or red color (depending on the type). Avoid cabbages with outer leaves that appear wilted or blemished.

➤ **Carrots** provide vitamin A, potassium, and fiber. Look for smooth, firm, well-formed carrots that have a rich orange color. Avoid roots that are discolored, soft, and flabby.

➤ **Cauliflower** provides vitamin C, folic acid, potassium, and fiber. Look for compact, firm curds (the edible creamy-white portion), and do not worry about green leaflets that may be scattered throughout a bunch. Although most grocers sell cauliflower without the outside jacket leaves, in the rare instance that they are left on, a nice green color reveals freshness. Avoid severe discoloration, blemishing, or spreading of the white curd.

➤ **Corn** provides vitamin A, potassium, and fiber. Although yellow-kernel is the most popular, there are varieties of white-kernel and mixed-kernel corn as well. Look for fresh green husks (the outer covering) and make sure that the silk ends are free from decay or worm injury. If the corn has already been husked (the outside covering removed), choose ears of corn that are heavily covered with bright yellow, plump kernels. Avoid kernels that appear dried or lacking in color.

➤ **Eggplants** provide potassium. Look for firm, heavy, dark-purple eggplants (although there are other colored varieties). Avoid any that are shriveled, soft, or lacking color or that reveal decay in the form of brownish spots.

➤ **Lettuce** comes in several varieties: iceberg, butter-head, romaine, and leaf lettuce. It provides vitamin C and folic acid. Look for bright color and crisp leaf texture when buying romaine. For other leafy variations, select succulent, tender leaves and avoid any serious discoloration or wilting.

➤ **Mushrooms** provide potassium, niacin, and riboflavin. Look for closed mushroom caps around the stems, with the underneath gills (rows of paper thin tissue located underneath the caps) colored pink or light tan. Avoid mushrooms with wide-open caps and dark, discolored gills.

➤ **Okra** provides vitamin A, potassium, and calcium. Look for bright green, tender pods that are under $4^{1}/_{2}$ inches long. Avoid stiff tips (those that resist bending) or pods with a lifeless, pale green color.

➤ **Onions** are not a significant source of nutrition, but they can certainly enhance the flavor of the foods you eat. With all types (red, white, and yellow), look for hard, dry onions that are free from blemishes. Avoid onions that are wet or mushy.

➤ **Peas** (green) provide vitamin A, folic acid, potassium, protein, and fiber. Look for a firm, fresh appearance with bright green pods. Avoid flabby, wilted pods, and any sign of decay.

➤ **Peppers** (sweet) provide vitamins A and C, potassium, and fiber. Although green peppers are the most common, other delicious varieties include yellow, orange, red, purple, and white. Look for firm peppers with deep characteristic color. Avoid very lightweight, flimsy peppers that have punctures or signs of decay on the outside.

➤ **Potatoes** provide potassium, most B-vitamins, vitamin C, protein, and fiber. Look for reasonably smooth, firm, and blemish-free potatoes. Avoid large bruises and soft spots and sprouted or shriveled potatoes.

➤ **Rhubarb** provides vitamin A, calcium, and potassium. Look for firm but tender stems with a decent amount of pink/red color. Avoid rhubarb that appears wilted or flabby.

➤ **Spinach** provides vitamin A, calcium, folic acid, potassium, and fiber. Look for healthy, fresh leaves that have a dark-green color. Avoid spinach leaves that appear wilted or show significant discoloration.

➤ **Squash** (summer) provides vitamins A and C, potassium, and fiber and includes several varieties such as yellow Crookneck, large Straightneck, the greenish-white Patty Pan, and the slender green zucchini. Look for firm, well-developed, tender squash. Check for a glossy (not dull) outside, which indicates the squash is tender. Avoid dull, tough, or discolored squash.

➤ **Squash** (winter) includes Acorn, Butternut, Buttercup, green and blue Hubbard, Delicious, and Banana, providing vitamins A and C, potassium, and fiber. Look for squash that is heavy for its size with a tough, hard outside rind. Avoid squash with any signs of decay including sunken spots, bruising, or mold.

➤ **Sweet potatoes** provide vitamins A and C, folic acid, potassium, and fiber. Look for firm, smooth sweet potatoes with uniformly colored skins. The moist type known as yams should have orange flesh, whereas dry sweet potatoes have a more pale appearance. Avoid discoloration, worm holes, and any other indication of decay.

➤ **Tomatoes** provide vitamins A and C and potassium. Look for well-ripened, smooth tomatoes with a rich red color. If you're not planning to eat them within the next few days, choose slightly less ripe, firm tomatoes with a pink/light red color. Only store fully ripe ones in the fridge because the cold temperature might prevent immature tomatoes from ripening. Avoid tomatoes that are over-ripened and mushy or show any signs of decay.

> *Moo!*
>
> **Overrated—Undercooked**
>
> Generally, canned vegetables tend to be loaded with salt. If you do buy cans occasionally, be on the lookout for labels that read "low-sodium" or "no added salt."

## Fabulous Fruits

For a quick nutritious snack, a deliciously healthy dessert, or even part of a creative meal, fruit rules. Similar to its neighbor in the produce section, fruit is naturally low in calories and fat (except for avocado and coconut), while chock-full of nutrients and fiber. Get in the habit of keeping a stash of fresh fruit. Although dried fruit is another tasty option, keep in mind that it is more concentrated in calories because it has less water than its fresh counterparts. Also, beware of canned (and sometimes frozen) fruit with "heavy syrup added"; they are packed with calories and sugar. When buying canned or frozen fruit, read labels and look for key phrases such as "no added sugar," "packed in its own juice," "packed in 100% fruit juice," or "unsweetened."

What about fruit juice? It's certainly not a substitute for whole fruit (in fact, even the brands with pulp added will be lacking in dietary fiber), but fruit juice does provide nutrients and is clearly better than colas, sweetened iced-teas, or fruit punch. Go ahead and put a couple of juice containers in your shopping cart; when available, opt for the brands with added vitamin C or the calcium-fortified varieties.

Here are some helpful hints for shopping for fresh fruits:

➤ **Apples** provide potassium and fiber and are available in a bunch of varieties, including Red Delicious, McIntosh, Granny Smith, Empire, Washington, and Golden Delicious. Although each kind differs in seasonal availability, taste, and appearance, some general shopping savvy is to look for crisp, firm apples with a rich color (depending upon the type). Avoid apples with bruising, soft spots, or mealy flesh.

➤ **Apricots** provide a lot of vitamin A, iron, and some potassium and fiber. Look for apricots that have a golden-orange color and appear to be plump and juicy. Avoid apricots that are dull-looking, mushy, or overly firm or that have a yellowish-green color.

➤ **Avocados** provide vitamin A, potassium, folic acid, and fiber. Look for avocados that are slightly tender to the touch if you plan to eat them immediately. Otherwise, buy firm avocados and let them ripen at room temperature for a few days. Avoid any with broken surfaces or dark prominent spots.

➤ **Bananas** provide a lot of potassium and some vitamin A and fiber. Look for firm bananas that are either yellow green (and will ripen in a few days) or fully yellow and ready to eat. In general, bananas have their best flavor when the solid yellow color is speckled with some brown. Avoid bananas that are bruised or have a gray appearance.

➤ **Blueberries** provide vitamin C, potassium, and fiber. Look for plump, firm blueberries that are dark blue in color. Avoid berries that are mushy, moldy, or leaking.

➤ **Cantaloupes** provide vitamins A and C and potassium. Look for cantaloupes with rough skin that are slightly soft and flexible when you press on the top or bottom and that have a sweet, fresh odor. Avoid extremely hard cantaloupes (unless you want to wait for them to ripen) and any with moldy spots.

➤ **Cherries** provide vitamin A and potassium. Look for cherries with a dark red color, plump surfaces, and fresh stems. Avoid cherries that appear dull, shriveled, or dried.

➤ **Grapefruits** provide vitamins A and C and potassium. Look for firm, compact grapefruits that are heavy for their size. Do not worry about slight discoloration or skin scars; this usually does not interfere with the quality of taste. Avoid grapefruits that look extremely dull and lack color.

➤ **Grapes** provide some fiber and come in several color varieties. Look for rich-colored, plump grapes that are tightly attached to the stem. Avoid grapes that are shriveled and soft or that have brown, brittle stems.

➤ **Kiwi fruit** provides a lot of vitamin C and potassium. Look for plump kiwi fruit that yields slightly to the touch; this means it's ripe. You can ripen firm kiwi fruit at home by leaving it at room temperature for a few days. Avoid kiwi fruits that are super-soft or shriveled.

➤ **Lemons** provide vitamin C. Look for firm lemons with a rich, glossy yellow color. Avoid lemons with mold, punctures, or a dull, dark-yellow coloring.

➤ **Mangos** provide vitamins A and C, potassium, and fiber. Look for orange-yellow to red mangoes that are well-developed and barely soft to the touch. Avoid mangos that are rock-hard or over-ripened and mushy.

➤ **Nectarines** provide vitamin A and potassium. Look for bright-colored, plump nectarines with orange, yellow, and red color combinations. Nectarines that are hard will ripen in a few days at room temperature. Avoid nectarines that are overly soft, lacking color, or show signs of decay.

➤ **Oranges** provide a lot of vitamin C, potassium, and folic acid. Look for firm, heavy oranges (because this indicates juiciness) with relatively smooth, bright-looking skin. Avoid oranges that are very light (no juice) or that have thick, coarse, or spongy skins.

➤ **Peaches** provide vitamin A and potassium. Look for peaches that are firm but slightly soft to the touch. Avoid greenish, hard peaches that are under-ripened and mushy peaches that are over-ripened.

➤ **Pears** provide potassium and fiber. Look for pears that are firm, but not too hard. The color depends on the variety. Bartletts are pale-yellow to rich-yellow, Anjou or Comice are light-green to yellowish-green, Bosc are greenish-yellow to brownish-yellow, and Winter Nellis are medium to light green. Avoid wilted or wrinkled pears with any distinct spots.

➤ **Pineapples** provide vitamin C and fiber. Look for pineapples that are plump, firm, and heavy for their size and that have a fragrant aroma. Avoid pineapples that appear dull, bruised, or dried or that have an unpleasant smell.

➤ **Raspberries** provide vitamin C, potassium, and fiber. Look for plump, tender berries with a rich, uniform scarlet color. Avoid berries that are mushy or have any mold.

➤ **Strawberries** provide a lot of vitamin C, along with potassium, folic acid, and fiber. Look for firm, red berries that still have the cap stem attached. Avoid berries that have large uncolored or seedy areas. Also avoid strawberries that have a shrunken appearance or any mold.

➤ **Tangerines** provide vitamins A and C. Look for deep yellow or orange tangerines with a bright luster (which indicates freshness and maturity). Avoid tangerines with a pale yellow or greenish color or punctures in the skin.

➤ **Watermelon** provides vitamin A and some vitamin C. For uncut watermelons, look for a smooth surface, well-rounded ends, and a pale green color. For cut watermelons, look for juicy flesh with a rich, red color that is free from white streaks. Avoid melons with a lot of white streaks running through pale-colored flesh and light colored seeds.

**Food for Thought**

Contrary to its name, buttermilk is actually a low-fat dairy product. In fact, buttermilk is simply skim or low-fat pasteurized milk with some added lactic acid. The consistency is thicker than regular milk and the sodium is also higher at 257 milligrams per 8 ounces (about double the amount of regular low-fat milk).

**Nutri-Speak**

**Pasteurized milk** is briefly heated to kill harmful bacteria and then is rapidly chilled.

**Homogenized milk** has been processed to reduce the size of milk fat globules so the cream does not separate and the milk stays consistently smooth and uniform.

# Aisle Two: Down Dairy Lane

Milk products supply you with calcium (responsible for healthy bones), along with providing protein, several B-vitamins, and vitamins D and A. The problem is that whole milk also contains a lot of saturated fat, which can increase your risk for heart disease, weight gain, and other serious illnesses. What can you do? Simple: When you're at home and have control over the type of dairy that goes into your cereals, recipes, and sandwiches, use the low-fat versions that are available in most supermarkets today.

Don't throw in the towel if you don't like some of the reduced-fat items; different brands have different tastes. Just try another brand or version the next time you shop. Another thing to keep in mind is that some of the "fat-free" dairy is literally "taste-free." (Some brands even resemble plastic.) You don't have to suffer with the fat-free if you can't stand the taste; low-fat is fine, with a mere 3–5 extra grams of fat.

Here's your low-fat dairy shopping list. Browse through the section and pick out the items that sound appealing:

1% low-fat milk

Non-fat yogurts (plain and flavored)

Skim milk (no fat)

Low-fat varieties of all cheese

Buttermilk

Non-fat varieties of all cheese

Non-fat dry milk

Part-skim varieties of all cheese

Evaporated skim milk

Reduced-fat cream cheese

Dry-curd cottage cheese

Reduced-fat sour cream

Low-fat cottage cheese

Low-fat/no-fat ice creams

Low-fat yogurts (plain and flavored)

Low-fat/no-fat frozen yogurts

# Aisle Three: Shopping for the Whole Grains

Here are some shopping tips for buying breads and cereals:

➤ Stick with whole-grain varieties, including whole wheat, multigrain, rye, millet, oat bran, oat, and cracked wheat. (This goes for all types of bread: sliced bread, pita, bagels, English muffins, crackers, and so on.)

➤ Although "wheat" bread might sound just as healthy as "whole-wheat" bread, don't be fooled; it's merely a blend of white and whole-wheat flour. A product labeled "whole-wheat" must be made from 100 percent whole-wheat flour.

➤ Check the label and choose breads with at least 2 grams of fiber per slice.

➤ If you're looking to save calories, try the whole-wheat, reduced-calorie bread (approximately 40 calories per slice with 2 grams of fiber).

➤ Don't forget to check the expiration date on the label.

➤ Take advantage of the fiber that some cereals pack in, and choose varieties that have at least 2 grams of fiber per serving. You can usually (not always) get a sense of whether a cereal has fiber from the name on the box (Bran Flakes, All-Bran, 100% Bran, Raisin Bran, Fiber-One, Shredded Wheat, and Corn Bran).

➤ Some cereals pack in more sugar and salt than most people realize. Check the Total Carbohydrates against the Sugars (on the nutrition label) to make sure sugar is not a main ingredient. In fact, opt for the brands that report 6 grams of sugar or less per serving. If your kids (or spouse) insist on the sugary brands, mix it with half a bowl of a healthier look-a-like (for instance, half Frosted Flakes and half Bran Flakes).

➤ Check the serving size. Some of the denser, heavier cereals only allot a miniscule amount for one serving. Take this into consideration if you plan to eat a normal size bowl (and you're watching your weight). Remember, double the serving size means double the calories.

➤ Don't forget to throw some hot cereal into your cart. Whether you opt for the instant or the kind that requires cooking, stick with unsweetened varieties of oatmeal, grits, cream of rice, and cream of wheat. You can sweeten them with some of the fresh fruit you bought in the produce section.

➤ Most cereals are low in fat with the exception of granola and others that add nuts, seeds, coconut, and oils. Read the label and choose cereals with no more than 2 grams of fat per serving.

➤ Read the list of ingredients on your cereal box and make sure that wheat, rye, corn, or oats are listed first. Items are listed in the order in which they are highest in quantity.

## Pasta, Rice, and More

Pasta is one of those American staple foods that everyone seems to enjoy. What's more, pasta is high in complex carbohydrates, easy to make, and inexpensive. Don't stop at the box of spaghetti; try the elbow macaroni, ziti, rigatoni, penne, fusilli, orzo, shells, bow ties, and lasagna noodles. If your supermarket has any whole-grain variet-ies, throw them in your basket; they're a great source of fiber.

Rice is another excellent source of complex carbohydrates and tends to be a popular standard in many homes. The most nutritious is brown rice, with a bit more fiber than the white varieties. Next in the nutrition line-up is polished white rice, and last is the instant white rice, with the fewest nutrients of all.

Try some of the not-so-common grains. Pile your cart with couscous, barley, buck-wheat, bulgur, kasha, millet, polenta, wheat berries, and cracked wheat. They are all brimming with complex carbohydrates—so jazz up your dinners and impress your family!

# Aisle Four: Best Bets for Protein

When buying beef, pork, lamb, and veal, look for lean, well-trimmed cuts. Meats are graded by the USDA (United States Department of Agriculture) according to their fat content and texture. *Prime* indicates the highest in fat (unfortunately, it's usually the most tender and juicy because of the marbled fat throughout); *choice* is moderately fatty; and *select* is the leanest. Lean meats provide a lot of high-quality protein, along with iron, B-vitamins, phosphorus, and zinc.

Your leanest beef choices are

| | |
|---|---|
| Top round | Top loin steak |
| Tenderloin | Chuck steaks |

| | |
|---|---|
| Lean T-bone | Lean rump |
| Lean porterhouse | Lean flank |
| Sirloin | Ground beef (only extra lean) |

Your leanest lamb and veal choices are

| | |
|---|---|
| Leg of lamb | Lamb roast |
| Foreshank | Arm chop |
| Lean loin chop | Veal roast |
| Veal loin chop | Veal cutlet |

Your leanest pork choices are

| | |
|---|---|
| Tenderloin | Top loin roast |
| Center loin chops | Canadian bacon |
| Lean ham | Rib chops |
| Sirloin roast | Shoulder blade steak |

## Poultry

Let's not forget about poultry. Poultry can be one of your leanest animal protein sources, but lose the skin—pure fat! You can buy poultry with the skin if it's more reasonably priced. You can even cook poultry with the skin for some added moistness; just be sure to remove it before eating.

Your leanest poultry choices are

Skinless chicken breast

Turkey breast (white meat, no skin)

Cornish game hen (no skin)

Ground chicken or turkey breast (look for white meat only/no skin added)

Duck and pheasant (no skin)

## Fish and Seafood

When choosing seafood, almost anything goes. Scout the aisle and pick up anything that looks fresh and appealing. Fresh fish and seafood should have bright skin, bulging eyes (for whole fish), firm flesh, and *no* fishy smell. You might have heard that some fish are fattier than others. It's true, but the amount of fat is so small that all fish and seafood remain great choices nutritionally. In addition, the type of fat found in fish is polyunsaturated (more specifically omega-3 fatty acid), which has been shown to do positive things in the fight against heart disease and cancer. What's more, all types of fish supply excellent high-quality protein, along with other vitamins and minerals.

Your leanest fish choices are

| | |
|---|---|
| Cod | Monkfish |
| Flounder | Perch |
| Sea bass | Tuna |
| Whiting | Mullet |
| Halibut | Swordfish |
| Red snapper | Mollusks (abalone, clams, mussels, oysters, scallops, and squid) |
| Shark | |
| Haddock | |
| Shellfish (crab, crayfish, lobster, and shrimp) | |

Fattier fish include

| | |
|---|---|
| Salmon | Albacore tuna |
| Mackerel | Bluefish |
| Herring | Shad |
| Eel | Catfish |
| Pompano | |

# Eggs

Eggs are a good source of high-quality protein, iron, and vitamin A—but they also provide a lot of cholesterol, about 213 mg, to get technical. Furthermore, there are approximately 5 grams of fat in just one yolk. Not bad if you only eat whole eggs occasionally. Otherwise, think about using only the whites of the eggs, or grab a carton of the egg substitutes (no cholesterol and low in fat) that are generally sold in the frozen section. Also, some supermarkets carry straight, pre-separated whites in refrigerated cartons.

# Legumes (Dried Beans, Peas, and Lentils)

Definitely add some legumes to your shopping list. Legumes supply protein, calcium, iron, zinc, magnesium, and B-vitamins. Most impressive is that dried beans, peas, and lentils are the only high-protein foods that provide ample amounts of fiber. Get creative and make a meatless meal a couple of times each week.

Look for these:

| | |
|---|---|
| Baked beans | Great northern beans |
| Pinto beans | Black beans |
| Kidney beans | Split peas |

Black-eyed peas             Lentils

Tofu                        Cannelloni beans

Lima beans                  Vegetarian chilis

Navy beans                  White beans

Garbanzo beans (chickpeas)

# Aisle Five: Frozen Meals, Canned Soups, and Sauces

As mentioned earlier, frozen and canned items can be convenient and tasty. Just remember to read the labels carefully and keep the following tips in mind:

➤ For full frozen meals, always read the label and look for *less* than 400 total calories, 15 grams of fat, and 800 milligrams of sodium.

➤ When choosing soups, avoid the creamy varieties unless you have the option of mixing in your own low-fat milk. Also buy soups that say "reduced-sodium," "low-sodium," or "no added salt." Some nutritious selections include minestrone, garden vegetable, chicken noodle, split pea, tomato rice, Manhattan clam chowder, and the lentil-bean combinations.

➤ To cut fat, buy sauces that are tomato or vegetable based. Check the labels and look for brands that have 3 grams (or less) of fat per serving.

# Aisle Six: Savvy Snacks

Most of us love to nibble in between meals. If you plan to stock up your kitchen, do so with these low-fat items:

Plain popcorn kernels for air poppers

Fruit and fig bars

"Lite" or "reduced-fat" microwave popcorn

Low-fat granola bars and chewy cereal bars

Pretzels and baked chips

Lower-fat whole-grain crackers

Animal crackers, ginger snaps, and graham crackers

Raisins and other dried fruit

Frozen fruit pops and sorbet

Trail mix

Flavored rice cakes

# Aisle Seven: Health-Conscious Condiments

The following low-fat condiments can help add pizzazz to your meals. But keep in mind that a lot of these flavor enhancers are also high in sodium. Salt-sensitive people need to pay close attention to the salt contents on the package:

| | |
|---|---|
| Ketchup | Cider vinegar |
| Mustard | Lemon juice |
| Jams | Fruit preserves |
| Low-sugar spreads | Worcestershire sauce |
| Soy sauce (low sodium) | Cocktail sauce |
| Teriyaki sauce (low sodium) | Chutney |
| Balsamic vinegar | Salsa |

# Aisle Eight: Heart-Smart Fats, Spreads, and Dressings

When purchasing fats, remember to stick with predominantly unsaturated. Also, opt for the reduced-fat or fat-free versions of the original dressings and spreads. You'll substantially cut down on your fat intake.

Here's a master list to select from:

**Monounsaturated**
Olive oil
Canola oil
Rapeseed oil
Peanut oil

**Polyunsaturated**
Safflower oil
Sunflower oil
Corn oil
Soybean oil

**Others That May Come in Handy...**
Nonstick cooking sprays
Fat-free and low-fat salad dressings
Low-fat dips, soft-tub margarines (regular and reduced fat)
Butter substitutes (sprays or granules)
Low-fat mayonnaise
Peanut butter (it may be high in fat, but it also provides a lot of protein)

## The Least You Need to Know

➤ The first step to a well-stocked kitchen begins with a comprehensive, healthy shopping list. Make sure to organize your list with individual food categories.

➤ Load up your cart with fresh vegetables and fruit, but only buy what you need because fresh produce is perishable. Frozen and canned fruits and vegetables are good options for people who do not shop frequently; just check to make sure there is not a lot of added fat, sugar, and salt.

➤ Buy low-fat dairy and lean cuts of meat, poultry, and fish, and don't forget about legumes for those meatless meals. Also, look in the freezer section of your market for egg substitutes; you'll save a lot of fat and cholesterol.

➤ Scout out the grains made with whole-grain flour. When choosing cereals, read the labels and select brands that are low in sugar and provide at least 2 grams of fiber per serving.

➤ Read labels on salad dressings, fats, and other spreads. Opt for products that are reduced-fat, low-fat, or fat-free.

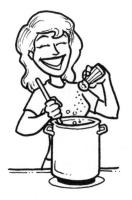

# Chapter 11

# Now You're Cooking

**In This Chapter**

➤ Simple cooking modifications

➤ Great recipes for breakfast, lunch, and dinner

➤ Finding a good cookbook

Mealtime is the perfect opportunity to bond with your family, converse with friends, relax in private, or impress your date with a knockout dish. The hardest part is already done: You've stocked your kitchen with the right ingredients. So grab some pots and pans and turn on some groovin' music; this chapter offers helpful hints for recipe remodeling, plus it provides you with easy-to-make, tasty meals for breakfast, lunch, dinner, and dessert.

## The Recipe Makeover: Remodeling Family Favorites

Skimming the fat in your recipe means more than just using leaner ingredients. It also means using healthful cooking techniques and tools. Here are some quick tips and tricks of the trade:

1. Use low-fat and no-fat cooking methods, such as steaming, poaching, stir-frying, broiling, grilling, microwaving, baking, and roasting as alternatives to frying.

2. Get a good quality set of nonstick sauce pans, skillets, and baking pans so you can sauté and bake without adding fat.

3. Use nonstick vegetable sprays or 1 to 2 tablespoons of defatted broth, water, juice, or wine to replace cooking oil.

4. Be aware that fat-free or reduced-fat cheeses have slightly different cooking characteristics than their fattier counterparts. For the most part, they don't melt as smoothly. To overcome this, shred these cheeses very finely. When making sauces and soups, toss the cheese with a small amount of flour, cornstarch, or arrowroot.

5. Trim all visible fat from steaks, chops, roasts, and other meat cuts before preparing them.

6. Replace one quarter to one half the ground meat or poultry in a casserole or meat sauce with cooked brown rice, bulgar, couscous, or cooked and chopped dried beans to skim the fat and add fiber.

7. Deciding to remove the skin from poultry before or after cooking depends on your cooking method. Skin helps prevent roasted or baked cuts from drying out, and studies have shown that the fat from the skin doesn't penetrate the meat during cooking. However, if you do leave the skin on, make sure any seasonings you've applied go under the skin or you'll lose the favor when the skin is removed.

8. Skim and discard the fat from hot soups and stews, or chill the soup or stew and skim off the solid fat that forms on top.

9. Use pureed cooked vegetables, such as carrots, potatoes, and cauliflower, to thicken soups and sauces instead of cream, egg yolks, or a butter and flour roux. Also, use soft tofu to thicken sauces.

10. Select "healthier" fats when you need to add fat to a recipe. That means replacing butter, lard, or other highly saturated fats with oils such as canola, olive, safflower, sunflower, corn, and others that are low in saturates. Remember, it takes just a few drops of a very flavorful oil, such as extra-virgin olive oil, dark sesame, walnut, or garlic oil, to really perk up a dish, so go easy.

11. Skim the fat where you won't miss it, but keep the characteristic flavor of fatty ingredients such as nuts, coconut, chocolate chips, and bacon by reducing the quantity you use by 50 percent. For example, if a recipe calls for 1 cup of walnuts, use $^1/_2$ cup instead.

12. Toast nuts and spices to enhance their flavor and then chop them finely so they can be more fully distributed through the food.

13. If sugar is the primary sweetener in a fruit sauce, beverage, or other dish that is not baked, scale the amount down by 25 percent. Instead of 1 cup of sugar, use $^3/_4$ cup. If you add a pinch of cinnamon, nutmeg, or allspice, you'll increase the perception of sweetness without adding calories.

14. In baked goods, add pureed fruit instead of fat. One of the reasons fat is included in baked products is to make them moist. The high concentration of natural sweetness in pureed fruit will actually help hold on to the moisture during the baking process.

Fat has flavor, but so does fruit. Fat adds liquid volume and moisture to bread or cake batter, but so does fruit. When making this substitution, if the recipe calls for 1/2 cup of fat, simply add 1/2 cup of pureed fruit. Use applesauce in apple bran muffins or cakes. Pureed, crushed pineapple works well in pineapple upside down cake. Here are some other tips:

➤ Dark-colored fruits, such as blueberries and prunes, are best used in dark-colored batters. You can add lighter colored fruits, such as pears or applesauce, to almost any batter without changing its color. Adding yellow-orange fruits, such as pureed peaches or apricots, can often add an appetizing yellowish crumb.

➤ You can use pears and apples nearly universally in baking because their taste is mild and unnoticeable. Apricots, prunes, and pineapple add a much stronger flavor. Bananas and peaches are somewhere in the middle, adding a little flavor, but never overwhelming. Here's a secret: If you don't have a food processor to use to puree your own fruit, use baby food. It is already pureed, has a mild flavor, and usually is made without sugar.

15. Beat egg whites until soft peaks form before incorporating them into baked goods. This will increase the volume and tenderness.

16. Make a simple fat-free "frosting" for cakes or bar cookies by sprinkling the tops lightly with powdered sugar.

17. Increase the fiber content and nutritional value of dishes by using whole-wheat flour for at least half of the all-purpose white flour. For cakes and other baked products that require a light texture, use whole-wheat pastry flour, available in some well-stocked supermarkets.

18. Vegetables can be fat replacements in other recipes, too. Try…

➤ Adding baby carrot puree, roasted red pepper puree, or mashed potatoes to your pasta sauce to replace olive oil.

➤ Replacing some of the fat in nut breads or cakes, such as carrot cake or zucchini bread, with vegetable purees or juices, such as carrot juice or pumpkin puree.

➤ Substituting pureed green peas for half the amount of mashed avocado in guacamole or other dips.

➤ Replacing fat in soups, sauces, muffins, or cakes with mashed yams or sweet potatoes.

➤ Using white potatoes to thicken lower-fat milks in cream soups and bisques.

➤ Substituting a layer of vegetables in your favorite lasagna to replace meat or sausage.

➤ Topping your pizza with vegetables instead of meat.

*Source: ADA. "Skim The Fat: A Practical and Up-to-Date Food Guide," 1995.*

## Top-10 List for Substitutions

Try some of these substitutions with your favorite recipes. They can help to reduce the fat while maintaining flavor.

1. Use non-fat plain yogurt instead of sour cream.
2. Use two egg whites instead of one whole egg.
3. Use 1% low-fat milk instead of whole milk.
4. Use $1/2$ the fat that a recipe calls for.
5. Use 3 Tbs cocoa powder and 1 Tbs oil instead of baking chocolate.
6. Use evaporated skim milk instead of cream.
7. Use fruit purees, fruit juices, or buttermilk to replace fat in a recipe.
8. Use non-fat yogurt or reduced-fat mayonnaise instead of regular mayonnaise.
9. Use diet margarine instead of regular margarine.
10. Use low-fat ricotta cheese or 1% cottage cheese instead of whole-milk cream cheese or ricotta cheese.

# Breakfast: Two Creative Morning Recipes

### French Toast a la Mode

*Serves three*

2 egg whites (or egg substitutes)

6 slices of wheat bread

$1/3$ cup of 1% low-fat milk

1 cup non-fat plain yogurt

$1/2$ tsp vanilla extract

1 cup fresh blueberries

1 Tbs reduced-fat margarine

Beat the eggs, milk, and vanilla in a bowl. Melt the margarine in a skillet over medium heat. Cut the bread into diagonal slices, and dip both sides evenly in the batter (made from the eggs, milk, and vanilla). Next, brown each side of the bread in the hot skillet by flipping the individual slices. Arrange the finished French toast on a plate (2 full slices or 4 halves per serving); top with a scoop of yogurt and fresh blueberries.

Nutrient Analysis for One Serving
Calories: 231
Total fat: 4 grams
Saturated fat: 0.7 grams
Fiber: 7 grams
Protein: 13 grams
Sodium: 467 mg
Cholesterol: 1 mg

*From the kitchen of Carol and Victor Bauer*

## Egg White-Veggie Omelet

*Serves two*

8 egg whites

$^1/_4$ cup chopped tomato

4 Tbs low-fat milk

2 ounces non-fat shredded cheddar cheese

$^1/_2$ cup sliced mushrooms

Non-stick vegetable spray

$^1/_2$ cup sliced onions

Pepper to taste

Mix the egg whites together with milk and some pepper; set it aside. In a separate dish, place the mushrooms, onions, and 2 Tbs of water. Cover and microwave the vegetables for approximately 2–3 minutes on high (depending on how soft you like your veggies). Drain vegetables, and mix in the chopped tomatoes and eggs. Apply nonstick spray to a large skillet, and cook the entire concoction over medium-high heat. When the eggs begin to set, sprinkle on the shredded cheese and allow it to melt. When the omelet appears cooked but moist, fold over one side and gently lift onto a plate. Round-off the meal with some whole-wheat toast and you're set.

<u>Nutrient Analysis for One Serving ($^1/_2$ large omelet)</u>
Calories: 161
Total fat: 1 grams
Saturated fat: 0.2 grams
Fiber: 2 grams
Protein: 26 grams
Sodium: 445 mg
Cholesterol: 1 mg

*From the kitchen of Debra, Steve, and Ben Beal*

# Lunch—Not the Same Old Sandwich Again!

## Greek Pasta Salad

*Serves four*

3 cups uncooked bowtie (or fusilli) pasta

1 cucumber, seeded and diced $^1/_4$ inch

3 ripe plum tomatoes, seeded and diced $^1/_4$ inch

$^1/_4$ cup chopped red onion

3 Tbs black diced olives

2 Tbs balsamic vinegar

1 grated lemon zest (the outer peel) and juice

2 Tbs fresh chopped mint leaves

Olive oil cooking spray

1 small head of Bibb or butter lettuce

Cook the pasta: Bring 2 quarts of water to a rapid boil over high heat. Add the pasta slowly, stirring constantly until all the pasta is in the pot. Bring back to a boil and reduce the heat to medium-high. Cook according to package directions or until pasta still has a slightly firm center (about 10–13 minutes). Drain in colander and rinse with cold water.

*continues*

*continued*

Make the salad: Combine all vegetables (except the lettuce), vinegar, lemon zest, and lemon juice in a mixing bowl. Toss in pasta and mint leaves and lightly spray with olive oil cooking spray. Toss again. Line four plates with lettuce leaves and divide pasta salad among them.

<u>Nutrient Analysis for One Serving</u>
Calories: 220
Total fat: 2 grams
Saturated fat: 0 grams
Fiber: 2 grams
Protein: 10 grams
Sodium: 150 mg
Cholesterol: 0 mg

## Open-Faced Tuna Melt

*Serves one*

1 whole-wheat English muffin, sliced in half  Sliced tomato

3-ounce can of water packed tuna (low sodium)  2 slices low-fat American cheese

2 tsp reduced-fat mayonnaise

Toast both halves of the English muffin and set aside. Drain and mash tuna, and then mix it with the low-fat mayonnaise. Spread tuna evenly over both pieces of the muffin, leaving the bread open-faced. Place a tomato and one slice of cheese on top of the tuna on each piece of bread. Put the opened-faced sandwich in the oven until the cheese is fully melted.

<u>Nutrient Analysis for One Serving</u>
Calories: 319
Total fat: 7 grams
Saturated fat: 1.5 grams
Fiber: 4 grams
Protein: 31 grams
Sodium: 530 mg
Cholesterol: 30 mg

*From the kitchen of Glenn and Erik Music (Castlebridge Recording)*

# Dinner: Recipes to "Wow" Your Taste Buds

## Shrimp and Pineapple Stir-Fry

*Serves four*

### Rice

1 1/2 cups instant brown rice

1 1/2 cups water

### Stir-Fry

Canola vegetable oil spray

1 cup assorted sweet peppers
(red, green, yellow), diced

1 cup sliced mushrooms

1/4 cup chicken broth

1/2 tsp red pepper flakes

1/2 Tbs cornstarch

12 ounces medium shrimp, peeled and deveined

1 Tbs light soy sauce

1/2 cup snow peas

1/2 cup crushed pineapple; drain and reserve juice

1 cup bean sprouts

Cook instant brown rice in microwave-proof, covered dish for 10 minutes on medium high power (80%) in your microwave.

Lightly spray a nonstick skillet with canola oil and heat over medium high. Sauté peppers until crisp-tender—about 2 minutes; add mushrooms and snow peas and allow to sauté until crisp-tender—about 2 minutes. Combine chicken broth, cornstarch, light soy sauce, and pineapple juice (reserved from drained, crushed pineapple) and add to skillet along with bean sprouts. Bring to a boil; add red pepper flakes and shrimp and cook until shrimp is done—about 1 or 2 minutes. Serve over hot cooked rice.

<u>Nutrient Analysis for One Serving</u>
Calories: 290
Total fat: 3 grams
Saturated fat: 0.5 grams
Fiber: 4 grams
Protein: 23 grams
Sodium: 290 mg
Cholesterol: 130 mg

*Copyright* Food for Health *newsletter, 1996. Reprinted with permission.*

## Chicken Paprika

*Serves six*

6 chicken breasts, skin removed
   (about 6 ounces each)

3–4 cloves of garlic, chopped

$1/2$ tsp ground black pepper

$1/2$ tsp paprika

2 onions sliced

1–2 peppers sliced (red, yellow, and green)

1–2 carrots, cut in half and sliced lengthwise

2 tsp olive oil

Season chicken breasts on all sides with garlic, pepper, and paprika; set aside. Heat olive oil in deep skillet with lid. Add onions and cook for 3–5 minutes over a medium heat. Add chicken and flip until all sides turn white. Add peppers and carrots; cover and simmer for $1^1/2$–2 hours. If you would like less sauce, remove the lid for the last 20 minutes.

Nutrient Analysis for One Serving
Calories: 252
Total fat: 13 grams
Saturated fat: 3 gram
Fiber: 1 grams
Protein: 27 grams
Sodium: 65 mg
Cholesterol: 118 mg

*From the kitchen of Frances Aaron*

## Jon's Terrific Turkeyloaf
## with Mashed Potatoes

*Serves eight*

### Turkeyloaf

2 lbs ground lean turkey breast (no skin)

1 cup onions, diced

3 slices whole-wheat bread, pulled apart

1 cup shredded fat-free cheddar cheese

2 cups whole cranberry sauce

6 crushed cloves of garlic

1 whole egg and 2 egg whites

5 fresh parsley sprigs

2 carrots, peeled and diced

### Mashed Potatoes

5 medium size potatoes, peeled and quartered

2 Tbs diet margarine

1 cup 1% low-fat milk

Preheat oven to 350°. Mix all turkeyloaf ingredients together in a bowl, and then place it into a loaf pan. Bake for $^1/_2$ hour; drain off oil.

In a separate pot, boil the 5 peeled, quartered potatoes. When soft (poke with fork), mash them and mix in the margarine and milk.

Now, for the finishing touch: Spread mashed potatoes across the top of the turkeyloaf and put the combination back in the oven for an additional 30 minutes (at 350°).

Nutrient Analysis for One Serving
Calories: 498
Total fat: 4 grams
Saturated fat: 1 gram
Fiber: 6 grams
Protein: 46 grams
Sodium: 325 mg
Cholesterol: 122 mg

*From the kitchen of Jon Cohen, Nancy Shapiro, and Camrin*

# Sensational Side Dishes

## Sautéed Italian Mushrooms

*Serves four*

1 10–12 ounce pack of white mushrooms (or 1 lb loose), sliced thickly

2–3 garlic cloves, sliced

Chopped parsley

1 tsp olive oil

Nonstick cooking spray

Fresh ground pepper to taste

Spray skillet with nonstick cooking spray and drizzle the olive oil into the pan. Brown garlic cloves over medium-high heat and add sliced mushrooms and chopped parsley. Add plenty of fresh ground pepper (according to your personal taste) and continue to sauté until mushrooms are brown and tender.

Nutrient Analysis for One Serving
Calories: 44
Total fat: 2 grams
Saturated fat: 0 grams
Fiber: 2 grams
Protein: 3 grams
Sodium: 5 mg
Cholesterol: 0 mg

*From the kitchen of Grace Leder*

## Cauliflower Soup

*Serves six*

1 cauliflower

1 sliced onion

2 medium carrots, sliced

1 stalk celery, chopped

5 cups of chicken stock, low-sodium

1 Tbs olive oil

Black pepper to taste

Blanche the whole cauliflower for a few minutes. Cook the sliced onion in the oil until it is transparent, and then add carrots, sliced cauliflower, and celery—and cook slightly. Add chicken stock and the seasoning. Simmer until the vegetables are just tender; then, puree the mixture. Return to the heat for a few minutes and adjust the seasoning.

Nutrient Analysis for One Serving
Calories: 78
Total fat: 3 grams
Saturated fat: 1 gram
Fiber: 2.5 grams
Protein: 4 grams
Sodium: 123 mg
Cholesterol: 3 mg

*From the kitchen of Frances Aaron*

## Tomato Zucchini Roast

*Serves four*

3 large, ripe plum tomatoes, diced medium

$1/2$ tsp Italian spice mix

1 medium zucchini, diced medium

Fresh cracked black pepper

$1^1/_2$ cups sliced mustard greens

Olive oil cooking spray

Preheat oven to 350°. Toss all ingredients together and place into suitable-sized glass or metal baking container. Bake 10–15 minutes uncovered until zucchini is tender. Stir well and serve.

Nutrient Analysis for One Serving
Calories: 35
Total fat: 0 grams
Saturated fat: 0 grams
Fiber: 2 grams
Protein: 2 grams
Sodium: 15 mg
Cholesterol: 0 mg

*Copyright* Food for Health *newsletter, 1996. Reprinted with permission.*

# Decadent Desserts

## Harvest Apple Cake

*Serves 12*

4 cups (1$^{1}/_{4}$ pounds) unpeeled, chopped
   Golden Delicious apples, divided

$^{1}/_{2}$ tsp salt

$^{1}/_{4}$ tsp each ginger and cloves

1 cup firmly packed brown sugar

$^{1}/_{4}$ cup vegetable oil

$^{3}/_{4}$ cup each all-purpose and whole-wheat flour

2 large eggs, lightly beaten

1 tsp baking soda

1 tsp vanilla extract

1 tsp cinnamon

1 Tbs confectioners' sugar

Combine 3 cups of the apples and the sugar in a bowl; let stand 45 minutes. Heat oven to 350°. Grease and flour a 6-cup fluted tube pan. Combine dry ingredients in a medium bowl. Combine oil, eggs, and vanilla in a small bowl; stir into the apple-sugar mixture. Stir in dry ingredients and remaining apples until blended. Pour into the prepared pan. Bake 40–45 minutes, until a toothpick inserted in the center of cake comes out clean. Cool in the pan on a wire rack 10 minutes; unmold cake and cool completely. Sprinkle with confectioners' sugar.

<u>Nutrient Analysis for One Serving</u>
Calories: 213
Total fat: 6 grams
Saturated fat: 1 gram
Fiber: 2 grams
Protein: 3 grams
Sodium: 212 mg
Cholesterol: 35 mg

## Angel-Devil Smoothie

*Serves four*

2 cups nonfat plain yogurt
2 chocolate nonfat brownies, broken into small pieces

2 cups frozen sliced strawberries
$1/4$ cup skim milk

Combine all ingredients in blender or food processor. Pulse until all is pureed fine. Serve immediately.

<u>Nutrient Analysis for One Serving</u>
Calories: 140
Total fat: 0 grams
Saturated fat: 0 grams
Fiber: 2 grams
Protein: 8 grams
Sodium: 135 mg
Cholesterol: 5 mg

*Copyright* Food for Health *newsletter, 1996. Reprinted with permission.*

## Banana-Health Split

*Serves one*

1 banana, peeled
$1/2$ cup vanilla fat-free frozen yogurt
2 Tbs granola cereal (low-fat)

Split the banana lengthwise down the middle, and line up the two pieces on either side of an ice cream dish. Scoop frozen yogurt in the middle and sprinkle granola on top. You've now got a guilt-free banana split!

<u>Nutrient Analysis for One Serving</u>
Calories: 243
Total fat: 1 gram
Saturated fat: 0 grams
Fiber: 2 grams
Protein: 5 grams
Sodium: 65 mg
Cholesterol: 0 mg

*From the kitchen of Pam and Dan Schloss*

# Start a Cookbook Library

Check with the following resources to begin your own collection of cookbooks. You can find healthy recipes in the following books:

*Cooking Light Cookbook 1996*
Oxmoore House Publishing
800-526-5111

*Cook Healthy Cook Quick*
Oxmoore House Publishing
800-526-5111

*Family Favorites Made Lighter*
Better Homes and Gardens
Meredith Books
800-678-8091

*The American Heart Association Cookbook*
Times Books/Random House
800-726-0600

*Healthy Favorites; From America's Community Prevention Magazine*
Rodale Press, Inc.
800-848-4735

*1,001 Low-Fat Recipes*
by Sue Spitler
Surret Books
800-326-4430

*Low-Fat Cook for Good Health*
by Gloria Rose
Avery Publishing Group
800-548-5757

*Secrets of Fat-Free Baking*
by Sandra Woodruff, R.D.
Avery Publishing Group
800-548-5757

*Quick and Healthy Recipes and Ideas*
by Brenda J. Pontichtera
ScaleDown Publishing
541-296-5859

**Overrated—Undercooked**

Be careful when cutting back on the amount of sugar in cakes, cookies, or other baked goods. Many times, reducing sugar will affect the texture or the volume.

*Everyday Cooking with Dr. Dean Ornish*
by Dean Ornish, M.D.
HarperCollins Publishers
Available at your local bookstore

*Kitchen Fun for Kids*
by Michael F. Jacobson and Laura Hill, R.D.
Center for Science in the Public Interest (CSPI)
800-237-4874

*Quick and Healthy Low-Fat Cooking*
edited by Jean Rogers, from the pages of *Prevention Magazine*
Rodale Books
800-848-4735

---

### The Least You Need to Know

➤ Simple ingredient substitutions can turn your favorite recipes into healthy, low-fat dishes.

➤ Stick with the healthier, lower-fat cooking techniques such as steaming, poaching, stir-frying, broiling, grilling, microwaving, baking, and roasting. Jazz up the flavor with non-caloric spices and seasonings.

➤ Use pureed, cooked veggies instead of cream, butter, and egg yolks to thicken soups and sauces. For baked products, add pureed fruit instead of butter, lard, and other oils. When a recipe calls for a large amount of sugar, scale it down by 25 percent.

# Chapter 12

# Restaurant Survival Guide

> **In This Chapter**
>
> ➤ Dining out healthfully
>
> ➤ Becoming a menu detective
>
> ➤ Best bets in ethnic cuisine

Too tired to cook, or just want to get out and socialize? Join the crowd! According to the National Restaurant Association, Americans spend an average of more than $800 million dollars a day on food away from home. Once considered a special occasion, eating out has become an everyday happening—and the food-service industry is growing by leaps and bounds. This chapter shows you that, along with convenience and atmosphere, restaurants can also provide healthy food. You just need to practice some defensive dining.

## Common Restaurant Faux Pas

First, the problem of overeating. Are you the type who needs to loosen your belt buckle a couple of notches after each course? Keep in mind that this is *not* the last meal of your life, and there's no need to lick your plate clean even though your stomach is ready to explode. When you feel comfortably full, either ask the waiter to take away your plate, or simply pack it up in a doggie bag and enjoy it the following day.

What about the actual food choices? Making healthy food choices requires planning, nutrition know-how, and compromise: *planning* during the day so you can budget your fat and calories; *nutrition know-how* so you can order the healthier, lower-fat items from your favorite ethnic cuisines; and the willingness to *compromise* between the foods you should be eating and the not-so-terrific foods you looooove to chow down.

Fortunately, due to the increasing emphasis on health, most places, from fast-food joints to fancy establishments, are making an effort to prepare and offer at least a few healthy alternatives. Quite often, you will even notice a *Spa Cuisine* section on the regular menu listing nutrition information underneath the lower-fat entrées. For the restaurants that don't provide this luxury, don't be shy or embarrassed: Speak up and ask for special requests such as "salad dressing or sauce on the side," "less oil and salt used during food preparation," and "substitute a baked potato or side salad instead of french fries." Remember, good food does not have to wear the price tag of cellulite.

# Become a Dining Detective

Go ahead and take on any type of restaurant. Ask yourself (and waiter) the following five key questions before ordering something on the menu:

1. **How is the food prepared?** The same methods I advised for your own personal recipes also apply to restaurants. Whether entrées or side dishes, scout out meals that are prepared by grilling, baking, poaching, roasting, boiling, blackening, steaming, broiling, or "lightly" stir-frying. If the menu doesn't indicate the cooking technique, ask your waiter or waitress. Don't assume that a food is not fried unless the menu clearly says it isn't.

2. **Are the cuts of meat lean?** Stick with the leaner cuts of meat. For instance, loin, round, flank, shoulder, leg, and extra-lean ground beef are the preferred choices when ordering red meat. Chicken and turkey breasts are two of the leanest choices to make, and of course, all fish and seafood can be terrific when prepared in a healthful manner. When you do occasionally order steak, ask whether the chef melts butter on top before cooking. Believe it or not, some establishments do this to make the meat seem more tender.

3. **What kind of sauces come with your meal?** Ask about the ingredients used for sauces. Generally, avoid hollandaise, butter, cheese, and cream sauces that come slathered over your meal. If you're not sure about something, or it sounds delicious and hard to pass up, get it on the side and enjoy it in smaller amounts.

4. **Are the ingredients loaded with sodium?** If you're on a sodium-restricted diet for medical reasons, it's especially important to avoid entrées and side dishes that are loaded with salt. Stay away from meats and fish that are smoked, cured, pickled, or canned. Also avoid sauces, seasonings, and marinades that use soy sauce, teriyaki sauce, dried stock, MSG, or plain old table salt during preparation.

5. **How can you balance out your meal?** If you order a pasta entrée, pass up the bread. If you know that you like to splurge on dessert, order a lean grilled fish for your main dish with a lot of vegetables. If the bread basket is your thing, skip the side starch that comes with your main meal and enjoy a few slices of fresh bread instead. If you like to use up calories on a few glasses of wine, skip the bread and get fresh fruit for dessert.

**Q & A**

Can you ever just "go whole hog" and order whatever you want without worrying about all the unhealthy ingredients?

Sure you can, but save it for occasional splurges—not everyday habit. In fact, some things are so obscenely scrumptious that if you didn't periodically indulge, I'd think you were nuts!

# Ethnic Cuisine: "the Good, the Bad, and the Ugly"

Take a quick trip around the world, and check out the best bets in French, Italian, Chinese, Japanese, Mexican, Indian, and American cookery. Be adventurous and excite your palate with exotic new flavors. *Bon appétit!*

## Chinese Food

Loaded with vegetables, rice, and noodles, the typical Chinese cuisine offers an assortment of healthy selections. Because most Chinese cooking is done in a wok (stir-frying), varying amounts of peanut oil are used. The good news is that peanut oil is unsaturated and won't clog up your arteries. The bad news is that excessive amounts of *any* oil can add a lot of fat calories. As you can imagine, some of the dishes have *startling* amounts.

If your thighs can't afford those extra fat calories, avoid anything fried. Try one of the steamed versions, or carefully drain off some of the fat in a stir-fried entrée by taking your portion from the serving plate drenched in sauce and transferring it to your dish with rice. Another idea, if you're dining with a friend, is to order one dish in sauce and a second steamed vegetable dish. Mix the two together, and you'll have half the sauce and double the vegetables.

Another problem with Chinese food can be sodium because a lot of the sauces are high in salt. If you're on a salt-restricted diet, you should probably stick with the plain steamed dishes.

| Lower-Fat Foods | Higher-Fat Foods |
| --- | --- |
| Hot and sour soup | Egg drop soup |
| Wonton soup | Egg rolls |
| Steamed dumplings (vegetable, chicken, and seafood) | Fried dumplings |

*continues*

*continued*

| Lower-Fat Foods | Higher-Fat Foods |
| --- | --- |
| Stir-fried or *steamed* chicken and vegetables | Fried won tons |
| Stir-fried or *steamed* beef and vegetables | Fried rice |
| Stir-fried or *steamed* seafood and vegetables | Egg fu yung |
| Stir-fried or *steamed* tofu and vegetables | Cold noodles with sesame sauce |
| Steamed whole fish | Moo-shu pork |
| | Sesame Chicken |
| | General Tsao Chicken |
| Moo-shu vegetables (with pancake rollups) | Sweet and sour pork |
| Steamed brown and white rice | Fried chicken and seafood dishes |
| Fortune cookies | Seafood with lobster sauce |
| Lychee nuts | Spareribs |
| Oranges and pineapple slices | |
| Low-sodium soy sauce (if available) | |
| Duck sauce and plum sauce | |

## French Food

Many positive changes (nutritionally speaking) have occurred in French food during the 20th century, from the classic *haute* cuisine that generally uses heavier cream sauces, to the newer *nouvelle* cuisine that uses a lighter and healthier approach to food preparation.

| Lower-Fat Foods | Higher-Fat Foods |
| --- | --- |
| Steamed mussels | Appetizers with olives, anchovies, or capers |
| Consommé | Quiche |
| Endive and watercress salads | French onion soup (with cheese) |
| Nicoise salads | Cream-based soups |
| Poached fish | Pate |
| Steamed fish | Fondue |
| Lightly sautéed vegetables | Crepes |
| Bouillabaisse | Brioche |
| Chicken in wine sauce | Duck or goose with skin |
| French bread and baguettes | Béarnaise sauce |
| Flambéed cherries | Hollandaise sauce |
| Peaches in wine | Béchamel sauce |

| Lower-Fat Foods | Higher-Fat Foods |
| --- | --- |
| Fresh and poached fruit | Mornay sauce |
| Fruit sorbet | Anything with the word "cream" or "au gratin" |
| Wine in moderation | Chocolate mousse |
| | Creme caramel |
| | Croissants |
| | Pastries and eclairs |

# Indian Food

As with most ethnic cuisines, there are pros and cons to Indian cookery. Beginning with the pros, Indian food emphasizes high carbohydrates such as basmati rice, breads, lentils, chickpeas, and vegetables, all accented with an array of spices. The most common veggies are spinach, cabbage, peas, onions, eggplant, potatoes, tomatoes, and green peppers. The con is that fat can easily find its way into many of the entrées, breads, and vegetable side dishes.

Scrutinize the menu and watch out for the word *ghee*, which is clarified butter used frequently in Indian cooking. Other oils that are used for sautéing and frying are sesame oil and coconut oil. Although sesame oil is unsaturated, it's quite the contrary for coconut oil—arteries beware! If salt is an issue, forego the soups, and ask the waiter to please prepare your meal without any added salt.

| Lower-Fat Foods | Higher-Fat Foods |
| --- | --- |
| Tamata salat | Anything made with ghee (clarified butter) |
| Mulligatawny soup (lentil, veggies, and spices) | Coconut soups |
| Chicken or beef tikka | Samosas (fried vegetable turnover) |
| Tandoori chicken, beef, or fish | Korma (meat with rich yogurt cream sauce) |
| Chicken, beef, and fish saaq (with spinach) | Curries made with coconut milk or cream |
| Chicken, beef, and fish vindaloo (with potatoes and spices) | Pakora (fried dough with veggies) |
| Shish kabob | Saaq paneer (spinach with cream sauce) |
| Gobhi matar tamatar (cauliflower with peas and tomatoes) | Creamy rice dishes |
| Matar pulao (rice pilaf with peas) | Fried breads |
| Steamed rice | Honeyed pastries |
| Papadum or papad (crispy, thin lentil wafers) | |

*continues*

*continued*

| Lower-Fat Foods | Higher-Fat Foods |
| --- | --- |
| Coriander, tamarind, and yogurt-based sauces | |
| Chapati (thin, dry whole-wheat bread) | |
| Naan (leavened, baked bread) | |
| Kulcha (leavened, baked bread) | |
| Mango, mint, and onion chutney | |

# Italian Food

Among my friends and family, Italian seems to be the one type of food that we can always agree upon. (It's amazing how quickly you can get into the mood.) Unfortunately, as with every other cuisine, if you take one wrong turn on the menu, you're headed for a nutritional nightmare. For instance, pasta can be a terrific meal if it is ordered with the right kind of sauce; stick with meatless marinara, red and white clam sauce, pomodora, white wine, and a light olive oil. On the other hand, a pasta entrée swimming in one of those cream sauces is a big zero. Also, watch out for super-cheesy entrées such as stuffed shells, manicotti, lasagna, and parmigiana. Of course, every once in a while, we are all entitled to indulge. Just make sure the rest of your day was pretty low-fat because some of this stuff can be lethal.

| Lower-Fat Foods | Higher-Fat Foods |
| --- | --- |
| Roasted peppers | Fried calamari and fried mozzarella |
| Mussels marinara | Garlic bread |
| Steamed clams | Caesar salads |
| Grilled calamari | Sausage and meatball heros |
| Minestrone soup | Calzones and pizza with pepperoni and sausage |
| Pasta with meatless marinara sauce | Antipasto salad with high-fat meats and cheese |
| Pasta primavera (not creamy) | Cheese- or meat-filled ravioli and manicotti |
| Pasta with red and white clam sauce | Meat lasagna and cheesy vegetarian lasagna |
| Pasta with marsala | Cannelloni and baked ziti |
| Chicken breast with red sauce | Chicken, veal, or eggplant parmigiana |
| Chicken cacciatore | Fettuccine alfredo and pasta carbonara |
| Shrimp, chicken, or veal in wine sauce | Shrimp scampi |
| Chicken and veal piccatta | Chicken or veal scaloppini |
| Pizza with fresh vegetable toppings | Cannoli, spumoni, and tartufo |

| Lower-Fat Foods | Higher-Fat Foods |
|---|---|
| Lightly marinated mushrooms | |
| Fresh Italian bread | |
| Fresh fruit or sorbet | |
| Italian ices | |
| Skim milk cappuccino | |
| Wine in moderation | |

## Japanese Food

The Japanese have perfected low-fat cooking with food-preparation methods that require little or no oil. Highlighting rice, vegetables, soybean-based foods, and small quantities of fish, chicken, and meat, these meals are artistic, healthy, and, best of all, delicious. What's more, once you master the art of using chopsticks, Japanese dining can be a lot of fun. The one drawback is the high-sodium marinades and traditional sauces, which include soy and teriyaki. Ask your waiter whether low-sodium soy sauce is available—and if it isn't, dilute the regular with some water.

| Lower-Fat Foods | Higher-Fat Foods |
|---|---|
| Miso soup (soybean-paste soup with tofu and scallions) | Vegetable tempura (battered and fried veggies) |
| Steamed vegetables | Shrimp tempura |
| Fish and vegetable sushi | Eel and avocado rolls |
| Sashimi (raw fish served with wasabi and dipping sauce) | Tonkatsu (breaded pork cutlet) |
| Hijiki (cooked seaweed) | Fried dumplings |
| Oshitashi (boiled spinach with soy sauce) | Fried bean curd |
| Yaki-udon | Oyako domburi (chicken omelet over rice) |
| Yakitori (skewers of chicken) | Chawan mush (chicken and shrimp in egg custard) |
| Su-udon | Yo kan (sweet bean cake) |
| Sukiyaki | |
| Sushi and sashimi (pieces and rolls) | |
| Nabemono (a variety of casseroles) | |
| Yosenabe (seafood and veggies in broth) | |
| Miso-nabe | |
| Shabu-shabu (sliced beef, vegetables, and noodles) | |
| Sumashi wan (broth with tofu and shrimp) | |
| Chicken, fish, or beef teriyaki | |
| Steamed rice | |

# Mexican Food

If your taste buds cry out for hot and spicy, Mexican food is probably high on your list of favorites. Unfortunately, some typical dishes on a Mexican menu can send you straight to nutrition jail. On a positive note, Mexican food can be healthy, especially because many dishes are high in complex carbohydrate and fiber; you just need to manage the menu. For example, those fried tortilla chips can be addictive. If you typically gobble down three baskets before your food even arrives, get them off the table. Stick with cheeseless entrées that include beans, rice, and grilled chicken or fish, and use plenty of salsa in place of high-fat sour cream and guacamole. (Although guacamole made from avocado is unsaturated, it still has a lot of fat.)

| Lower-Fat Foods | Higher-Fat Foods |
|---|---|
| Gazpacho | Tortilla chips |
| Corn tortillas with salsa | Nachos with cheese |
| Chicken fajitas | Chorizo (sausage) |
| Enchiladas | Carnitas (fried beef) |
| Camarones de hacha (shrimp sautéed in tomato coriander sauce) | Refried beans |
| Arroz con pollo (chicken breast with rice) | Quesadillas with cheese |
| Cheeseless burritos | Beef tacos |
| Grilled fish or chicken breast | Burritos with cheese |
| Frijoles a la charra | Beef and cheese enchilada |
| Borracho beans and rice | Chimichangas |
| Soft chicken taco | Sour cream and guacamole |
| Chicken tostada | Sopapillas (fried dough with sugar) |
| Salsa, pico de gallo and cilantro | Frozen margaritas and piña coladas |
| Jalapeno peppers | |
| Ceviche (raw fish cooked in lime or lemon juice) | |

# American Food

American-style restaurants borrow an assortment of ethnic dishes from around the world. Of course, we *are* responsible for salad bars, steak and potatoes, chicken and ribs, a bunch of sandwiches, and good ol' American apple pie, but the typical American menu usually resembles the United Nations.

For example, you can usually expect to find chicken teriyaki from Japan, a stir-fried dish from China, chicken fajitas from Mexico, and a pasta dish from Italy on the spread. The nice part about such a comprehensive menu is that it offers something for everyone (even finicky kids). Placing heavy emphasis on appetizers, salads, and sandwiches, American food can certainly swing both ways. When you're in the mood for a sandwich, stick with the unadulterated versions such as turkey, roast beef, and chicken breast. Beware of breads and buns that are pre-buttered before they reach your table (such as the buttery grilled cheese sandwich). Ask your waiter to substitute a side salad for those greasy french fries, and stay clear of large salad entrées that pack in more fat than you want to know about. (Read the descriptions and go easy on bacon, avocado, shredded cheese, olives, and dressings.) For standard entrées, look for the usual green-light words (grilled, broiled, and blackened); you know the routine by now.

| Lower-Fat Foods | Higher-Fat Foods |
| --- | --- |
| Shrimp/seafood cocktails | Creamy soups |
| Tossed salads with light vinaigrette | Caesar salads |
| Broth and vegetable-based soup | Salads with avocado, bacon, and creamy dressings |
| Turkey, roast beef, and grilled chicken sandwiches | Buffalo/chicken wings |
| Broiled, blackened, and grilled fish and chicken | Fried zucchini and mushrooms |
| Plain hamburgers, turkey burgers, and veggie burgers | Cheeseburgers |
| Grilled chicken on salad | Grilled cheese sandwiches |
| Grilled vegetable plates over rice | Philadelphia cheese steaks |
| Chicken kabobs and rice | Reuben sandwiches and tuna melts |
| Baked potatoes with Dijon mustard, ketchup, marinara, salsa, or small amount of butter | Tuna salad, egg salad, and chicken salad |
| Pasta with tomato-based sauce | Fried chicken or fish |
| Steamed or lightly sautéed vegetables | Hot dogs |
| Frozen yogurt, fruit ice or sherbet | French fries and potato salad |
| Fresh fruit | Fruit pies, cookies, cakes, and ice cream sundaes |
| Angel-food cake | |

## Fast Food

The restaurants might lack ambiance, but fast food is certainly one hopping business! It's quick, convenient, and cheap. The nice thing about fast food today is that most places offer an assortment of healthy alternatives due to the growing number of nutrition-conscience customers. Try your best to keep things simple. Generally, the items with complicated names are laden with high-fat meats and "special sauces." For example, the Bacon Double Cheeseburger Deluxe at Burger King has a whopping 39 grams of fat with 16 grams from saturated fat. Be sure to also skip the fried chicken and all sandwiches smothered with cheese. Also, don't ever assume that fish automatically gets a nutrition gold medal. Did you know that McDonald's Filet-O-Fish (breaded and fried) contains 18 grams of fat, compared to the plain hamburger, which only has 9 grams? Stick with the healthier choices to make the best of your fast-food outings.

| Lower-Fat Foods | Higher-Fat Foods |
| --- | --- |
| Bagel with jelly | Biscuits and danish |
| Hot cakes (no butter) | Egg sandwiches with sausage or bacon |
| Grilled chicken sandwiches | Cheeseburgers |
| Plain hamburgers | Jumbo burger combinations |
| Turkey burgers | Fried chicken sandwiches and fried chicken nuggets |
| Veggie burgers | Fried fish filets |
| Vegetable pizza | Pepperoni or sausage pizza |
| Vegetable salads with "lite" dressings | French fries |
| Chunky chicken salads | Baked potatoes with butter, sour cream, or cheese |
| Turkey sandwiches (no mayo) | Nachos with cheese |
| Lean roast-beef sandwiches (no mayo) | Onion rings and fried vegetables |
| Chicken fajitas | Apple pie and milkshakes |
| Mashed potatoes | |
| Baked potatoes with vegetables, salsa, ketchup, or vegetarian chili | |
| Grilled or steamed veggies | |
| Fruit salads and fresh fruit | |
| Frozen yogurt cones | |
| Juice or low-fat milk | |
| Ketchup, mustard, barbecue, and honey mustard sauce | |

Your best bets in fast food:

➤ At McDonald's, try the McLean Deluxe, side salad with "lite" vinaigrette, and some orange juice.

➤ At Domino's, try a plain pizza with vegetable toppings, a side salad with "lite" dressing, and a tall glass of water.

➤ At Wendy's, try the grilled chicken sandwich on a multi-grain bun, or a baked potato with plain broccoli (or chili), and a salad tossed with "lite" dressing. Wash it down with some water or juice.

# Going Out for Breakfast or Brunch?

Master the following do's and don'ts.

*Do* order pancakes and waffles with plenty of fresh fruit and just a touch of syrup. Choose egg-white omelets stuffed with various veggies, Canadian bacon, unsweetened cereals with skim milk, and fresh fruit. Other healthy alternatives are hot oatmeal, cream of wheat and rice (made with low-fat milk), English muffins, bagels, and whole-grain breads with some jam and low-fat yogurt. To wash it all down, opt for some fresh juice and low-fat milk.

*Don't* make it a habit to start your day with an unhealthy catastrophe, such as scrambled eggs, bacon, sausage, hashbrowns, cheese omelets, biscuits, croissants, bagels with butter, large cake-like muffins, donuts, pancakes and waffles smothered in butter and syrup, deep-fried french toast, or steak and eggs.

### Overrated—Undercooked

Don't let the words "salad bar" fool you. There are just as many high-fat pickings displayed on the buffet as there are low-fat ones. Survey the situation and load your plate with fresh vegetables, beans, whole grains, and low-fat dressings. On the flip side, watch out for the high-fat mayonnaise traps (such as tuna, egg, seafood, and chicken salads), and take it easy on the creamy dressings, bacon bits, high-fat cheeses, olives, nuts, and seeds.

### The Least You Need to Know

➤ Once considered a luxury, dining out has become commonplace for most all Americans today.

➤ Remember that "eating out" does not mean "pigging out." Don't give yourself the license to overeat just because you are in a restaurant. Eat slowly and selectively, and stop when you are comfortably full.

➤ With the proper planning, nutrition know-how, and willingness to compromise, you can fit almost any ethnic restaurant into a healthy low-fat eating plan.

➤ Become a dining detective and examine the menu carefully. Look for lean cuts of meat, poultry, and fish that have been prepared by low-fat cooking methods. Ask your waiter about the type of sauce that accompanies your meal. If salt is an issue, watch out for high sodium marinades.

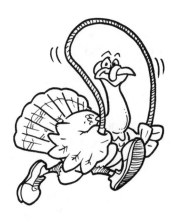

# Chapter 13

# Trimming Down the Holidays

### In This Chapter

➤ Slicing fat and calories out of your holiday season

➤ Healthy menu alternatives for each major holiday

➤ Some great-tasting recipes

We all love holidays. There are family, friends, gifts, days off from work, and more delicious treats than we know what to do with. Doesn't it seem like we can eat whatever we want—with no consequences in the morning?

Unfortunately, over-indulging leaves most of us feeling heavy, sluggish—and guilty. And suddenly you don't fit into your pants. The fact is, holidays are hard when it comes to making smart food choices, but there are ways to make it work.

## Staying on Track on Holiday

No matter how much you expect to eat at Grandma's, stick with your regular meals. Skipping breakfast and barely eating lunch will only make you more ravenous and prone to overeating at a holiday party. Just because your holiday agenda involves sitting around, telling stories, and eating doesn't mean you have to stop your regular exercise routine. The more active you are around holiday season, the better you'll feel, and hence, you'll be more likely to feed your body in a healthy manner. What's more, exercise doesn't have to mean hitting a gym: You can do little things such as parking your car a little further from your destination, taking the stairs instead of the elevator, or taking a quick walk around the block.

It's also important to be selective with your food choices. Survey the spread *before* you dive in and eat everything. Figure out what you really want, and then monitor everything else so you can balance it out. Don't deprive yourself! If you want a piece of cake, have some, but remember that quality is more important than quantity.

Follow these simple holiday menus to help cut your calories and fat intake down from one holiday to the next. Keep in mind that the nutritional info was based on real-life, *generous* holiday portions.

# Easter

The spirit of Easter is all about new beginnings. It's the onset of spring; there are flowers blooming and birds returning. As the days start to get longer and the sunshine gets warmer, it's time to shed those winter doldrums, peel off those big winter sweaters, and add some spring to your step...and your meal.

Your Easter meal doesn't have to be heavy and filling; it can be light and airy, like the holiday. Just revamp your traditional menu, and lose half the calories and one third of the fat; besides, it'll leave a little room for those sweet marshmallow chicks.

### Traditional Meal
Poached salmon with cucumber dill sauce
Baked ham with pineapple, drenched in syrup
Potato and cheese gratin
Peas with black olives and hard boiled eggs
Buttery biscuits
Vanilla ice cream
Easter candy

### Nutrition Information
Calories: 1,532
Total fat: 77 grams
Saturated fat: 37 grams
Cholesterol: 366 mg
Sodium: 1,381 mg
Dietary fiber: 9 grams
Protein: 69 grams

### Healthier Meal
Poached salmon with honey mustard dill sauce
Baked ham with fresh pineapple
Wild rice salad with chopped dried fruit
Asparagus with shallot vinaigrette
Whole-grain bread
Coconut sorbet
Chocolate fondue (small bowl of chocolate syrup or any other ice cream topping with strawberries, orange slices, and banana chunks for dipping)

### Nutrition Information
Calories: 867
Total fat: 27 grams
Saturated fat: 7 grams
Cholesterol: 138 mg
Sodium: 523 mg
Dietary fiber: 11 grams
Protein: 60 grams

# Passover

One of the oldest and most continuously celebrated holidays, Passover commemorates the Jewish exodus from Egypt after years of suffering and slavery. It is the tradition of the Jewish people to remember their ancestors with a big meal! Well, with a few minor changes to the menu, you can still indulge in Passover with all the taste and a lot less fat and calories. What's more—the extra fiber in the healthier version can help to declog all of that matzo meal.

**Traditional Meal**

Matzo ball soup
Gefilte fish
Brisket
Roast chicken
Potato kugel
Chopped broccoli casserole
Tzimmis
Chocolate Passover cake
Macaroons

**Nutrition Information**

Calories: 2,086
Total fat: 101 grams
Saturated fat: 35 grams
Cholesterol: 734 mg
Sodium: 1,768 mg
Dietary fiber: 17 grams
Protein: 116 grams

**Healthier Meal**

Matzo ball soup (Substitute kosher olive oil for chicken fat and use seltzer instead of liquid to get your matzo balls fluffy.)
Gefilte fish on green salad with lemon and olive oil vinaigrette (Use salmon instead of white fish; it's a great source of Omega 3 fatty acids.)
Rock Cornish game hens stuffed with dried fruit and tomatoes
Sweet potato and carrot tzimmis
Artichokes stuffed with herbed matzo
Large fruit salad
Chocolate Passover cake

**Nutrition Information**

Calories: 1,575
Total fat: 56 grams
Saturated fat: 11 grams
Cholesterol: 454 mg
Sodium: 1,715 mg
Dietary fiber: 27 grams
Protein: 84 grams

# Fourth of July

Think fun-filled barbecues with your friends and busting out your summer attire. It's about soaking up the sun and being comfortable in your body, not feeling bloated and so heavy that you'd rather cover up and stay inside. The best way to keep yourself looking good and feeling groovy is to cut down on those heavy, high-fat foods and splurge on the fresh fruits and veggies that are in season. The traditional menu has a whopping 2,099 calories and 116 grams of fat, but the healthier menu has 985 calories less and 40 percent of the fat—so you can say goodbye to that beer gut and greet some great abs without feeling the least bit deprived.

<u>**Traditional Meal**</u>

Grilled hamburgers and hot dogs on buns
Cold fried chicken
Potato salad
Macaroni salad
Cole slaw
Potato chips
Brownies
Watermelon
Ice cream bars

<u>**Nutrition Information**</u>

Calories: 2,099
Total fat: 116 grams
Saturated fat: 40 grams
Cholesterol: 381 mg
Sodium: 3,741 mg
Dietary fiber: 10 grams
Protein: 72 grams

<u>**Healthier Meal**</u>

Turkey or veggie burgers on buns
Grilled tuna, salmon, or chicken filets
Pasta salad with tomato basil vinaigrette
Grilled vegetables
Health salad
Baked potato chips
Low-fat brownies
Watermelon
Frozen fruit pops

<u>**Nutrition Information**</u>

Calories: 1,411
Total fat: 55 grams
Saturated fat: 10 grams
Cholesterol: 110 mg
Sodium: 1,640 mg
Dietary fiber: 14 grams
Protein: 47 grams

# Thanksgiving

It's supposed to be about giving thanks and feeling grateful for all the positive things in your life. But come on, we know it's really about the fine art of American gluttony: mounds of turkey, rich gravy, starchy stuffing, cranberry sauce, four kinds of potatoes, veggies soaked in butter and oil, pumpkin pie, apple pie, and going in for round two a few hours after your stomach finally settles. Then, there's all those leftovers: Thanksgiving eating goes on for days!

Keep your family traditions and indulge. If you make minor alterations in your meal, you'll feel a whole lot better in the morning—and maybe even have the energy to make it outside for your own game of football instead of just watching it on the tube.

<u>**Traditional Meal**</u>

Roast turkey
Stuffing with onions and sausage
Yams with marshmallows
Green bean casserole
Creamed onions
Cranberry jelly
Vanilla ice cream
Pumpkin pie

<u>**Nutrition Information**</u>

Calories: 1,713
Total fat: 59 grams
Saturated fat: 21 grams
Cholesterol: 246 mg
Sodium: 2,904 mg
Dietary fiber: 13 grams
Protein: 79 grams

**Healthier Meal**
Roast turkey (no skin)
Cornbread stuffing with apples,
celery, and cranberries
Baked yams
Mashed potatoes made with buttermilk
and roasted garlic
Roasted vegetables (drizzled with olive oil)
Cranberry chutney
Cinnamon frozen yogurt
Pumpkin chiffon pie

**Nutrition Information**
Calories: 1,090
Total fat: 39 grams
Saturated fat: 9 grams
Cholesterol: 143 mg
Sodium: 1,238 mg
Dietary fiber: 18 grams
Protein: 72 grams

With Thanksgiving leftovers coming out of your ears, here are some creative ways to have seconds and thirds:

**Ready-Made Menu**

➤ Turkey and cranberry risotto

➤ Turkey and roasted vegetables stuffed in a pita

➤ Turkey and rice soup

# Hanukkah

For the kids, the festival of lights is all about the presents, but for us adults, it seems to be all about the scrumptiously fried food (and of course, commemorating the Maccabean victory over Antiochus of Syria and how the Maccabees created a miracle and lit the menorah with a drop of oil that lasted for eight long nights). Today, we're a lot more nutritionally enlightened; we realize that fried foods aren't a good base for any meal, holiday or not. With a few minor adjustments to the traditional menu, you can take the healthy route, cutting 644 calories and your fat in half, and still get your potato latkes. (A Hanukkah without them would be sacrilegious, wouldn't it?)

**Traditional Meal**
Chicken soup
Brisket
Potato latkes
Applesauce
Green salad with vinaigrette
Jelly donuts
Hanukkah gelt

**Nutrition Information**
Calories: 2,038
Total fat: 105 grams
Saturated fat: 27 grams
Cholesterol: 520 mg
Sodium: 2,896 mg
Dietary fiber: 8 grams
Protein: 114 grams

**141**

**Healthier Meal**

Chicken soup

Roast chicken breast, no skin

Potato latkes

Applesauce

Green salad with vinaigrette

Fresh fruit salad

Apple Streusel pot pie (see recipe)

**Nutrition Information**

Calories: 1,393

Total fat: 53 grams

Saturated fat: 11 grams

Cholesterol: 322 mg

Sodium: 1,959 mg

Dietary fiber: 13 grams

Protein: 76 grams

---

### Low-Fat Apple Streusel Pot Pie

*Serves six*
*Calories/serving: 300*

8 sheets phyllo dough

Canola oil

Honey

8 cup apple, slices

$^1/_2$ cup golden raisins

$^1/_2$ cup brown sugar, packed

$^1/_2$ tsp nutmeg, ground

1 tsp cinnamon, ground

Lemon juice

Vanilla extract

In a small bowl, combine equal parts honey and canola oil. Remove 4 sheets of phyllo dough, not separating leaves. Place on even surface and carve outline of serving bowl with a paring knife. Remove phyllo round to a non-stick sheet pan, and brush the top with oil/honey mixture. Place in oven and bake for about 10 minutes. (Do not let rounds get too dark.) Remove from onion, gently flip, and brush the dry side with oil/honey mixture. Bake for 2 more minutes and remove from oven.

In a large bowl, combine apple slices, spices, brown sugar, vanilla, and 1 Tbs canola oil. Mix well. Put in saucepan and cook over low heat, covered, for 20 minutes or until apples are soft.

Remove apples with slotted spoon and place in serving bowls. Whisk cornstarch into remaining liquid and bring to a boil. Add thickened liquid to apple mixture in bowls. Top with phyllo round and let it cool before serving.

---

# Kwanzaa

Kwanzaa, from the African language Kiswahili, means "first fruits of the harvest"—contrary to how we celebrate this holiday, with foods that are high in fat and low in fruit content. As this is a relatively new holiday, now is the time to start some healthy traditions and indulge in a festive meal (with 400 fewer calories and 35 percent of the fat) that's good for you, too.

**Traditional Meal**

Peanut soup
Sweet potato fritters
Southern fried okra
Kale with bacon
Black-eyed peas with ham
Jerk chicken
Sweet potato pie
Benne cakes

**Nutrition Information**

Calories: 1,979
Total fat: 90 grams
Saturated fat: 26 grams
Cholesterol: 349 mg
Sodium: 3,933 mg
Dietary fiber: 28 grams
Protein: 101 grams

**Healthier Meal**

African tomato-avocado soup (see recipe)
Winter squash and yams
Kale with garlic
Black-eyed peas with ham
Jerk chicken
Sweet potato souffle (see recipe)
Benne cakes

**Nutrition Information**

Calories: 1,568
Total fat: 59 grams
Saturated fat: 18 grams
Cholesterol: 215 mg
Sodium: 2,795 mg
Dietary fiber: 28 grams
Protein: 95 grams

## African Tomato-Avocado Soup

*Serves six*
*Calories/servings: 111*

1 cup buttermilk
2 cups V8 Bloody Mary mix
2 cups chopped tomatoes
1 Tbs lime juice

1 whole Haas avocado, peeled and pitted
$1/2$ cup cilantro leaves
$1/2$ cup low-fat plain yogurt

In a saucepan, combine buttermilk, Bloody Mary mix, and chopped tomatoes. Heat gently; do not boil.

In a small food processor or in a bowl with a fork, mash avocado, cilantro, yogurt, and lime juice.

Serve soup in individual bowls, topped with a tablespoon of the avocado mix.

## Sweet Potato Souffle

*Serves four*
*Calories/serving: 125*

1 cup sweet potato, canned

1 tsp nutmeg, ground

1 tsp cinnamon, ground

2 Tbs lemon juice

5 egg whites, raw

$^1/_2$ tsp cream of tartar

2 Tbs white granulated sugar

Preheat oven to 400°. Spray four 1-cup ramekins with spray cooking oil, sprinkle with sugar, and set aside.

Combine sweet potatoes, nutmeg, cinnamon, and lemon juice. Set aside.

Beat egg whites with cream of tartar until they form soft peaks. Slowly add sugar and continue beating until stiff peaks form.

Slowly fold whites into sweet potato mixture. Spoon mixture into ramekins and place on sheet pan. Bake 10 to 12 minutes. Serve immediately.

# Christmas

With homemade Christmas cookies, creamy veggie dishes, and what always seems like 24 hours of nibbling, you'll be praying to open up boxes of oversized sweaters from under the tree. What better way to hide all the pounds we tend to pack on during the chilly season of decked halls and tons of parties? Well, you can still splurge on warm, rich comfort foods that are good for the soul, but if you lighten up your menu just a tad, you'll be indulging in yummy eats that are good for the arteries, too. See, it can still look a lot like Christmas with almost half the calories and 20 percent of the fat!

### Traditional Meal
Oyster stew
Roast beef with gravy
Yorkshire pudding
Oven-roasted potatoes
Creamed spinach
Chocolate mousse
Christmas cookies

### Nutrition Information
Calories: 1,915
Total fat: 122 grams
Saturated fat: 56 grams
Cholesterol: 717 mg
Sodium: 2,516 mg
Dietary fiber: 7 grams
Protein: 107 grams

## Healthier Meal

Manhattan oyster chowder
Beef tenderloin with horseradish yogurt sauce
Potato and carmelized onion gratin (see recipe)
French green beans, tied with leek bow
Chocolate angel-food cake
Peppermint frozen yogurt

## Nutrition Information

Calories: 1,068
Total fat: 25 grams
Saturated fat: 6 grams
Cholesterol: 130 mg
Sodium: 1,620 mg
Dietary fiber: 10 grams
Protein: 66 grams

### Potato and Onion Gratin

*Serves eight*
*Calories/serving: 134*

4 cups onion, sliced

1 Tbs Canola Oil

1 balsamic vinegar

4–5 large Idaho potatoes

1 tsp table salt

1 tsp mixed dried herbs

3 Tbs sun-dried tomatoes, chopped

$^3/_4$ cup fat-free chicken broth

Preheat oven to 350°. Carmelize onions; in a large nonstick saute pan, heat oil and add onions. Cook over medium heat, stirring frequently, for about $^1/_2$ hour or until onions are very soft and beginning to brown. Add 1 Tbs balsamic and cook for another few minutes. Set aside.

Slice potatoes $^1/_4$" thick and put in a large bowl with 1 tsp salt and 1 tsp mixed dried herbs. Do not rinse or soak potatoes in water.

In a casserole dish, sprinkle $^1/_3$ of the carmelized onions and $^1/_3$ of the sun-dried tomatoes on the bottom of the pan. Shingle $^1/_3$ of the potatoes on top of that and then repeat this process two more times. Add $^3/_4$ cup chicken stock and cover with foil.

Bake for 1 hour, remove foil, and bake for 15 more minutes.

The holidays are about celebration and rejoicing—not overeating and gaining weight. Remember to exercise, eat something before going to a party, and eat smaller portions of the higher-fat entrees and desserts. Also, try some of my menu ideas and recipes at your next holiday gathering. You and your family will enjoy the tradition with a lot less fat and calories.

---

### The Least You Need to Know

➤ Trim down your Easter meal by using honey mustard dill sauce on the poached salmon. Also, trade in those biscuits for some fresh whole-grain bread.

➤ For Passover, forget brisket and go with some gourmet Cornish game hens. You can also substantially cut your saturated fat by making your matzo ball soup with kosher olive oil instead of chicken fat. Sure, you can have potato latkes on Hanukkah; just balance it out by serving roast breast of chicken instead of the brisket.

➤ On the Fourth of July, say goodbye to red meat and hot dogs and hello to turkey and veggie burgers.

➤ Reduce the traditional Thanksgiving meal by switching from pumpkin pie to pumpkin chiffon pie—and using plain baked yams instead of mashed yams with marshmallows.

➤ For Kwanzaa, nix the peanut soup and serve African tomato-avocado soup. Also, substitute sweet potato souffle for sweet potato pie.

➤ For Christmas, have beef tenderloin instead of roast beef with gravy—and lighten your dessert load by enjoying chocolate angel-food cake topped with peppermint frozen yogurt.

# Part 3
# The ABCs of Exercise

*Exercise goes hand in hand with eating well. It can make you feel more energetic, increase your mental outlook, your balance, and your coordination, help to prevent certain diseases, and enable you to look and feel terrific. With all that in mind, this section provides you with the inspiration and know-how to get you moving and keep you moving. It's a crash course on becoming physically fit.*

*In the following chapters, I supply vital information on how to get started on an exercise program that's right for you. You'll hear the lowdown on strengthening your heart and lungs through aerobic exercise and get tips to buff your bodacious bod through proper weight-conditioning techniques. In addition, you'll get the education you need to enter a gym with confidence and learn how to properly fuel your body— whether for casual exercise or competitive sport.*

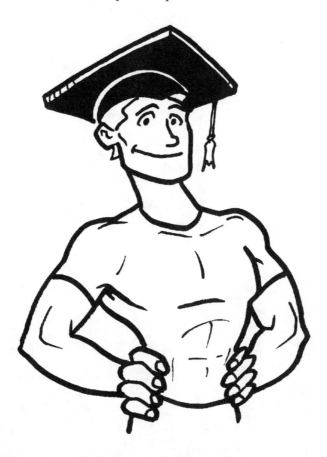

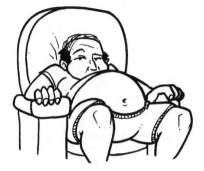

# Chapter 14

# Getting Physical

## In This Chapter

➤ All the great stuff exercise can do for you

➤ How to properly warm up, cool down, and stretch

➤ All about aerobic exercise

➤ Getting started on a weight-training program

➤ Some great ideas for your personal workout plan

Throughout history, health professionals have promoted the notion that folks who regularly exercise have better overall health, improved physical functioning, and increased longevity. Even dating back to 400 B.C., the Greek physician Hippocrates (known as the *father of medicine*) addressed exercise in one of his works by writing, "Eating alone will not keep a man well; he must also take exercise." Same thought, different century!

What is exercise anyway? Exercise is formally defined as physical activity that is planned, structured, and repetitive—with the objective of improving or maintaining a level of physical fitness. Simply stated, *exercise whips your body into shape*. Put down the TV remote and say adios to the sofa; this chapter offers concrete guidelines and information on becoming physically active.

Of course, if you have any medical conditions, check with your physician before plunging full-force into any type of exercise program.

# Why Bother Exercising?

Simply put, exercise...

➤ Makes you feel better physically.

➤ Improves self-esteem and provides a more positive mental outlook.

➤ Makes you look better and helps to control your weight.

➤ Increases your balance, coordination, and agility.

➤ Helps prevent osteoporosis, cardiovascular disease, and non–insulin-dependent diabetes.

➤ Makes you feel invigorated and more energetic.

➤ Strengthens bones and muscle, giving you the functional strength for everyday living.

Before you begin, there are some things to consider:

➤ **Have realistic expectations.** For all you beginners, don't expect to turn into Arnold Schwarzenegger or Cindy Crawford overnight. (The majority of us never will.) It's great to have a hero, but understand that people come in all shapes and sizes, and genetics plays a major role in your body makeup and proportion. Rule #1: Exercise is about looking and feeling *your* best—not somebody else's best.

➤ **Set reasonable goals for yourself.** Plan reachable short-term goals each week that will not leave you overwhelmed or set you up for failure. An example of a reasonable goal is, "I will work out four days this week and eliminate all high-fat desserts."

Not a reasonable goal: "I will work out two hours every day and lose 10 pounds in three weeks."

➤ **Work exercise conveniently into your day.** You know the story: Unless exercise sessions are planned during realistic time slots, your "workouts" ain't gonna "work out." Take into consideration your schedule. Are you a morning person or a night owl? Some people are lucky enough to have leisurely lunch breaks and can sneak in a quickie during their day.

➤ **Rise and shine.** Studies show that exercisers who work out in the morning are 50 percent more likely to stick with it. Basically, get it out of the way before the day wipes you out. (What's more, it can also save you an extra shower later.) If you have the capacity to endure a grueling day at the office and then *shake, rattle, and roll* in the gym—more power to you.

➤ **Keep it short and sweet.** Most people have hectic lifestyles and cannot afford to dedicate hours each day to the gym. And they shouldn't! Each workout should be short and efficient. The *consistency* of regular physical activity is as important as duration and intensity. Without any of these three elements, exercise is simply not effective. Furthermore, people who get carried away usually wind up with injuries or exercise burnout.

# What's an Appropriate Exercise Program?

An effective exercise program has three main parts: the before, the middle, and the after. The *before* includes a brief warm-up; the *middle*, or bulk of the workout, involves aerobic activity plus weight conditioning; and the *after* consists of a cool-down and stretch. Let's take a closer look at each.

## Warming Up

A warm-up literally *warms up* the body. By increasing your internal temperature and preparing muscles for the activity ahead, a proper warm-up can help prevent injury to muscles, joints, and connective tissue. Further, a quick 5–10 minute warm-up will increase the blood flow to the primary muscle groups so that they are ready to go.

When you think of a warm-up, do you visualize yourself sitting in a straddle position on the floor, moaning loudly while reaching for your left toe (which feels like it's somewhere south of the equator)? You're not alone. But contrary to what most people think, a warm-up doesn't necessarily involve stretching exercises. Actually, 5–10 minutes of light aerobic activity is an effective warm-up (such as biking, rowing, walking, or even marching in place). More specifically, warm up with a lighter version of the exercise you will be engaging in.

For instance, runners can start with a 5–10 minute brisk walk, and swimmers can warm up with a couple of easy, slow laps in the pool. Even take a 5–10 minute walk on a treadmill (and include arm circles) before hitting the weight room.

## The Cardiovascular Workout: Challenge Your Heart and Lungs

*What are aerobics*? If you think that aerobics are just jumping around to bad disco music, dust off your sneaks; you're way behind the times. The term *aerobic* literally means *with air*. Therefore, the exercises in which your muscles require an increased supply of air (more specifically, the *oxygen* within air) are termed aerobic. Aerobic activity is also known as cardiovascular activity (or cardio) because it most definitely challenges your heart and lungs. Think about this: When you jog, the large muscles of your lower body are continuously working over an extended period of time and therefore require more than their usual supply of oxygen. Because your heart and lungs are the key players in retrieving and circulating oxygen, they go into overdrive to increase oxygen delivery. Therefore, in addition to working out the large exterior muscles, aerobic activity also provides one heck of a workout for your heart and lungs.

Normally, aerobic exercise should last for 20–60 minutes, depending upon how much time you have and how fit you are. People who are fit can work longer and harder than those who are not, simply because they can handle the increased demand for oxygen. For all you beginners, don't let a few discouraging workouts get you down. Doing aerobics is like playing the piano; the more you practice, the better you get.

**Nutri-Speak**

**Aerobics**, which is also known as *cardio*, are the exercises in which your muscles require an increased supply of oxygen.

Walking briskly, biking, jogging, stair-climbing, cross-country skiing, jumping rope, and, yes, aerobic dance are all examples of aerobic activity. Generally speaking, anything involving weights and machines or a fair amount of standing in place is *not* considered aerobic activity.

What can aerobics do for you?

➤ Burn calories and help with weight management. (Most people are happy to hear that one.)

➤ Improve the functioning of your heart and lungs, therefore, making you less likely to suffer from serious problems involving these key organs.

➤ Improve your circulation.

➤ Improve your sleep patterns

➤ Improve your state of mind.

➤ Intense aerobic activity can release endorphins, in other words, the "natural" or "runner's" high—legal in all states, with no nasty side effects the day after.

## How Long, How Much, How Hard?

The following guidelines are set by the American College of Sports Medicine:

➤ **How long:** 20–60 minutes of aerobic activity per session

➤ **How much:** 3–5 times per week

➤ **How hard:** Low-to-moderate intensity or 60–90 percent of your maximum heart rate

Beginners should start with a modest game plan. In fact, beginners need to shoot for 40 percent of their maximum heart rate and work up from there. As you improve, you can do more activity by going longer, harder, or more frequently. But keep in mind that you should only increase the length, frequency, and intensity one at a time. Increasing all three at once is the perfect recipe for injuries and exercise burnout.

## Cooling Down

The goal of a cool-down is to gradually stop the activity, allowing your heart rate, blood pressure, and body temperature to slowly return to normal. Think about how rapidly your heart is pounding and blood is pumping following an intense bout of exercise—*not* a good time to hit the shower. In fact, stopping an intense workout abruptly is a sure way to get dizzy and feel terrible after a workout. Furthermore, cooling down properly can help prevent serious health risks for older or out of shape participants. Take an extra 5–10 minutes and slowly reduce the intensity of the exercise you've been working on. Your body will thank you.

## Stretching

Stretching is definitely important for maintaining and increasing flexibility, which in turn makes it easier for you to move around. The best time to stretch is when your body is warm, either after you have done a light aerobic warm-up *or*, more preferably, at the end of your workout following a cool-down period. Proper stretching allows the muscles to relax and lengthen, and it can even help alleviate some built-up body tension. What's more, it *might* also aid in the removal of waste products, such as lactic acid. This can prevent injury and improve muscle tone.

Some general stretching guidelines include

➤ Always get your blood pumping and body warmed up before you stretch.

➤ Stretch *all* your major muscle groups (not just the ones you think were used).

➤ Hold each stretch for at least 15 seconds; never bounce. You can still feel a good stretch with slightly bent knees.

➤ Only stretch to the point of mild tension, not agonizing pain!

➤ Ask a qualified trainer to show you the correct stretching techniques; there's a lot more to it than touching your toes.

# Are You Working Hard Enough?

Let's check it out. A couple of easy ways to tell whether you are working hard enough during an aerobic workout include taking your heart rate (the number of times your heart beats per minute) and the talk test.

Follow this mathematical equation to check whether you are working in your training zone (also called the target heart rate zone). Generally, your training heart rate falls between 60 and 90 percent of your *maximum heart rate* (the maximum times your heart can beat in one minute). Although this formula only provides an estimate, it's a great indication of whether you are working too hard or not hard enough:

**Training heart rate formula: (220 – your age) × .60 and .90**

Let's break it up and take it step-by-step:

| | |
|---|---|
| Step 1 | Calculate your estimated maximum heart rate (220 – your age). |
| Step 2 | Multiply your maximum heart rate × .60 for lower range. |
| Step 3 | Multiply your maximum heart rate × .90 for upper range. |

Here's the training zone for a 35-year-old man:

$(220 - 35) \times .60 = 111$ Lower range

$(220 - 35) \times .90 = 167$ Upper range

Therefore, his target zone would range between 111–167 beats per minute. This means if it's lower than 111, he needs to step on the accelerator, and if it's more than 167, he needs to slightly ease up.

## Test Your Heart Rate and Your Math Skills

Now that you know the math, take some time during your workout and give it a whirl. Place two fingers (your pointer and middle finger) on the inside of your wrist (just to the thumb side of the large cords you feel) *or* on your neck (below and off to the side of your chin). If you can't find your pulse, ask for assistance. (Don't worry, you're alive.) Once you locate it, look at the second hand of your watch or a clock and count the beats in a 15-second span; then, multiply that number by four. That's your working heart rate. Just make sure it falls within the range you've calculated as your training zone—not slower, not faster.

## Try the "Talk" Test

Here's a *much* easier way to tell whether you're working at an appropriate level. Can you comfortably carry on a conversation while exercising? If the answer is yes, you're doing fine. If you're so out of breath that you can't say, "Yippee! I'm rich," when someone announces you've won the lottery, you need to slow down. On the other hand, if you can belt out the chorus to "YMCA" by the Village People, you'd better step it up. In the final analysis, you should feel like you're working, but not to the point of a cardiac explosion.

# Hit the Weights and "Pump Some Iron"

Let's clear something up: Weight training is *not* the same as body building. Weight training is about improving muscle strength and muscle tone. For men, who have naturally higher levels of testosterone, it usually does mean an increase in muscle size, *hypertrophy*. On the other hand, women tend to increase the tone without significantly increasing the muscle size. Typically, muscle conditioning uses dumbbells and barbells (called free weights) and various types of weight machines (usually referred to by brand names such as Cybex and Nautilus).

What can weight training do for you?

➤ Stronger muscles can improve your posture and help keep your body in balance.

➤ Stronger muscles can prevent injuries.

➤ Weight training helps to tone, lift, firm, and shape your body.

➤ Stronger muscles can help with your everyday activities such as lugging shopping bags, moving furniture, lifting kids and strollers, and so on.

➤ Weight training can help prevent osteoporosis.

➤ Weight training can help to *reshape* problem areas such as your sagging arms and your butt. Unfortunately, there is no such thing as "spot reducing"—zapping off fat from specific body parts. But don't fret because the combination of a low-fat diet and aerobic activity burns *total fat* from all over your body, and chances are it will eventually come off your personal pudge.

➤ Weight training can increase your lean body mass and therefore increase your metabolism.

**Nutri-Speak**

**Hypertrophy** is an increase in muscle size.

## *Your Weekly Weight-Training Routine*

Your weekly schedule is just as important as the exercises themselves. Set aside time for two to three muscle-conditioning workouts per week, targeting all of your major muscle groups. A major warning here is *not* to work the same muscles on consecutive days. Leave a day of rest in between to allow all those important biological changes to take place. In fact, *resting is just as important as the workout itself.* For instance, if you'd like to work all of your muscle groups on the same day, an effective schedule is Monday/Thursday/Saturday.

Another option is doing *split routines*. In this case, you can lift more often simply because you split up the muscles being worked over the week. In other words, train your upper body one day and your lower body the next. For those truly gung-ho types, train your chest, triceps, and shoulders on one day and your legs, back, and biceps on the next. Go ahead and plug in your abdominal exercises whichever day you like. Chest and triceps are involved in pushing-type activities, and your back and biceps are involved in pulling activities; therefore, they should be worked in pairs if you

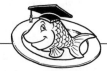

**Food for Thought**

When training with weights, your three sets should be 6–15 repetitions or 70–90 percent of the maximum weight you can lift.

want to split up the upper-body workouts. One reason people prefer a split-routine workout is that they can devote more energy to the muscles worked on a particular day.

## Cardio and Weight Training: the Perfect Combination

Some people ask, "Which is more important, cardio or weight work?" The answer is both. You need the combination of aerobic and weight training for overall fitness. As one of my clients once said, "Weights make it hard; cardio gets rid of the lard."

### Q & A

Cardio or muscle conditioning: Which comes first?

If you want to do cardio and weights on the same day, that's fine. It's also fine to alternate days, whichever you fancy. There is not, as of yet, a definite rule on which you should do first—merely personal preference. Some folks like to be good and sweaty before they hit the weights, whereas others prefer to get the weight training out of the way and then loosen up with cardio afterwards. The choice is yours.

## Top-Five Exercise Myths

This list will help to debunk the common misconceptions floating around the gym. Read on and learn the whole truth.

1. **No pain, no gain.** Bogus statement! It is true that both weight training and cardiovascular exercise usually involve *some* type of minor discomfort, such as feelings of slight burning or fatigue and moderate to heavy breathing. However, pain is entirely different. If you feel pain when you work out (particularly joint pain), you're doing something wrong. Stop exercising immediately, and have it checked by your physician. Pushing through agony can lead to serious trouble. If it checks out okay, seek the assistance of a qualified trainer; something is probably wrong with your exercise program or technique.

2. **Eating extra protein builds muscle.** We already went over this one in the protein chapter, but allow me to drive the point home. The increase in muscle size, known as hypertrophy, has nothing to do with eating a lot of protein. Muscles get bigger when you overload them via weight training—*not* kilos of tuna. The recommended daily amounts for protein remains about 15 percent of total calories, regardless of whether you are Mr. Rogers or Mr. Universe.

3. **Weight training will give you bulky muscles.** After reading that weight training causes muscles to increase in size, it's no wonder some women are hesitant to lift weights. Fear not: Your lower testosterone levels cause increases in strength and tone without all that increase in size. Incidentally, even men have to have a genetic predisposition to getting bigger. Some guys can cut and bulk quickly, whereas others work their tails off without much visible result. Stick with a moderate weight-training program, and you'll be fine.

4. **You only burn fat working cardio at a slower pace.** This myth got a lot of play back in the '80s, with exercise classes actually slowing down the pace to "burn more fat." In terms of weight loss, that's just not the case. The crucial factor for losing weight is *the total amount of calories burned*, and it doesn't matter whether it comes from carbs, protein, or fat. For instance, a 130-pound woman doing a high-intensity workout (such as jogging) for 30 minutes will burn approximately 350 calories; that same woman will only burn 140 calories at a low-intensity workout (such as walking).

   What if you're just starting out and can't sustain a fast pace for more than 5 to 10 minutes? In that case, you're certainly better off doing something at a slower pace for a longer length of time. Again, the reason is that you'll burn more total calories in the end.

5. **Sit-ups can burn fat off your waist.** Not a chance! Remember, there is no such thing as spot reducing or burning the fat off a particular body part. Fat comes off the body as a whole (through aerobic activity and proper nutrition) and, unfortunately, not always in the places you want it to come from first (such as "the incredible shrinking bra"). You can buy every tummy-tucker and blubber-blaster on the market. Abdominal-toning exercises *only* strengthen the tissue underneath; they don't zap off that mid-section fat (contrary to what they might say). Look on the bright side: Below all the flub, you probably have some dynamite muscles—something to look forward to when you lose that outer layer.

# How to Get Started: Your Personal Plan of Attack

Before embarking on an exercise program, figure out what type of plan will best fit your personality and schedule. Take a paper and pen and answer the following questions:

1. What type of activities do you enjoy doing?
2. What are your time restraints?
3. Are you a morning person or a night owl?
4. Do you like to work out alone or with people?
5. Do you prefer the indoors or outdoors?
6. What's the weather like in your neck of the woods?

7. Do you want to travel to a facility, or does the privacy of your own home sound more appealing?

8. What is within your budget?

# A Million Things You Can Do to Stay in Shape

Now that you've answered the previous questions, you should have a pretty good idea of your personal preferences and limitations. Read through the possible exercise options and determine which ones are feasible. Be sure to focus on both categories: aerobic (3–5 times per week) and muscle conditioning (2–3 times per week). Remember, nothing is set in stone; mix and match often to avoid getting bored or burnt out.

## Aerobic Suggestions

| Activity | Where You Can Do It |
| --- | --- |
| Walking | Outside or treadmill (gym or at home) |
| Running | Outside or treadmill (gym or at home) |
| Biking | Outside or stationary bike (gym or at home) |
| Swimming | Outside or indoor pool at the gym |
| Skating | Outside or indoor rink |
| Stair climbing | Indoor staircase or stair-climbing machine (gym or at home) |
| Cross-country skiing | Outside or machine (home or gym) |
| Rowing | Outside or rowing machine (gym or home) |
| Aerobic classes | At the gym or home (using videos):<br>Low-impact<br>Multi-impact<br>Step<br>Spinning<br>Jazz<br>Tap<br>Funk<br>Hip-hop<br>African dance<br>Boxing |

## Muscle Conditioning Suggestions

| Activity | Where You Can Do It |
| --- | --- |
| Body sculpting | Classes in the gym or videos at home |
| Circuit/interval workouts | Classes in the gym or videos at home |
| Weight training | Gym or home equipment |
| Weight machines | Gym or home equipment |
| Free weights | Gym or home equipment |

# When Formal Exercise Is Just Not Your Thang!

Not into planned sweat? Only read this far to humor yourself? Well you're not hopeless yet; you can still cash in on some of the benefits. In fact, everyday activities can *also* substantially benefit your health, even if they are done *intermittently* throughout the day. For example, take the stairs instead of the elevator (you live on the 25th floor—great!), walk short distances instead of driving the car, join your kids in a game of tag, do some gardening, rake the leaves, shovel the snow, and let's not forget how physical housecleaning can be. Whatever your style, formal exercise *or* increasing plain old daily activity, make your only life a healthy and active one.

Whether you are 18, 50, or 70 years old, invest the time to becoming more physically active. Regular exercise will help you to feel your best and keep you fit—while increasing bone strength, reducing your risk of disease, and helping to maintain an ideal body weight. Keep in mind, that the perfect compliment to properly fueling your body is *moving* your body.

Take a look at the amount of calories you can burn doing everyday chores:

Moo!

**Overrated—Undercooked**

Pushing your body more often than the experts recommend (unless you are in an athletic training program) can and usually *does* lead to injuries from over-used muscles, tendons, and joints. What's more, *varying* your exercise intensity and duration is also important to prevent overtraining. For example, some days, you should work hard and long, but on other days, make it short and sweet. Pay attention to your body's cues and make exercise an enjoyable part of your life.

| Activity | 130-Pound Person | 183-Pound Person |
| --- | --- | --- |
| Car washing | 123 | 171 |
| Housecleaning | 111 | 153 |
| Raking leaves | 96 | 135 |
| Shoveling snow | 150 | 213 |
| Wallpapering | 84 | 120 |
| Weeding | 96 | 135 |
| Window cleaning | 105 | 147 |

---

### The Least You Need to Know

➤ Exercise reduces your risk for certain diseases, helps you control your weight, provides you with strength and vigor for everyday activities, and makes you feel *great* both mentally and physically.

➤ The important parts of an exercise program include the warm-up, aerobic activity and weight training, cool-down, and total-body stretch.

➤ Aerobic exercise (also known as *cardio*) is any continuous activity that requires increased oxygen and therefore challenges your heart and lungs.

➤ How long, how much, and how hard should you do aerobic activity? The experts recommend 3–5 days each week for 20–60 minute sessions at a low–moderate intensity.

➤ Don't forget about your muscles! A proper weight-training program 2–3 times per week can increase your strength, reduce the risk of osteoporosis, enhance your posture, and help to reshape your body.

➤ Select activities that complement your personality and time schedule, and vary your routine often to avoid exercise burnout.

---

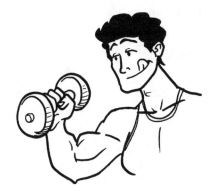

# Chapter 15

# The Gym Scene

---

**In This Chapter**

➤ Acquainting yourself with the health–club scene

➤ Translating gym jargon into English

➤ Popular exercise equipment for cardio and weight training

➤ Your muscles and some exercises to work 'em out

---

Now that your body is rarin' to go, you might want to join a local health club. Be sure to prepare yourself for more than a physical experience: Between the language barrier, high-tech equipment, scantily clad women, and members strolling around with biceps bigger than their heads, going to the gym can feel like traveling to a foreign land or outer space. But don't be intimidated. The gym scene can be terrific. Where else can you have such a tremendous variety of workout choices? There's always someone available for instruction, encouragement, and motivation. Check out the health clubs in your area and browse through the basics before hitting the locker room.

## Gym Jargon 101

Here's the gym terminology you'll need to hang with the muscle-heads; it's sure to make your conversations with the locals a bit easier:

➤ **Reps**—Short for repetitions, meaning the number of times you do an exercise. Usually 6–15 reps make a set.

➤ **Sets**—A group of repetitions. Usually you do 1–3 sets per exercise. (A man working on bicep curls might do 3 sets of 10 reps. This translates to 3 full rounds of 10 bicep curls each.)

➤ **"He's/she's ripped"**—A major compliment about a guy or gal's defined physique.

➤ **"You've really got great definition in your..."**—A tired but effective gym come-on. Sort of gym slang for "Wow" (drool, drool).

➤ **Being cut**—Having well-defined muscles.

➤ **Being pumped**—A temporary increase in the size of a muscle due to increased blood flow during exercise.

➤ **"Can I work in?"**—Someone wants to use the weight machine you are using, and she is asking whether she can alternate sets with you. Because the gym is usually crowded, it's normal practice to share equipment. For example, you do a set of eight reps, then someone else changes the weight to do a set, then you again, and so on. This only makes sense when you have a bunch more to go. If you only have one more set left, reply, "This is my last set"—gym slang for "Hold your horses, fella, I'm almost done."

➤ **"How many more sets do you have here?"**—Someone is getting antsy to use the weight machine and doesn't particularly want to "work in" with you. This is a polite way of saying, "Are you planning on staying here all day? Perhaps I could order you a cappuccino."

➤ **"Can I get a spot?"**—Basically, someone is asking you to help him do an exercise with an amount of weight he is nervous about. Politely pass on this one if you don't know how to spot the exercise. Things could get ugly if a bad spot ruins his set (or worse, the weight lands on his head).

➤ **Juice**—Slang for steroids. If muscle-heads are said to be "juicing," you can be sure they're not talking about fresh produce.

# A Tour of the Equipment

Health clubs are loaded with amazing machinery. With all the high-tech, futuristic equipment that's available, it can almost feel like you're on *The Jetsons*. ("Hey Jane, how long you been on that Stairmaster?") Take advantage and try them all. Don't get stuck in that "same machine day-in day-out" routine. Swap around from week to week and keep your workouts interesting and fun.

## *Get to Know the Aerobic Contraptions*

All cardiovascular exercise equipment is designed to get large muscles pumping in a rhythmic fashion—to increase the heart rate and blood pressure and burn calories. What's the best piece of cardio equipment? The answer: Any machine you'll use. Pop some jammin' tunes in your Walkman, read the paper, or watch TV (*Good Morning America*, *The Flintstones*—whatever grabs ya), and you'll be surprised how quickly the time flies:

➤ **Treadmills**—Cardiovascular equipment that presents light-to-moderate impact on your joints, depending on whether you're walking or running. Walking on a flat grade is a good starting place for beginning exercisers. As fitness and confidence builds, you can fool around with increasing the incline and speed.

➤ **Stairclimbers**—Cardiovascular equipment that provides a challenging workout with some potential stress to your knees and lower back. (Listen carefully to your body.) This is a more advanced piece of machinery due to the importance of technique, and therefore, you need a base level of stamina and strength to use this machine, even on lower levels.

➤ **Stationary bikes**—Now, they come in two flavors—the upright bike (like a regular outdoors bicycle) and the recumbent bike (legs out in front with high bucket seats lending more support for people with lower back pain). Both types provide aerobic workouts that give your joints a break because they are non–weight-bearing activities. Make sure the tension isn't too high and the seat isn't too low. If you're a beginner, ask a trainer to help you get into the proper position. When you're ready to pump up the intensity, increase your speed before increasing the tension.

➤ **Cross conditioner/cross-country ski machines**—A great aerobic exercise that uses the entire body and burns tons of calories without any jarring impact. It's also good for quick warm-ups because it gets the whole body going. There is, however, one catch: Learning the movement can be tricky for some people, and let's just say the term "poetry in motion" takes on a whole new meaning.

➤ **Rowing machines**—Another good "total-body" workout (and warm-up machine) without any impact. Be sure to get some pointers on technique; there's an easy way and the *right* way to do it. Obviously, the right way requires more energy, concentration, and muscular effort.

### Overrated—Undercooked

Do something too much, too hard, or too often, and sooner or later it'll get stale. Don't be afraid to vary your activities and change your program. In fact, I encourage it. Try inline skating instead of using the treadmill. Use weight machines instead of free weights. Attend an exercise class instead of riding the Life Cycle. Hey, if you want to dance around naked, I say go for it. (Just keep it at home, and close the window shades.)

## Become Familiar with the Weight-Training Tools

Weight-training equipment can be super high-tech (multi-muscle machinery) or super low-tech (a pair of dumbbells and a box). Don't be fooled into thinking that something more complicated means a better workout. That's not the case at all:

➤ **Weight-training machines**—In general, machines are a good starting point for beginners. They remove a lot of the guess work; you just move from machine to machine. (Adjust your seat, stick in a pin, and you're ready for action.) Several machine variations include weight stacks with pulleys and cords (such as Universal and Cybex), metal rod systems (such as Cybex and Med-X), cams and chains (such as Nautilus), or air pumps (such as Kaiser). Just name the nut and bolt, and there's a machine out there that has it. Test them all and find the one you're most comfortable with.

➤ **Free weights**—These, on the other hand, require a fair amount of coordination, strength, and skill because they heavily depend on your balance and body control. Although weight training with barbells and dumbbells (free weights) might seem significantly harder at first, some people claim free weights yield greater gains than machines. When embarking on a free-weight program, consult with a qualified trainer for tips on proper form and technique. *Bad* habits lead to *bad* injuries.

**Q & A**

**Do I really need to buy all of the belts, wraps, and straps associated with weight training?**

No. In fact, the only peripheral equipment you might need is a pair of gloves to help protect against calluses.

# Learn Your Muscles and "Buff that Bod"

This section provides a quick rundown on the major muscles that conscientious gym folks tend to work out. Of course, your body is action-packed with hundreds more. Browse through the list, and become familiar with your muscles *and* the exercises that work them out. Be sure to ask a qualified trainer to personally show you the correct form and technique for each and every exercise.

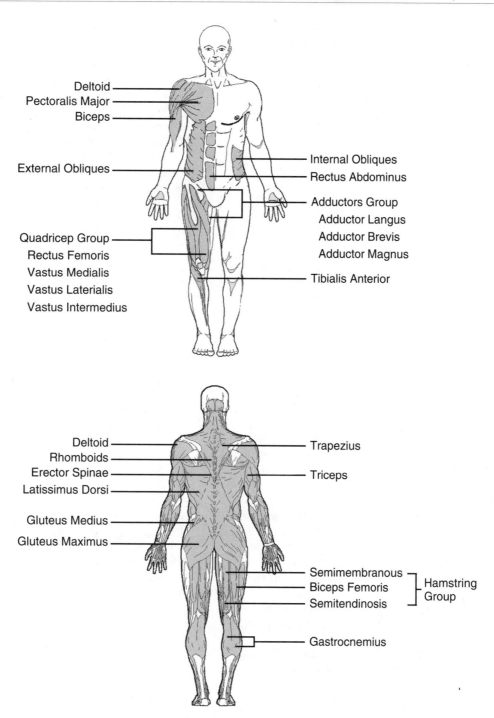

Deltoid
Pectoralis Major
Biceps

External Obliques

Internal Obliques
Rectus Abdominus

Adductors Group
Adductor Langus
Adductor Brevis
Adductor Magnus

Quadricep Group
Rectus Femoris
Vastus Medialis
Vastus Laterialis
Vastus Intermedius

Tibialis Anterior

Deltoid
Rhomboids
Erector Spinae
Latissimus Dorsi

Trapezius

Triceps

Gluteus Medius

Gluteus Maximus

Semimembranous
Biceps Femoris
Semitendinosis

Hamstring
Group

Gastrocnemius

165

| Gym Slang | Muscle Group | Exercises That Work 'Em |
|---|---|---|
| Traps | Trapezius | Upper traps: shoulder shrugs<br>Mid traps: reverse flys, seated rows<br>Lower traps: dips |
| Delts | Deltoids | Anterior delts: frontal raises<br>Medial delts: lateral raises<br>Posterior delts: reverse flys |
| Midback | Rhomboids<br>Mid trapezius | Seated rows<br>Reverse flys |
| Pecs | Pectoralis major | Dumbbell bench press<br>Dumbbell flys<br>Push-ups<br>Dips |
| Lats | Latissimus dorsi | Lat pulldowns<br>Seated row pulley rowing |
| Lower back | Erector spinae | Lower back lifts (on a mat)<br>Opposite arm/leg lifts on all fours |
| Bis | Biceps | Bicep curls<br>Supination curls with dumbbells |
| Tris | Triceps | Tricep dips<br>Tricep pulldowns |
| Abs | Abdominal group:<br>*internal obliques*<br>*external obliques*<br>*rectus abdominis* | Stomach crunches<br>Oblique twist<br>Side crunches |
| Butt | Gluteus maximus | Leg press/squats<br>Hip extension (with a low pulley cable) |
| Outer hips | Abductor group:<br>*gluteus medius*<br>*gluteus minimus* | Abductor machine<br>Side leg lifts (with a low pulley cable) |
| Inner thighs | Adductor group:<br>*adductor longus*<br>*adductor brevis*<br>*adductor magnus* | Adductor machine<br>Inward leg lifts (with a low pulley cable) |
| Quads | Quadricep group:<br>*rectus femoris*<br>*vastus medialis*<br>*vastus lateralis*<br>*vastus intermedius* | Leg press<br>Leg extension (also includes squats, lunges, and step ups with dumbbells) |
| Hams | Hamstring group:<br>*biceps femoris*<br>*semitendinosus*<br>*semimembranosus* | Leg press<br>Leg curl |

| Gym Slang | Muscle Group | Exercises That Work 'Em |
|---|---|---|
| Calves | Gastronemius soleus | Heel raises straight leg |
| | | Toe presses straight leg |
| | | Heel raises bent leg |
| | | Toe presses bent leg |
| Shins | Tibialis anterior | Toe taps |
| | | Toe backs |

# Do You Need a Personal Trainer?

Some people decide to hire a personal trainer to help them get into shape. Although some exercisers require a personal trainer only for a single "show you the ropes" session, others enjoy continual weekly appointments that help keep them focused and motivated. If you decide to work with a trainer, be selective about whom you hire because the unfortunate truth is that *anyone* can call himself a personal trainer.

Consider hiring a personal trainer if you fall into any of the following categories:

➤ You are completely out of shape and haven't the slightest idea how to begin an exercise program. A trainer can acquaint you with all of the up-to-date exercise techniques and available aerobic and weight machinery.

➤ You are in a *huge* exercise rut and have been doing the same old routine for as long as you can remember. A trainer can show you variations on your day-to-day workout and make exercising more efficient and effective.

➤ You just plain lack the "umph" to exercise on your own. A trainer can help to push, motivate, and whip your butt into shape.

Seek out somebody with a B.S. (better yet, a masters degree) in exercise physiology, physical education, or kinesiology. You can also look for a *certified* fitness trainer, which means she has studied for and passed a comprehensive training exam. Some of the most reputable organizations that provide certifications include

➤ ACSM (American College of Sports Medicine)

➤ ACE (American Council on Exercise)

**Food for Thought**

Studies report that arthritis sufferers who regularly participate in strength training and stretching programs can greatly improve their balance, speed, and ability to walk, as well as reduce joint pain and fatigue. Check it out with your doctor first to be sure there's not too much joint inflammation.

For more information, contact the Arthritis Foundation at 800-283-7800, and ask about its Aquatics and PACE program (People with Arthritis Can Exercise).

➤ NSCA (National Strength and Conditioning Association)

➤ AFAA (Aerobics and Fitness Association of America)

➤ NASM (National Academy of Sports Medicine)

Other comprehensive fitness certifications are offered at various universities. Most of these organizations offer a variety of certifications (aerobic instructor, yoga, and so on). Make sure your trainer is specifically certified in *personal training* or *fitness instruction* and that his or her certification is up-to-date.

Interview a trainer before you actually set up an appointment to be sure you feel comfortable with his or her workout philosophy, personality, and fee scale. Rates vary tremendously, anywhere from $20 to $80 per workout. They can even run more than $100 if you're looking for a "trainer to the stars."

---

### The Least You Need to Know

➤ Joining a local gym can be an invaluable tool in your pursuit of that "body beautiful." Take advantage of the variety of workout choices and the qualified staff of trainers who can help instruct, motivate, and encourage you.

➤ Some of the popular aerobic equipment commonly found in most gyms includes treadmills, bikes, stairclimbers, rowing machines, and cross-country ski machines. Weight-training equipment generally involves either multi-purpose machinery (Cybex, Nautilus) or free weights (barbells and dumbbells).

➤ Because bad form and technique can lead to injuries, seek the assistance of a qualified trainer before embarking on any type of program.

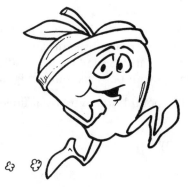

# Chapter 16

# Sports Nutrition

---

**In This Chapter**

➤ Super-fueling your body with carbohydrates

➤ Where to find high carbohydrate foods

➤ Increased protein requirements for athletes

➤ What to eat before, during, and after exercise

---

If you've read this far, you know the basics of sports nutrition. Contrary to what some people think, there isn't any "magic" ingredient that helps optimize exercise and training (such as instant-muscle shake concoctions or endurance potions). In fact, the same healthy-eating guidelines you read about in the earlier chapters apply for competitive sport and casual exercise. You know the story: high on the carbs, low on the fat, and moderate amounts of protein. You might just need to increase your total calories to compensate for the amount you're now burning with all that activity.

Just because you're familiar with the Egyptian triangle on your cereal box, don't stop reading: There's a lot more to "sport-specific nutrition," and this chapter clues you in. Stay tuned for a mouthful of information that can help enhance your athletic performance and secure that competitive edge.

## Carbohydrates: Fuel of Choice

Carbohydrate is literally the high-octane fuel for exercise and should provide at least 55 percent of an athlete's total daily calories. To get a bit more technical, you should consume approximately 3.0 to 4.5 grams of carbohydrate per pound of body weight. Where do you fit in? If your sport is pretty low key—not a lot of nonstop running around—you should approximate 3.0 grams. On the other hand, if you participate in a super-endurance sport that involves hours of heavy training each day, you should approximate 4.5 grams.

What does that mean, anyway?

Math time—grab a calculator. Take your weight in pounds and multiply it by 3.0 grams (for moderate intensity sports) and 4.5 grams (for strenuous endurance training). Obviously, these are two extremes; most exercisers and athletes fall in the middle. In fact, give yourself a range; play around and see where your body feels most vigorous.

For example: Here's the carbo requirement for a 150-pound *elite* runner training several hours each day:

150 pounds × 4.5 grams = 675 grams of carbohydrate

Because 1 *gram* of carbohydrate = 4 calories, we can now convert 675 carb grams into carb calories by using the following equation:

675 × 4 = 2,700 carbohydrate calories

Now, let's look at a typical 150-pound health club member, working out at a moderate intensity (approximately 45 minutes), 4–5 days a week:

150 pounds × 3.0 grams = 450 grams of carbohydrate

Now, convert into carb calories:

450 × 4 = 1,800 carbohydrate calories

**Food for Thought**

Without question, carbohydrate-rich foods are the fuel of choice for athletes. Carbs provide the muscles with ongoing energy in the form of glucose and help maintain prolonged endurance and optimal performance.

As you can see, a more intense endurance exercise program will demand more carbohydrate. But keep in mind that the proportion of carbs, protein, and fat pretty much remain the same as in the previous chapters (about 55 percent carbs, 15 percent protein, and less than 30 percent fat) because in the end, you're taking in more of everything.

# Develop Your Own High-Carb Diet

Need to boost your carbs? Take a look at the variety of foods you can choose from, and watch how fast you can rack up the grams.

## The Starchy Carbs

Generally speaking, breads, grains, and other starchy foods contain approximately 15 grams (give or take a few) of carbohydrate per serving (1 slice bread, 1/2 cup pasta, 1 serving of cereal). These foods receive top billing for endurance athletes simply because it's easy to eat multiple servings in one sitting. For instance, a pasta entree can easily total five grain servings, and because one pasta serving contains about 20 grams of carb, five servings supplies a whopping 100 grams of carbohydrate. Clearly, this is the reasoning behind marathon runners "packing in the pasta" before the lengthy 26-mile run.

## Fruits

Next up are fruits, also providing about the same 15 grams of carbohydrate per serving (1 medium fresh fruit, 1 cup berries/melon, $^1/_2$ cup fruit juice). Why are they second? Athletes looking to load up on carbs can eat 10+ servings of grain more comfortably than 10+ servings of fruit. Remember, fruit has a lot of fiber and tends to fill you up more quickly. (You might be "bursting with fruit flavor" in more ways than one!) Incorporate a lot of fresh fruit into your regimen, but don't skimp on the grains and rely *solely* on fruit. You'll probably get a stomach ache and more than likely *toot* your way to the finish line.

## Milk Products

Milk products contain about 12 grams of carbohydrate per serving (1 cup milk, 1 cup yogurt) and can certainly boost your total carbs together with the starchy foods, fruits, and vegetables. What's more, milk pumps you with calcium, a key ingredient for maintaining strong, athletic bones.

## Vegetables

Veggies provide approximately 5 grams of carbohydrate per serving (1 cup raw or $^1/_2$ cup cooked) and are certainly packed with vitamins and minerals. Although veggies alone can't supply enough concentrated carbohydrate for increased requirements, they can sure jazz up your meals and add tremendous amounts of nutrition to your table.

| Common High-Carb Foods | Carbohydrate Grams |
| --- | --- |
| Medium bagel | 45 |
| 2 slices whole-wheat bread | 23 |
| 1 cup oatmeal | 25 |
| 1 cup cereal (ready to eat) | 16 |
| 10 crackers | 21 |
| 1 cup of pasta (cooked) | 40 |
| 1 cup rice | 35 |
| Granola bar | 16 |
| 1 ounce pretzels | 21 |
| 2 fig cookies | 23 |
| Power bars | 42 |
| Banana | 27 |
| Glass of O.J. (8 ounces) | 26 |
| Medium baked potato | 51 |

*continues*

*continued*

| Common High-Carb Foods | Carbohydrate Grams |
|---|---|
| $^1/_2$ cup peas | 11 |
| $^1/_2$ cup corn | 17 |
| 1 cup low-fat milk | 12 |
| 1 cup low-fat yogurt (plain) | 18 |
| 1 cup low-fat yogurt | 43 |
| 1 cup beans | 41 |

Note that the carbohydrate grams are calculated for serving sizes that are *commonly eaten*, not the standard *single* serving sizes frequently listed throughout the book and on the Food Guide Pyramid.

**Food for Thought**

You can take in more than 100 grams of carbohydrate by eating 4 bananas, or $2^1/_2$ power bars, or 3 cups pasta, or 6 medium pancakes, or $2^1/_2$ cups Raisin Bran cereal, or 2 medium–baked potatoes, or 8 fig cookies and a glass of milk.

**Nutri-Speak**

**Muscle Glycogen** is the stored carbohydrate within the muscles. Athletes can use the "energy stores" during prolonged exercise.

# All About Muscle Glycogen

*Muscle glycogen* is stored carbohydrate in your muscle. Imagine this: After you eat and digest a meal, the amount of carbohydrate that you immediately need will get used as fuel, but the rest (up to a point) will be stored in your muscles for *future* fuel. Athletes in ultra-endurance sports such as soccer, basketball, hockey, and distance running rely on high-octane muscle fuel for energy. In fact, between the grueling practice sessions and vigorous competitions, serious endurance athletes are *constantly* depleting and restoring their muscle glycogen stores, so they require much more carbohydrate-rich foods than athletes involved in less aerobic activity (golf, archery, and martial arts).

Just because you don't compete in an ultra-endurance sport doesn't mean you can fumble in the carb department. Think about all of the laborious *practice* sessions that wrestlers, divers, or short-distance swimmers put in during the week. Bear in mind, it's not just the actual competition that matters, but the intensity of your training as well.

What happens if you don't replenish your muscle-glycogen stores? Simple: If you run out of glycogen, you run out of energy. The amount of muscle fuel you have determines how long you can exercise. As a car needs a full tank of gas before heading out on a long trip, an endurance athlete requires sufficient "muscle gasoline" to sustain the pace and go the distance. Always tired or run down? Obviously, a vigorous training schedule alone is enough to make you feel that way. You might also want to look into your carbohydrate consumption. Keep a food log and do the math; there could be an easy solution to your problem.

# What's Carbo-Loading About?

Carbo-loading is just that—loading your body with gargantuan amounts of carbohydrate before an event. Athletes who compete in *extreme* endurance events such as marathons and triathlons can actually manipulate their exercise and eating schedule to help heighten their amount of stored muscle glycogen. You see, during intense, prolonged aerobic activity, your muscle-glycogen stores can become severely depleted and cause you to slow down, or worse, drop out. Picture that car running out of gas: *putt, putt, pshh.* By super-saturating your muscles with carbohydrate beforehand, an athlete can ensure that her stores are maximally loaded.

**Overrated—Undercooked**

For you non-athletes who decided to browse through the chapter, not everyone is a candidate for overdosing on carbs. Active people might continuously burn loads of carbohydrate calories, but your muscles can only store a certain amount of carbohydrate. If you're not using what is already there, you'll just end up putting on weight.

Start this program six days before your event:

| Exercise Schedule | | % of Carbs in Daily Diet |
|---|---|---|
| Day 1 | 90 minutes | 50 |
| Day 2 | 40 minutes | 50 |
| Day 3 | 40 minutes | 50 |
| Day 4 | 20 minutes | 70 |
| Day 5 | 20 minutes | 70 |
| Day 6 | Rest | 70 |
| Day 7 | Get out there and master your event! | |

# Personal Protein Requirements

Remember back in the old days when athletes would eat a huge slab of steak with some scrambled eggs for breakfast and then head off to play ball? *Protein power, gotta keep up that strength.* Boy, have things changed.

It's true that athletes do need more protein than sedentary folks, but because most people already take in far more protein than the RDA, chances are you're A-OK. (You're okay unless you're one of those "carb-o-holics" who live on the "cereal-bagel-pasta" program, or you're trying so hard to carbo-load that you forget the other key ingredients for optimal performance. *Wake up and smell the Gatorade!*)

Athletes do need protein for that competitive edge. You learned the vital roles of protein in Chapter 3, "The Profile on Protein," but let's get sport-specific for a minute.

Protein is essential for building and maintaining muscle tissue, as well as repairing the muscle damage you endure during hard workouts. Remember, dietary protein does *not* automatically build bigger muscles: *You* build bigger muscles through regular exercise and training. Dietary protein simply allows all your hard work to pay off. Go ahead and take the credit; it had nothing to do with all the protein powder you shoveled in each day.

Following are the recommended daily intakes for protein. You'll see that athletes do have greater requirements than the RDAs for the general population (also in Chapter 3). But keep in mind that your total proportion should still be high in carbs, moderate in protein, and low in fat. This is because you're taking in more of everything (especially carbohydrate).

Find your exercise category, and then multiply your weight (in pounds) by the number of grams to the right. After you do the math and know your personal daily requirements, keep a food log for a week and tally up your daily protein totals by checking your foods in the chart located in Chapter 3.

| Exercise Category | Recommended Daily Protein (Grams per Pound) |
|---|---|
| Sedentary folks | .36 |
| Moderate exercisers | .36–.5 |
| Endurance athletes | .5–.8 |
| Strength athletes | .6–.8 |
| Growing teenage athletes | .6–.9 |

Here are some examples:

➤ A 200-pound bodybuilder needs between 120 and 160 grams of protein daily.

➤ A 150-pound triathlete needs 75 to 120 grams of protein each day.

➤ A 14-year-old elite gymnast weighing 92 pounds needs 55 to 83 grams of protein each day.

➤ A casual 120-pound health-club member needs 43 to 60 grams of protein each day.

Notice that even though the growing gymnast might require more protein per pound than the bodybuilder, bodybuilders usually weigh a lot more and therefore tend to have greater protein requirements.

# Food Before, During, and After Exercise

This section investigates favorable food choices for your pre-event meal, *plus* the recovery foods to help your body bounce back after an intense workout. It also lays out the guidelines for fueling your system throughout prolonged periods of exercise.

# Pre-Event Meals

Let me begin by saying that the most outstanding meal before your sporting event won't make up for a week's worth of potato chips, french fries, and cookies! With that in mind, study the following guidelines and help make your pre-event meal a "winning beginning":

➤ Make your large meal (approximately 600–800 calories) at *least* 3–4 hours prior to an event. This will provide adequate time for your food to digest. (You don't want to feel heavy or nauseous, or have indigestion, while you're running around on the field.)

➤ Stick with carbohydrate-rich foods and moderate amounts of lean protein. The carbs are both loaded with energy and easy to digest. Avoid eating a lot of high-fat stuff; it takes much longer to leave your stomach, and you don't want food bouncing along for the ride.

➤ Avoid super high-fiber foods that can cause annoying stomach gurgles, *or* send you running to the bathroom right before kickoff.

➤ Also limit gaseous foods such as beans, Brussels sprouts, grapes, broccoli, and anything else you think might give you a gassy stomach.

➤ Liquid meals are also fine, especially if you have "pre-game jitters" and can't stomach solid food. Some athletes prefer liquid supplements because they don't leave you feeling as full as a large meal of equal calories does. In fact, they leave your stomach quicker than solid food.

➤ Also, lay off the salt. As you read in the salt chapter, some people tend to retain a lot of fluid, which can lead to puffiness and discomfort.

➤ Never eat something completely new before an important competition. *Always* test it during training and see how it settles in your stomach.

➤ Reduce the size of your food intake as you approach the time of your event. For example, 3–4 hours before, you can have a large meal (approximately 600–800 cals); 2–3 hours before, you can have a smaller meal (approximately 400–500 cals); and less than 2 hours before, you can grab some lighter snacks (cereal bars, fruit, flavored rice cakes, fruit juice, yogurts, and so on).

What time is your sporting event? Which meal will be your pre-event send-off: breakfast, lunch, or dinner? Check out the sample menus and get an idea of the foods you should choose. Keep in mind that you should *always* have a well-balanced, carbo-rich meal the night before, especially because on game day, you might get fidgety and lose your appetite.

## Ready-Made Menu

**Breakfast:**
(For a late morning or an early afternoon competition)
Bowl of cereal with low-fat milk
Sliced bananas
Bagel with jam
Glass of orange juice

**Lunch:**
(For a late afternoon or evening competition)
Turkey sandwich on whole-wheat bread
Salad with light dressing
Frozen yogurt with sliced strawberries
Glass of low-fat milk or juice

**Dinner:**
(For an early morning or "any time the next day" competition)
Grilled chicken
Pasta with marinara sauce
Broccoli and carrots
Fruit salad
2 fig bars
Glass of low-fat milk

## Q & A

**Is there really such a thing as "winning meals" or "winning foods" that can enhance your performance?**

Yes! You see, if a particular food or meal makes you *mentally* feel at your best, then for you, that is a winning meal.

# Fueling Your Body During Prolonged Endurance Activity

Some sports are so lengthy they require feedings *throughout* the event, to help supply your body with glucose when glycogen stores are running low. For example, marathon runners (and other endurance athletes such as soccer players) need to take about 30–60 grams of carbohydrate per hour, which translates into a mere (but important) 120–240 calories. Although it's a minuscule amount, these calories should be spread out over each hour. The simplest method is to drink one of the popular sports drinks during the event. You can "hydrate" and "*carbo*-hydrate" your body at the same time.

## Recovery Foods

Now for the last piece of the puzzle—the aftermath nourishment. First, understand that recovery foods are not just for recovering after a competition or game. They're equally important after practice as well. In fact, athletes who regularly train long and hard should replace emptied glycogen stores, fluids, and potassium lost through sweat on a daily basis. What's more, carbohydrate and fluid repletion should begin immediately, within 30 minutes after exercise, to promote a quick recovery. Sound unrealistic? Just grab a fruit juice or sports drink while you make your congratulatory "high-fives." When you can focus on a real meal, enjoy whatever you fancy; just make sure to include the following essentials:

➤ Plenty of fluids: water, fruit juice, sports drinks, soups, and watery fruits and veggies (watermelon, grapes, oranges, tomatoes, lettuce, and cucumbers).

➤ A lot of carbohydrate-rich foods: pasta, potatoes, rice, breads, fruits, yogurts, and so on.

➤ Moderate amounts of lean protein.

➤ Potassium-rich foods such as potatoes, bananas, oranges, orange juice, and raisins.

➤ Do *not* attempt to replenish lost sodium by smothering your food in salt *or* by popping dangerous salt tablets. A typical meal, moderately salted, supplies enough sodium to replace the amount lost through sweat.

As you have read, food can make or break your athletic performance. While, training hard is incredibly important, you'll never reach your full potential without paying close attention to balanced food choices. Remember to focus on the right mix of carbohydrate and protein, and preplan your pre-event and recovery meals. You'll feel great, and you'll have more energy and strength for a winning performance.

## The Least You Need to Know

➤ Athletes need carbohydrate-rich foods such as grains, pasta, rice, fruits, and veggies. Carbohydrates supply energy for both grueling practice sessions and competitions.

➤ Athletes have greater daily protein requirements than sedentary folks—roughly .5–.8 grams per pound of body weight. However, this is easily met because their greater caloric intake usually provides proportionately more protein.

➤ Your pre-event meal is important, and you need to reduce your food intake as you get close to your event.

➤ During prolonged exercise, your body requires about 30–60 grams of carbohydrate per hour, which translates into 120–240 calories.

➤ Help your body recover after a grueling workout with plenty of fluids, carbohydrate, and potassium-rich foods.

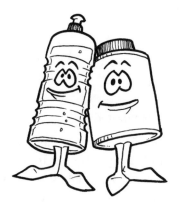

# Chapter 17

# Going That Extra Mile: Fluids and Supplements

## In This Chapter

➤ All about fluids and proper hydration

➤ The nutritional content of popular sports bars

➤ The lowdown on so-called exercise enhancers

Grab your water bottle and guzzle down. In fact, exercise places such great demands on fluid replacement that proper hydration before, during, and after intense physical activity is critical. Think about the numerous tasks that depend on fluid: Your *blood* needs fluid to transfer oxygen to working muscles, your *urine* needs fluid to funnel out metabolic waste products, and your *temperature regulating system* needs fluid to dissipate heat through sweat.

You might feel wet, gross, and disgusting on the outside, but sweating helps keep you at a comfortable working temperature. You need to *continuously* replace the fluids lost through sweat so that you can prevent your body from becoming dehydrated and overheated. What's more, athletes who fail to keep up with their water requirements not only jeopardize performance, but also place themselves at risk for serious heat conditions (heat cramps, heat exhaustion, and heat stroke).

## Guidelines for Proper Hydration

Unfortunately for athletes, the thirst mechanism is an unreliable indicator. First, by the time you feel thirsty, you could already be on your way to dehydration; second, the amount of fluid that quenches your thirst might not be enough to quench your body. To ensure adequate hydration, you need to follow a drinking schedule. Here's what's recommended:

➤ 16 ounces (or 2 cups) 2 hours prior to exercise

➤ 8–16 ounces (1–2 cups) 15–30 minutes *before* exercise

➤ 5–10 ounces (or $^2/_3$–$1^1/_3$ cup) every 15 minutes *during* exercise

➤ 16 ounces (or 2 cups) for every pound lost *after* exercise

Here are two quick ways to tell whether you are properly hydrated:

➤ **Weigh in before and after:** Hop on the scale before and after you exercise. For each pound of fluid lost (it's just fluid, *not* fat), drink 2 cups of water (or other fluid) to properly *rehydrate* your body. You don't have to gulp it all down at once; just make sure you're fully hydrated by the next day. For example, a soccer player weighs 165 pounds before the game and 162 pounds after the game. Therefore, he must drink 6 cups of water to replace the 3 pounds of lost fluid.

➤ **Check your urine:** The color of your urine is also a good indicator of hydration. If your urine is voluminous and clear to pale yellow, you're doing just fine. On the other hand, if your urine is dark and concentrated, keep chugging that fluid; you've got a ways to go.

**Nutri-Speak**

Alcohol, coffee, and tea might cause dehydration because they act as **diuretics**—substances that cause you to urinate and therefore lose water.

## Sports Drinks Versus Water

Plain old $H_2O$ is cheap, effective, and just fine for most athletes, but in some instances, you'll benefit from the added carbohydrate in a sports drink (Gatorade, PowerAde, AllSport, Boost, and so on). Spring for the loaded stuff when continuous exercise lasts longer than 60 minutes or when you're exercising in extremely hot weather. You see, water can provide straight hydration, but sports drinks can also provide some electrolytes and carbohydrate—just enough to keep you moving and grooving during those exceptionally long or hot workouts.

## The Bar Exam

Sports bars can be convenient and advantageous for athletes trying to increase calories, carbohydrates, and protein (depending upon the brand). Here's the nutritional profile on a variety of popular bars on the market. Because most brands carry an assortment of flavors, the information might slightly vary from the list. Also, be sure to sample several brands before you formulate any taste opinion; they vary tremendously!

**Clif Bar**
Calories: 250
Fat: 3g (.5g saturated fat)
Chol: 0mg
Carbs: 51g (fiber: 3g, sugars: 15g)
Protein: 4g

**Balance Bar**
Calories: 200
Fat: 6g (3g saturated fat)
Chol: <5mg
Sodium: 220mg
Carbs: 22g (fiber: 1g, sugars: 17g)
Protein: 14g

**Tiger's Milk**
Calories: 145
Fat: 5g (1g saturated fat)
Chol: 0mg
Sodium: 70mg
Carbs: 18g (fiber: 1g, sugars: 13g)
Protein: 7g

**Pure Protein**
Calories: 280
Fat: 7g (3g saturated fat)
Chol: 5mg
Sodium: 80mg
Carbs: 9g (fiber: 0g, sugars: 6g)
Protein: 33g

**MET Rx**
Calories: 340
Fat: 4g (.5g saturated fat)
Chol: 0mg
Sodium: 135mg
Carbs: 50g (fiber: 0g, sugars: 29g)
Protein: 27g

**Power Bar**
Calories: 230
Fat: 2.5g (.5g saturated fat)
Chol: 0mg
Sodium: 110mg
Carbs: 45g (fiber: 3g, sugars: 20g)
Protein: 10g

**Ultimate Protein Bar**
Calories: 280
Fat: 6g (3.5g saturated fat)
Chol: 0mg
Sodium: 50mg
Carbs: 19g (fiber: 0g, sugars: 12g)
Protein: 32g

**Myoplex**
Calories: 340
Fat: 7g (1.5g saturated fat)
Chol: <5mg
Sodium: 230mg
Carbs: 44g (fiber: 0g, sugars: 36g)
Protein: 24g

**PromaxBar**
Calories: 280
Fat: 5g (4g saturated fat)
Chol: 14mg
Sodium: 200mg
Carbs: 35g (fiber: 1g, sugars: 23g)
Protein: 20g

**PR Ironman**
Calories: 230
Fat: 8g (1.5g saturated fat)
Chol: 0mg
Sodium: 280mg
Carbs: 23g (fiber: 0g, sugars: 17g)
Protein: 16g

**Steel Bar**
Calories: 330
Fat: 6g (3g saturated fat)
Chol: 20mg
Sodium: 160mg
Carbs: 52g (fiber: 0g, sugars: 28g)
Protein: 16g

**Source One (by MET Rx)**
Calories: 190
Fat: 3g (2.5 saturated fat)
Chol: 0mg
Sodium: 70mg
Carbs: 29g (fiber: 0g, sugars: 4g)
Protein: 15g
(Also provides 50% calcium)

# What's the Story on Ergogenic Aids?

People make outrageous claims regarding substances that can help enhance performance. The word *ergogenic* literally means "work producing," and, unfortunately, there are always cockamamie advertisements selling nutritional pills and potions claiming to beef up performance. To date, there are only a few scientifically sound ergogenic aids, including a proper diet, carbo-loading, a well-trained body, a determined soul, and the right equipment.

Here's what you need to know about ergogenic aids in food and supplement form.

## *Thumbs Up*

To date, the following substances have been shown to improve athletic performance. Of course, this doesn't mean you should start popping pills. In fact, scientists are constantly coming up with new information (good and bad), so stay on top of the current research if you decide to go with one of these supplements. Naturally, *always* check with your physician before embarking on anything new:

➤ **Antioxidants** (C, E, beta carotene, and selenium)
**Claim:** Protects against the tissue damage from free radical formation induced by exercise.
**Fact:** Might protect against tissue damage following prolonged endurance exercise but doesn't improve performance while you are actually exercising. Although the quantities of antioxidants found in food are somewhat small, they do help to stop the production and spread of harmful substances.

➤ **Caffeine**
**Claim:** Improves endurance.
**Fact:** Consuming 3–6 mg of caffeine per kg (your weight in pounds divided by 2.2) one hour before exercise improves endurance performance without raising urinary caffeine levels above the International Olympic Committee standards. Side effects of high caffeine consumption include nausea, muscle tremors, palpitations, and headache. Not a good idea if you have a sensitive system.

➤ **Creatine**
**Claim:** Increases the creatine phosphate content in muscles, improves high-power performance, and increases muscle mass.
**Fact:** Research has suggested that consuming 20 grams of creatine per day (5 grams four times daily) for 5 days might improve performance in brief, maximal exercise lasting less than 30 seconds. After this loading dose, a maintenance dose of 5 grams per day should suffice. However, not all studies have found that creatine improves strength, sprint performance, or lean muscle mass—so it might not improve all high-power activities.

➤ **Sodium bicarbonate**
**Claim:** Counteracts the build-up of lactic acid in the blood and improves anaerobic (without oxygen) performance.
**Fact:** Several studies conducted on sprinters have supported improved anaerobic performance with bicarbonate supplementation. Taking 0.3 grams per kg (your body weight in pounds divided by 2.2) of sodium bicarbonate with water over a two- to three-hour period might improve sprinting time by several seconds. However, as many as half of those individuals using sodium bicarbonate experienced urgent diarrhea 30 minutes after soda loading. Obviously, caution is strongly advised.

➤ **Phosphates**
**Claim:** Improve endurance.
**Fact:** Phosphate loading might increase $VO_2$ max (your oxygen capacity) and decrease the rise of lactic acid during intense exercise. The dose is 1 gram of sodium phosphate 4 times a day for 3 days. More research on phosphate loading is needed.

## Thumbs Down

The following exercise enhancers do not have any solid scientific data to back them up. Needless to say, they won't improve your athletic performance:

➤ **Amino acids** (arginine, ornithine, and lysine)
**Claim:** Stimulates the release of human growth hormone, promotes muscle growth, and increases strength.
**Fact:** These oral amino-acid supplements do *not* increase the growth hormone levels or muscle mass. Studies have shown that weightlifting and endurance sports alone (without the extra amino acids) both significantly increase growth-hormone levels.

➤ **Bee pollen**
**Claim:** To improve physical performance.
**Fact:** It has no magical quality. It is composed of the same nutrients found naturally in food: starch, sugars, protein, and a small amount of fat. For some, taking this substance results in an allergic reaction. Anyone with kidney disease or a predisposition for gout should avoid it.

➤ **Brewer's yeast**
**Claim:** Improves athletic performance (among many other claims).
**Fact:** Although it is a great source of certain B-vitamins, there's no evidence that it enhances exercise performance.

➤ **Boron**
**Claim:** Increases serum testosterone levels to enhance muscle growth and strength.

**Fact:** These claims were based on a USDA study that showed that Boron supplementation increased the levels of testosterone in post-menopausal women. Normal male testosterone is about 10 times that of post-menopausal women— and in the case of the male population, Boron has no effect on testosterone levels, lean body mass, or strength in strength-trained athletes.

➤ **Carnitine**
**Claim:** Causes an increase in the metabolism of fat, thus promoting a decline in total body fat.
**Fact:** Carnitine facilitates the transfer of fatty acids into the mitochondria (the location in each cell where metabolism takes place) to be used for energy. There is no evidence that carnitine supplementation promotes increased use of fatty acids during exercise or a decrease in body fat.

➤ **Choline**
**Claim:** Increases strength and causes a decrease in body fat.
**Fact:** There is no evidence that choline supplementation increases strength and reduces body fat.

➤ **Chromium picolinate**
**Claim:** Increases muscle mass, decreases body fat, and promotes weight loss.
**Fact:** Nutrition Research Centers in Beltsville, MD, and Grand Forks, ND, found that a daily supplement of chromium picolinate coupled with weight training for 8–12 weeks did *not* increase strength or muscle mass or decrease body fat. In fact, in November 1996, the Federal Trade Commission ordered all supplement companies to stop making unsubstantiated weight-loss and health claims for chromium picolinate.

➤ **Coenzyme Q10**
**Claim:** Optimizes ATP (our body's energy) production to increase vigor, energy, and stamina.
**Fact:** There is no dietary requirement for this substance. According to current literature, supplementation with coenzyme Q10 does *not* improve endurance performance, nor does it improve your oxygen capacity.

➤ **Gamma-oryzanol**
**Claim:** Increases serum testosterone and growth-hormone levels, enhancing muscle growth.
**Fact:** Oryzanol is a plant sterol and has a similar structure to cholesterol. Numerous claims have been made that these plant sterols (oryzanol one of them), like cholesterol, can be converted to testosterone. However, oryzanol is *not* anabolic because it cannot be converted to testosterone by the human body and therefore does not promote muscle growth.

➤ **Glandular extracts**
  **Claim:** Enhances the function of the same gland in the body. For example, testes extract enhances testosterone production.
  **Fact:** The glandular extracts are inactive, therefore worthless, when absorbed. They contain no hormones and cannot exert any effect.

➤ **MCT (medium chain triglycerides)**
  **Claim:** Promotes muscle growth and body fat loss.
  **Fact:** MCT is an inefficient energy source during aerobic exercise. There is nothing in the research to prove that MCT meets its claims in strength-trained athletes. Consuming large amounts can cause gastrointestinal distress and diarrhea.

➤ **Smilax**
  **Claim:** Increases serum testosterone levels, muscle growth, and strength. Also indicated to be a legal alternative to anabolic steroids.
  **Fact:** Smilax does contain saponins—substances that serve as precursors for the semi-synthetic production of certain steroids. But this conversion takes place only in the laboratory, and there is no evidence that Smilax functions as a "legal replacement" for anabolic steroids. What's more, saponins have a strong diuretic action and possible laxative effect and might also intensify your perspiration.

➤ **Succinate**
  **Claim:** Metabolic enhancer; reduces lactic-acid production and maintains energy production.
  **Fact:** Succinate is an intermediate in the aerobic pathway (where our bodies produce energy for exercise). However, supplementation will *not* increase the process of aerobic metabolism or ATP (energy) production; these actions are controlled by enzymes within the pathway.

➤ **Vitamin B-12**
  **Claim:** Enhances DNA synthesis; increases muscle growth.
  **Fact:** Vitamin B-12 is essential in the synthesis of DNA. However, there is no evidence that *extra* B-12 promotes muscle growth or enhances strength.

➤ **Yohimbe**
  **Claim:** Increases serum testosterone levels to enhance muscle growth and strength. Also claims to reduce body fat—and have an aphrodisiac effect.
  **Fact:** There is no proof in the current research to show that yohimbe is anabolic, so its ability to increase muscle growth is questionable. (Its value as an aphrodisiac is also inconclusive.) The FDA has declared yohimbe unsafe and ineffective for over-the-counter sale.

The appeal for magic pills promising bigger muscles and faster speeds are tremendous. However, it's important to know that very few supplements have scientific backup—in fact, most of the sport enhancers offer nothing but misleading labels. Without a doubt, the best investment for top performance is the old fashioned mix—good eats and plenty of hard training.

---

### The Least You Need to Know

➤ Proper hydration is essential for maintaining prolonged activity *and* for optimal performance.

➤ Water is the perfect fluid replacement for exercise lasting under 60 minutes. However, ultra-endurance athletes, and anyone exercising in extremely hot weather, will benefit from the added carbohydrate and electrolyte content in the popular sports drinks.

➤ Don't be misled by ads claiming to sell exercise enhancers in the shape of a pill. The way to optimize performance is to eat smart and train hard!

➤ Sports bars can be convenient and advantageous for athletes trying to increase calories, carbohydrates, and protein (depending upon the brand). Sample several brands before you form a taste opinion; they vary tremendously.

---

# Part 4
# Beyond the Basics: Nutrition for Special Needs

*There are so many sub-specialties within the world of nutrition. New research comes along all the time and offers us exciting information regarding specialized areas. Among them, I've selected four interesting topics that appear to get a lot of attention; diet and cancer, vegetarian food plans, herbal remedies, and food sensitivities.*

*Whether you are interested in reducing your cancer risk, feasting purely on plants, wanting to learn some Chinese medicine, or simply tired of bolting for the bathroom after ingesting dairy, stayed tuned.*

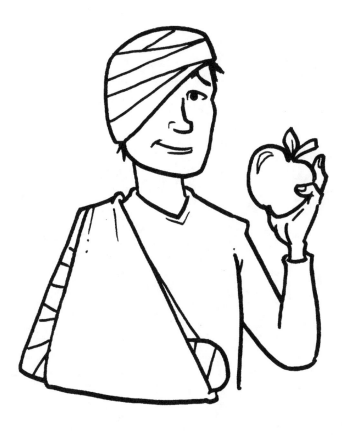

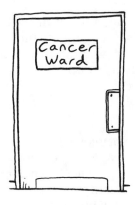

# Chapter 18

# Diet and Cancer

## In This Chapter

➤ Foods that might decrease your risk of contracting certain cancers

➤ Omega 3s—and how they can help

➤ Eating the right fish and getting the most from flaxseed

➤ Your best bets in vegetables and fruit

➤ The many benefits of soy

Over the years, there's been a lot of speculation and controversy over how eating certain foods might prevent cancer. You certainly don't need a Harvard oncologist (or a New York City nutritionist) to tell you that if you eat in a healthy manner, your body will be stronger, your immune system and organs will be in good shape, and therefore, you might be more likely to be cancer free. But just eating tons of fruits and veggies and the right kind of nutrients isn't a foolproof way to avoid the wrath of cancer. Unfortunately, there is no exact science linking food and cancer prevention, although we are constantly researching and studying the subject in search of some answers.

Nonetheless, while scientists and doctors learn, you can take a proactive approach to feeding your body well, giving it fuel to fight disease, and doing whatever you can to ward off this horrific illness. Even though there is no hardcore proof about which foods offer the best protection against malignancy, research has uncovered how certain foods can get in the way of a tumor's growth.

## Which Fats Can Help

For years, there has been an incredible amount of hype over fat. Fat clogs your arteries, fat increases your cholesterol, fat causes weight gain—fat is the root of all evil. However, some kinds of fat are not just okay to eat—but are actually good for you. To date,

### Nutri-Speak

The **Omega-3 Fats** (also known as linolenic fatty acids) are polyunsaturated—meaning their structural makeup is lacking several hydrogen atoms. Eating foods rich in Omega-3 Fats has been shown to have beneficial effects, such as lowering triglycerides and cholesterol, lowering blood pressure, helping alleviate arthritic pain, aiding with digestive problems, and possibly reducing the risk of certain cancers.

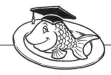

### Food for Thought

You can buy flaxseed by mail order; Flax Council of Canada 877-BUY-FLAX.

Moo!

### Overrated—Undercooked

Alcohol is not recommended—but if you must, limit your consumption to no more than one drink per day.

the best type of fat is polyunsaturated and called the Omega 3s. The Omega 3 fats might have the potential to lower the risk of cancer and heart disease as well as help ease the pain of rheumatoid arthritis. It is found in flaxseed, canola oil, and fish.

## The Fatty Fish

Seafood lovers, rejoice! Epidemiological studies have shown a lower rate of cancer in people who eat a lot of fish. The best advice is to have a few servings of tuna, mackerel, sardines, bluefish, striped bass, herring, trout, and salmon—the fish dishes with a rich concentration of Omega 3 fats. In fact, eat them at least three times each week (even more if you can).

## Flaxseeds and Flaxseed Oil

Flaxseed, the light brown seed from the flax plant, has received a lot of attention for its potential to protect against breast and other hormone-related cancers (in addition to lowering cholesterol and relieving constipation). Rich in Omega 3s, antioxidants, lignans-phytoestrogens (which you'll read about later in this chapter), and soluble and insoluble fiber, this impressive seed has been growing in popularity.

You can buy whole flaxseed in most health-food stores and grind them with a coffee grinder as needed. Mix them into in your cereals, salads, yogurts, cookies, muffins, pancakes, omelets, and even casseroles. Flaxseed oil is effortless, quick, and ready to pour on salad, but you'll miss out on the lignans and fiber found in the whole flaxseed. For more information visit the Web site www.flaxcouncil.ca.

# Fight Back with Antioxidants

Unfortunately, harmful agents called *free radicals* are produced when we breathe and process oxygen. In fact, these destructive bad guys can also be produced as a result of pollution, stress, pesticides, asbestos, x-rays, preservatives, exhaust fumes, tobacco smoke, and injury. As discussed in a previous chapter, free radicals trek all over the body and actually destroy the cell's DNA—a cancer-promoting activity. The good news is that we naturally protect ourselves by forming antioxidants, substances that help our body's defense system fight off free radicals and preserve healthy cells. Furthermore, we know that certain foods are rich in nutrients that act as *powerful* antioxidants and might intensify the body's ability to degrade free radicals into harmless waste products that get eliminated before they do any damage.

The following sections form a list of some cancer-fighting ingredients to regularly include in your diet.

# Vitamins C and E, and Beta Carotene

Vitamins C and E and beta carotene (a form of vitamin A) are chock-full of antioxidants. You can find them in fruits and vegetables. Your best bets with each are the following:

**Foods Rich in Vitamin C**
Citrus fruits (oranges, grapefruits, and so on)
Melons
Berries
Tomatoes
Potatoes
Broccoli
Kiwi
Mango
Papaya
Yellow peppers

**Foods Rich in Vitamin E**
Vegetable oils
Margarine
Salad dressings
Whole-grain cereals
Green leafy vegetables
Nuts and seeds
Peanut butter
Wheat germ

**Foods Rich in Beta Carotene**
Cantaloupe
Carrots
Sweet potato
Winter squash
Spinach
Broccoli

## Green Tea

Green tea is a traditional Asian brew, the chicken soup, cure-all remedy that Japanese grandmas swear by—and it contains potent chemical antioxidants called polyphenols, so drink up. In fact, research has shown that green tea might actually interfere with cancer-causing agents' ability to bind to our DNA—therefore stopping cancer activity. It's no wonder the Japanese, who far surpass the Americans in tea consumption, have a much lower cancer rate.

Further, you'll want to take it easy with the amount of milk that you pour into your mug because milk proteins might bind with the antioxidants, making them unavailable to your body. For those who prefer lemon and sugar, you're in luck because they both appear to be perfectly fine. Unfortunately, herbal teas do not work in the same protective manner that the green teas do.

**Food for Thought**

Folic acid (400 milligrams per day) has been shown to reduce the risk of colon cancer.

## Tomatoes

Tomatoes contain lycopene, which is actually the pigment that gives tomatoes their blush hue. The catch is that tomatoes must be cooked to make the lycopene available to the body. Grill 'em up, stew them, simmer in soups, or make a mean marinara sauce—but don't forget to season it with a little garlic. (The allyl sulfides in garlic, chives, and onions might help the body process cancer-causing chemicals more safely.) Also, add a touch of olive oil because a bit of fat will help the lycopene move through your body.

# Can't Get Enough of Those Fruits and Veggies

Everyone knows the nutritional value of fruits and vegetables; that's why at least five servings a day are recommended. I've already pointed out that certain plant foods are loaded with C, E, and beta carotene—helpful vitamins and antioxidants our bodies need to fight disease and stay strong. In addition, plant foods have been shown to play a significant role in the fight against most cancers because they contain phytochemicals and Cox-2 inhibitors—a compound that can stop the growth of new blood cells, which would ultimately impede the growth of a tumor. Let's not forget about the fiber bonus; that's the icing on the cake, if you will.

**Food for Thought**

Include plenty of whole grains in your diet. The insoluble fiber in wheat bran can increase the transport of waste products and cancer-causing agents through the gut and lower intestines. The less time waste products spend in your system, the less risk of certain types of cancer such as colon and rectal.

Cruciferous veggies such as broccoli, cauliflower, cabbage, bok choy, kale, brussel sprouts, collards, mustard greens, and turnip greens can also help reduce the risk of cancer by increasing the production of certain enzymes that help carry potential carcinogens out of the body. Make sure you load your stir-fry dishes and salads with the all-mighty cruciferous ones!

# Phytochemicals, Phytonutrients, and Phytoestrogens

They sound confusing but they're really quite understandable:

➤ **Phytochemicals**—Phytochemicals (meaning plant chemicals) is another group of compounds in plant foods—legumes, veggies, fruits, and whole grains—that might positively affect your body. They're naturally produced by plants to protect themselves against viruses, bacteria, and fungi. The term phytochemical includes hundreds of naturally occurring substances such as carotenoids, flavonoids, indoles, isoflavones, capsaicin, and protease inhibitors.

Their exact role in promoting health is still uncertain—but research has suggested that they might help protect against certain cancers, heart disease, and other chronic illnesses.

➤ **Phytonutrients**—Phytonutrient is a term typically used on a supplement bottle to denote that certain botanical supplements extracted from vegetables and other plant foods have been added.

There isn't enough scientific evidence to know whether supplement manufacturers have picked the "right" active substance, because there can be thousands to choose from, or if the amount contained in the pill actually offers any benefits.

➤ **Phytoestrogens**—Phytoestrogens are plant hormones similar to, but weaker than, human estrogens. They are believed to reduce the risk of breast cancer and prostate cancer; they also might minimize mood swings and hot flashes associated with menopause. Some medical researchers think that phytoestrogens might one day take the place of conventional ERT (estrogen replacement therapy).

Phytoestrogens, now identified in some 300 plants, are grouped as

**Coumestans:** bean sprouts, red clover, sunflower seeds

**Lignans:** rye, wheat, sesame seeds, linseed, flaxseeds

**Isoflavones:** many fruits and veggies but, most of all, soybeans and soy products

**Food for Thought**

Rosemary, turmeric, and red grapes contain Cox-2 inhibitors—compounds that can prevent tumor growth.

**Nutri-Speak**

**Isoflavones** are hormone-like substances, which are similar to estrogen and are found in plants.

**Food for Thought**

Make a soy-fruit smoothie: In a blender mix soy-protein powder with fruit juice, fresh fruit, and some crushed ice.

# The Story on Soy Products

Substituting steaks, burgers, and franks with tofu, tempeh, miso, and veggie burgers can work to your advantage. (You vegetarians are definitely on to something.) That's because soy foods contain phytoestrogens called *isoflavones*, weak estrogens that help fight against certain hormone-related cancers, such as breast, uterine, prostate, and possibly ovarian. These weak estrogens bind to the receptors that would otherwise get filled by stronger estrogens—stronger estrogens that have the potential to promote tumor growth.

Although the research is preliminary regarding the amount we should consume, everyone can benefit by shifting from an animal-based to a plant-based diet. The best soy sources include soybeans, tempeh, tofu, soy protein isolate (dry), textured soy protein (TVP), dry soy concentrate, and soy milk.

Diet won't eliminate cancer—but we can say that in certain circumstances the foods we eat can help reduce the risk. Try to adopt a cuisine that incorporates some or all of the foods previously discussed, and you will be taking a proactive step toward improving your overall health.

## The Least You Need to Know

➤ Your mom knew what she was talking about when she pushed you to eat your veggies; plant foods are especially good for reducing the risk of cancer because they contain compounds that inhibit the growth of tumors.

➤ Not all fats are taboo; flaxseed, canola, and fish oils are known as Omega 3s, which can actually play a role in the fight against cancer.

➤ Drinking green tea, stewing up tomatoes, and eating foods with a high concentration of vitamins C and E and beta carotene will help fight harmful agents called free radicals and therefore preserve healthy cells and reduce the risk of cancer.

➤ A diet rich in fiber might help decrease your risk of colon and rectal cancer. Insoluble fiber, found in whole grains, wheat bran, and most fruits and veggies, can help the body dispose of waste products and cancer-causing agents from the gut and lower intestines.

➤ Consume more tofu, miso, tempeh, and soy beans; they all contain soy, which can help fight against hormone-related cancers, such as breast, uterine, prostate, and possibly ovarian.

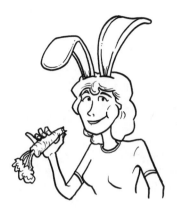

# Chapter 19

# Going Vegetarian

### In This Chapter

➤ The reasons people go vegetarian

➤ Difference between vegans, lacto-vegetarians, and ovolacto-vegetarians

➤ Great vegetarian protein and iron sources

➤ What's soy protein all about?

➤ Meatless recipes to tantalize your taste buds

Vegetarian diets are becoming popular, with more and more Americans jumping on the "tofu bandwagon." Like every other prudent diet, people following vegetarian food plans must eat well-balanced, varied meals and include fruits, vegetables, nuts, seeds, low-fat dairy (depending upon your vegetarian restrictions), legumes, and plenty of whole grain products. Although a typical vegetarian eating plan tends to be super-low in saturated fat and cholesterol, it's not automatically low in *total* fat and sugar. Therefore, veg-heads, like meat-heads, need to limit their intake of fatty foods, oils, spreads, and sweets.

## The Vegetarian Food Guide Pyramid

Similar to the Food Guide Pyramid used as the mainstream standard, the vegetarian version provides recommended guidelines for the "meatless" population.

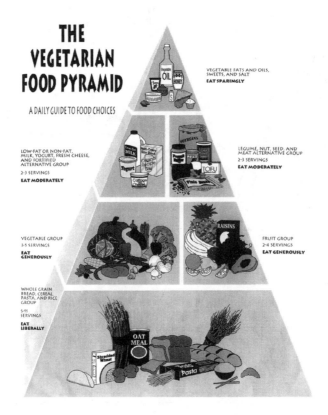

*Source: The Health Connection, 800-548-8700. To order poster or handouts, call the toll-free number or 301-790-9735.*

# The Various Types of Vegetarians

A vegetarian diet, when properly followed, can be one of the healthiest diets out there. Benefits of the vegetarian diet include

➤ **Decreased obesity:** Vegans are rarely obese and on the average, ovolacto-vegetarians are leaner than those who eat meat. However, being vegetarian doesn't guarantee a slim figure. If you eat foods that are high in fat, you can consume as many or more calories than meat eaters.

➤ **Less risk of Coronary Heart Disease (CHD):** Vegetarians tend to have lower blood cholesterol levels and diets with lower overall saturated fat content.

➤ **Lower rates of hypertension:** The reason for this is still unknown, but researchers think it might be related to increased potassium, magnesium, polyunsaturated fat, and fiber intake. All the same, more research is still needed to determine whether the diet itself has anything to do with the lower levels.

Vegetarian eating covers broad territory and can run the gamut from people who avoid *all* animal products to people who simply refrain from eating a few select animal foods. Here's a look at the assortment of vegetarian-style eaters:

➤ **Vegans**—This is the strictest type of vegetarian (sort of the pope of all vegetarians). Vegans abstain from eating or using *all* animal products, from eating meat, dairy, and eggs, to wearing wool, silk, or leather. If you're a vegan, you'll need to be extra careful about getting adequate protein, iron, calcium, vitamin D, vitamin B-12, and zinc.

➤ **Lacto-vegetarians**—This group eliminates meat and eggs but includes all dairy products.

➤ **Ovolacto-vegetarians**—This group eliminates all meat (red meat, poultry, fish, and seafood); however, they do include dairy products and eggs.

➤ **Semi-vegetarians**—This group does not eat red meat but eats most chicken, turkey, and fish, along with all dairy and eggs.

➤ **"Pseudo"-vegetarians** This group will not eat meat on the days they decide they're vegetarian but will, however, inhale hamburgers and steak sandwiches when they get a craving.

# How to Ensure an Adequate Protein Intake

All vegetarians can easily meet their protein needs. Protein doesn't discriminate; it's found in both animal and plant foods. Low-fat dairy and eggs can provide generous amounts of protein for vegetarians who dare to eat them, and the vegans in the crowd should become close pals with tofu, nuts, seeds, lentils, and tempeh. Flip back to Chapter 3, "The Profile on Protein," to refresh your memory on complementary proteins—that is, making a complete protein (a protein containing all of the essential amino acids) by combining two or more incomplete plant proteins.

**Food for Thought**

Although tofu and other soy proteins contain some fat, it's very low in saturated fat and contains no cholesterol. For more information and free brochures on soy protein, call 800-TALK-SOY.

## *The Many Faces of Soy Protein*

Decades ago, soy foods were one of the world's best kept secrets. Finally out of the closet and raring to jump into just about any recipe, soy protein can boost protein, calcium, and the iron content of almost any dish. Go ahead and experiment by incorporating some of the following varieties into your meals, and remember that unflavored soy will take on any flavor you cook or marinate with:

➤ **Soymilk**—Start your day with a glass of soymilk, or pour it over your cereal for breakfast. Soymilk provides about 4–10 grams of protein per one cup serving and can be found in low-fat and flavored varieties.

➤ **Isolated soy protein**—This powdery substance is literally 90 percent pure protein because most of the fat and carbohydrate have been discarded. It's made from defatted soy flour and can be strategically blended into muffins, pancakes, and cookies to help boost your daily protein. A 1-ounce serving (approximately 4 Tbs) contains between 13 and 23 grams of protein.

➤ **Soy flour**—Here's another great way to hike up the protein in your baked products. Soy flour can be used for quick breads, muffins, cookies, and brownies, and $^1/_2$ cup serving supplies 22 grams of protein.

➤ **Textured soy protein (TSP)**—Also called textured vegetable protein (TVP), this is made from defatted soy flour and takes on a granular, flake, or chunk characteristic. TSP comes both plain and flavored and can be mixed into chili, tacos, veggie burgers, vegetarian casseroles, and stews. When mixed with water, 1 cup prepared provides 22 grams of protein.

➤ **Vegetable-type soybeans**—These dry, mature soybeans are loaded with 14 grams of protein per $^1/_2$ cup serving. What's more, they also contain fiber—double bonus. Tasting both sweet and buttery, their flavor makes them a nice addition to stir-fry dishes, salads, and soups.

➤ **Tempeh**—This cultured soyfood has a tender, chewy consistency that makes it a great candidate for grilled sandwiches, chunky soups, salads, casseroles, and chili. A 4-ounce serving provides 17 grams of protein, about 80 milligrams of calcium and 10 percent of your daily iron.

➤ **Tofu**—Just about anything goes with this soy protein. "I'll have a tofu a la mode!" It's made from soymilk curds and can be blended, scrambled, stir-fried, grilled, baked; you name it, chances are it can be done with tofu. There are three types of tofu:

> **Firm tofu** is stiff, dense, and perfect for stir-fry dishes, soups, or anywhere that you want tofu to maintain its shape. A 4-ounce serving of firm tofu supplies 13 grams protein, 120 milligrams calcium, and about 40 percent of your daily iron.

> **Soft tofu** provides 9 grams protein, 130 milligrams calcium, and a little less than 40 percent of your daily iron from a 4-ounce serving. Soft tofu is good for dishes that require blended tofu (commonly used in soups).

> **Silken tofu** is creamy and custard-like and therefore also works well in pureed or blended recipes such as dips, soups, and pies. Silken tofu doesn't provide as much calcium as the more solid tofu varieties (only 40 milligrams), but it is the lowest in fat and is packed with $9^1/_2$ grams of protein per 4-ounce serving.

## *Ironing Out the Plant Foods*

Unfortunately for this less-carnivorous crowd, the *heme iron* found in animal foods is much more absorbable than the *nonheme* iron supplied from plants. But that's okay; just go out of your way to eat an abundance of iron-rich plant foods and you'll meet your quota. Foods rich in iron include dried beans, spinach, chard, beet greens, blackstrap molasses, bulgur, prune juice, and dried fruits. You might also find that your favorite breakfast cereals are fortified with this mineral. Another trick of the trade is to boost the amount of iron absorbed at a meal by including a food rich in vitamin C (tomatoes, orange juice, and so on). For further information on increasing iron, see Chapter 8, "Mighty Minerals: Calcium and Iron."

## *Searching for Non-Dairy Calcium*

For the lactos and ovolactos, low-fat dairy is brimming with calcium. On the other hand, for all you vegans, it takes some planning, but you too can meet your daily calcium requirements by including collard greens, broccoli, beans, kale, turnip greens, calcium-fortified orange juice, calcium-fortified grains, and, of course, your calcium-fortified soymilk products (including tofu, soybeans, and tempeh).

## *Have You Had Enough B-12 Today?*

Getting enough vitamin B-12 can also be an obstacle for strict vegans, simply because B-12 is derived primarily from animal foods. Once again, you lactos and ovolactos are off the hook because dairy and eggs provide enough to satisfy your daily requirements. The vegan gang has to dig a little deeper. Buy food products that are B-12 fortified: cereals, breads, some soy-analogs, and possibly tempeh. You might also want to pop a B-12 supplement providing 100 percent of the RDA, just to be safe.

## *Don't Forget the Kitchen Zinc*

Not only do you have to get all of the necessary RDA of calcium, protein, B-12, and other nutrients, yet another concern for the strict vegetarian is getting a fair share of zinc. Although this mineral is found in whole-grain products, tofu, nuts, seeds, and wheat germ, our bodies absorb much less "plant zinc" than "animal zinc." This is because *phytic acid* (a substance in the fiber) combines with the zinc and prevents it from being fully absorbed. Therefore, vegetarians need to pay particular attention to getting an abundance of this mineral.

**Food for Thought**

Vegans who don't eat dairy and aren't regularly out in the sun should buy foods fortified with vitamin D or speak with their doctors about vitamin D supplementation.

### A day in the life of a vegan.

**Menu 1**

Breakfast
Amaranth flakes with soy milk
Fresh blueberries and raspberries
English muffin topped with peach preserves

Lunch
Peanut butter and banana sandwich
Cup of vegetarian chili topped with scallions
Glass of low-fat soymilk

Snack
Mixture of dried fruit and walnuts
Glass of juice or soymilk

Dinner
Vegetable-tempeh stir-fry (carrots, broccoli, cauliflower, and tempeh) with brown rice
Sweet potato
Steamed kale sprinkled with sesame seeds
Glass of soymilk

Dessert
Rice Dream (ice cream substitute)
Sliced bananas

**Menu 2**

Breakfast
Scrambled tofu (see recipe) with whole-wheat toast
Bowl of oatmeal with chopped dates and almonds
Glass of cranberry-orange juice

Lunch
Bowl of lentil soup with sourdough rolls
Carrot sticks with humus dip
Glass of juice or soymilk

Snack
Piece of banana bread
Glass of soymilk

Dinner
Whole-wheat tortilla stuffed with beans, salsa, and arugula
Spinach salad drizzled with olive oil and red wine vinegar

Dessert
Baked apple with maple syrup and chopped walnuts

## Tips for the Vegetarian Dining Out

Whether you're dining out to be social or because you just don't feel like cooking, if you're trying to stick to a vegetarian diet, it can be tough to get satisfied, let alone nourished. Here are some tips to get through a night out without starving:

➤ When your dining buddies won't have anything to do with a vegetarian restaurant, suggest Chinese, Vietnamese, Thai, or Italian. There's always a bunch of vegetarian entrees on the menu.

➤ If there aren't any vegetarian entrees, make up a full meal by selecting a few side dishes. For example, have a baked potato or a house salad and ask whether they'll serve a side of beans. Better yet, request a special vegetarian entree. Most restaurants can be pretty accommodating.

➤ Soup can be a great option in any type of restaurant. Remember to ask whether the soup is meat-based or vegetable-based.

➤ Feel free to make substitutions and special requests. For instance, change a bacon, lettuce, and tomato sandwich to a cheese, lettuce, and tomato sandwich, or change an order of chicken fajitas to veggie fajitas.

### Q & A

**Help, I'm in love with a meat-eater! What do I do?**

Relax, get with the '90s; mixed marriages are in! If cooking is a major hassle because you and your partner don't eat the same foods, plan some neutral meals that you'll both enjoy. For example, make a large dish of stir-fry vegetables and brown rice. You take a portion and toss in tofu; he or she takes a portion and throws in chicken or beef.

## Remarkably "Meatless" Recipes

Order some of these award-winning vegetarian cookbooks:

*Skinny Vegetarian Entrees*
Phyllis Magida and Sue Spliter
Surrey Books
800-326-4430

*New Vegetarian Cuisine*
Linda Rosensweig, from the pages of
*Prevention Magazine*
Rosdale Books
800-848-4735

*The Enchanted Broccoli Forest*
Mollie Katzen
Ten Speed Press
800-841-2665

*The Vegetarian Times Cookbook*
Macmillan Publishers
800-428-5331

### Food for Thought

Pregnant vegetarians need to pay extra attention to their diets. For some further reading, pick up

*Vegetarian Pregnancy*
by Sharon Yntema
McBooks Press
888-BOOKS11

Bringing up kids in a veggie household? For further reading, pick up

*Vegetarian Children*
by Sharon Yntema
McBooks Press
888-BOOKS11

## Cajun Red Beans and Rice

*Serves four*

1 cup long-grain white rice

2 cups water

1 15$^{1}$/$_{4}$ oz. can kidney beans, drained and rinsed

2 tsp Paprika

1 cup canned, crushed tomatoes

1 tsp Worcestershire

$^{1}$/$_{2}$ onion, peeled and diced $^{1}$/$_{4}$ inch

Pinch cayenne pepper

1 green bell pepper, diced $^{1}$/$_{4}$ inch

$^{1}$/$_{4}$ tsp garlic powder

2 bay leaves

4 Tbs chopped green onion

Place all ingredients (except for the chopped, green onions) in a large saucepan; cover and bring to a boil. Reduce heat and simmer 15–20 minutes until rice is tender and liquid is evaporated. Top each portion with 1 Tbs of chopped green onion. Balance out this meal with a dark, leafy green salad tossed with nonfat Italian salad dressing.

Nutrition Analysis for One Serving
Calories: 290
Total fat: 1 gram
Saturated fat: 0 grams
Dietary fiber: 7 grams
Protein: 10 grams
Sodium: 170 mg
Cholesterol: 0 mg

*Copyright* Food for Health *newsletter, 1996. Reprinted with permission.*

## Vegetarian Spinach Lasagna

*Serves eight*

2 lbs. low-fat ricotta cheese

1 whole egg + 2 egg whites

4 cups skim milk mozzarella cheese, shredded

3/4 tsp pepper

1 32 oz. jar of tomato/marinara sauce (low-sodium)

Garlic and basil to taste

1 package lasagna noodles, uncooked

Nonstick cooking spray

2 10–12 oz. boxes of frozen spinach, chopped

1 cup water (for cooking only)

$^{1}$/$_{4}$ Tbs oregano

Cook and drain spinach well, and then set aside. Mix together ricotta cheese, eggs, pepper, garlic, oregano, basil, and only half of the mozzarella cheese. Add in spinach and mix again thoroughly. Coat lasagna pan with nonstick spray and preheat oven to 350°. Cover the bottom of pan with tomato sauce and then place a layer of the uncooked lasagna noodles. Next, spread $^{1}$/$_{2}$ of the spinach-cheese mixture evenly on top, and repeat the layers (noodles and then the remaining spinach-cheese mixture). Place on top one more layer of noodles (total of 3 noodle layers) and pour on the remaining tomato sauce. Sprinkle on the other half of the mozzarella cheese. Last, pour the water around the edge of the pan (this will cook the noodles) and cover tightly with tin foil. Bake for 1 hour and 15 minutes, until the cheese is bubbling. Let stand and cool for 15 minutes before slicing.

Nutrition Analysis for One Serving
Calories: 243
Total fat: 7.5 grams
Saturated fat: 3 grams
Dietary fiber: 3 grams
Protein: 19 grams
Sodium: 479 mg
Cholesterol: 43 mg

*From the kitchen of Ellen Schloss*

## Chunky Vegetarian Chili

*Serves six*

$^1/_2$ cup texturized vegetable protein (TVP)

2 medium celery stalks, chopped

$^1/_4$ cup boiling water

1 green bell pepper, seeded and chopped

$^1/_2$ Tbs olive oil

8 ounces mushrooms, quartered

1 large onion, diced

Juice of one lemon

3 cloves garlic, minced

$^1/_2$ tsp dried basil

2 medium carrots, chopped

$^1/_2$ tsp dried oregano

$^1/_8$ tsp red pepper flakes

1 15-ounce can kidney beans

$1^1/_2$ tsp chili powder

1 28-ounce can crushed tomatoes

$1^1/_2$ tsp ground cumin

1 Tbs tomato paste

1 large tomato, chopped

$^1/_2$ Tbs Marsala wine (optional)

1 15-ounce can pinto beans

2–4 Tbs fresh chives and/or parsley (optional)

Combine the TVP and boiling water in a bowl and set aside. Meanwhile, heat oil in a large stock pot; add onions and sauté until soft (about 3 minutes). Next, add garlic, carrots, celery, pepper, mushrooms, lemon juice, and spices. Cook over medium heat covered for 5 minutes.

Stir in TVP, beans, chopped tomato, and crushed tomatoes. Bring to a simmer. Cook uncovered over low heat for 15 minutes, stirring occasionally. Add Marsala wine and tomato paste, and simmer again for an additional 5 minutes. Remove pot from heat and stir in fresh herbs. Ladle the chili into bowls and garnish with a dollop of low-fat sour cream and chopped red onion. Serve with a fresh loaf of whole-grain bread.

*continues*

*continued*

<u>Nutrition Analysis for One Serving (Chili Only)</u>
Calories: 330
Total fat: 2.4 grams
Saturated fat: 0 grams
Dietary fiber: 14 grams
Protein: 22 grams
Sodium: 400 mg
Cholesterol: 0 mg

*From the kitchen of Meredith Gunsberg M.S., R.D.*

## Scrambled Tofu

*Serves four*

16 ounces of firm tofu

Dash of ground cumin

5 Tbs of water

Dash of garlic powder

2 Tbs mellow barley light miso

Fresh ground pepper to taste

$1/2$ tsp Tumeric

Mash tofu in a small saucepan. In a separate bowl, whisk together all remaining ingredients. Heat tofu over medium flame, and immediately add in the miso mixture. Stir constantly until the scrambled tofu mixture is heated through. Serve hot with toast and ketchup if desired.

<u>Nutrition Analysis for One Serving (Tofu Only)</u>
Calories: 82
Total fat: 4 grams
Saturated fat: 1 gram
Dietary fiber: 0 grams
Protein: 8 grams
Sodium: 32 mg
Cholesterol: 0 mg

*From the kitchen of Meredith Gunsberg M.S., R.D.*

## Cucumber Yogurt Dip

*Serves four*

1 large cucumber, peeled, seeded, and grated

2 cloves garlic, pressed

1 cup nonfat plain yogurt

Juice of one small lemon

1 Tbs fresh dill, chopped fine

1–2 tsp fresh chives, chopped fine

Combine all ingredients (except chives and dill), and mix thoroughly. Sprinkle chives on top before serving. Serve with pita bread and plenty of raw vegetables. Yields just over 1 cup.

Nutrition Analysis for One Serving ($1/4$ of Dip)
Calories: 32
Total fat: 0 grams
Saturated fat: 0 grams
Dietary fiber: 0 grams
Protein: 3 grams
Sodium: 270 mg
Cholesterol: 0 mg

*From the kitchen of Meredith Gunsberg M.S., R.D.*

If you're thinking of becoming a vegetarian, you now know the basics. If you are already a vegetarian, check your food with the guidelines presented in this chapter and see how you stack up. And if you simply read this chapter because it was between Chapters 18 and 20—try substituting some of your meat meals with plant-based meals. Vegetarian entrees can offer food variety, interest, and perhaps a unique experience for your taste buds.

### The Least You Need to Know

➤ *Vegans* are the strictest and avoid all meats, dairy, and eggs. Lacto-vegetarians eat dairy but avoid all meat and eggs. Ovolacto-vegetarians eat dairy and eggs but avoid all meat.

➤ Vegetarians (especially vegans) need to be extra responsible about getting enough protein, calcium, vitamin D, vitamin B-12, iron, and zinc.

➤ A lot of non-animal foods provide protein. Nuts, seeds, legumes, and soy-based products are all great sources. The less strict lactos and ovolactos can also obtain protein from dairy products and eggs. The key for the vegetarian is to eat plenty of complementary proteins to get all that are required.

➤ Soy protein can help boost the protein, calcium, and iron content of almost any meal.

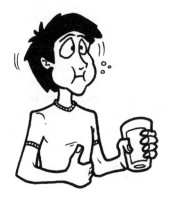

# Chapter 20

# Food Allergies and Other Ailments

> **In This Chapter**
>
> ➤ The lowdown on food allergies
>
> ➤ Diagnosing a true food allergy
>
> ➤ Different food sensitivities
>
> ➤ Living with a lactose intolerance
>
> ➤ Learning about celiac disease

Do you break out in hives at the mere mention of a peanut? Do you bolt for the bathroom after ingesting anything made with milk? Does the smell of seafood make your stomach churn? Hey, even my Grandma Mary sneezes repeatedly after devouring her favorite ice cream.

For millions of Americans, symptoms such as these turn the pleasurable act of eating into an uncomfortable and sometimes dangerous situation. In fact, an estimated two out of five American adults have some type of food sensitivity, ranging from severe food allergies to less serious (but often still bothersome) food intolerances. This chapter provides an inside look at the variety of food hypersensitivities and sorts through the confusion, controversy, and skepticism in the world of tasty offenders.

## Understanding Food Allergies

A true *food allergy* is a hypersensitive reaction that occurs when your immune system responds abnormally to harmless proteins in food. That is, your body misinterprets something good as an intruder and produces antibodies to "halt" the invasion. Remember the episode of *Three's Company* when Jack sneaked in late one night, and Chrissy and Janet mistook him for a robber and clobbered him over the head? It's the same thing with food allergies, only you're the one who gets clobbered.

The most common food culprits linked to allergic reactions are wheat, shellfish, nuts, soybeans, corn, the protein in cow's milk, and eggs. Furthermore, the organs most commonly affected are the skin (symptoms include skin rashes, hives, itching, and swelling), the respiratory tract (symptoms include difficulty breathing and "hay fever"), and the gastrointestinal tract (symptoms include nausea, bloating, diarrhea, and vomiting). Some allergic reactions are so severe they can even provoke anaphylactic shock, a life-threatening, whole-body response that requires immediate medical attention.

Here's a list of terms to know:

➤ **Food sensitivity** is a general term used to describe any abnormal response to food or food additive.

➤ **Food allergy** is an overreaction by the body's immune system, usually triggered by protein-containing foods (such as cow's milk, nuts, soybeans, shellfish, eggs, and wheat).

➤ **Anaphylactic shock** is a life-threatening, whole-body allergic reaction to an offending substance. Symptoms include swelling of the mouth and throat, difficulty breathing, drop in blood pressure, and loss of consciousness. In other words, get help fast!

➤ **Food intolerance** is an adverse reaction that generally does not involve the immune system (such as lactose intolerance).

➤ **Food poisoning** is an adverse reaction caused by contaminated food (micro-organisms, parasites, or other toxins).

➤ **Antibodies** are large protein molecules produced by the body's immune system in response to foreign substances.

**Food for Thought**

Statistics report that up to 7 percent of all infants and small children are allergic to certain foods, a much higher incidence than among American adults (less than 2 percent).

**Nutri-Speak**

The word **allergy** comes from the Greek words *allos*, meaning other, and *ergon*, meaning working. In other words, the immune system is working other than normally expected.

# Diagnosing a True Food Allergy

Many folks view this whole food-sensitivity business as faddism and quackery, and unfortunately, we have earned this mindset. Did you know that out of the gazillions of people who think they have a food allergy, less than 2 percent of the American adult population actually have one? Why does the idea of a food allergy get so recklessly thrown around? One reason may be that people are often quick to blame physical ailments on food. Another aggravating reason for all the misdiagnoses are those so-called "allergy quacks" that grab your hard-earned money and diagnose you with the "allergy of the month."

In today's world, a true food allergy can be properly diagnosed with scientifically sound testing. If you think you might suffer from an allergic response to certain foods, get it checked out. The first step is to find a qualified and reputable physician who has been certified by the American Board of Allergy and Immunology. Ask your primary doctor for a referral, *or* call the American Academy of Allergy and Immunology at 800-822-2762, and it'll set you up with a physician in your area. Next, schedule an appointment. Here's what you can expect:

➤ **Thorough medical history:** You'll give a detailed history of both your and your family's medical background. Special attention will be given to the type and frequency of your symptoms, along with when the symptoms occur in relation to eating food.

➤ **Complete physical examination:** You'll have a routine physical exam, with special focus on the areas where you experience the suspected food-allergy symptoms.

➤ **Food-elimination diets:** The doctor will probably have you keep a food diary while you eliminate all suspicious foods from your diet. The allergist might then tell you to slowly, one at a time, add these foods back to your diet so you can specifically identify which foods might cause an adverse reaction.

➤ **Skin tests:** An extract of a particular food is placed on the skin (usually arm or back) and then pricked or scratched into the skin to look for a reaction of itching or swelling. This isn't 100-percent reliable because people who aren't allergic can develop skin rashes. On the other hand, some people don't show skin reactions but do have allergic responses when they eat the food.

➤ **RAST test (radioallergosorbent test):** This test involves mixing small samples of your blood with food extracts in a test tube. If you are truly allergic to a particular food, your blood will produce antibodies to fight off the food extract. One advantage is that this test is performed outside your body, so you don't have to deal with the itching and swelling if the test is positive. Note: This test will only foretell an allergy, not the extent of sensitivity to the offending food.

➤ **Double-blind food-challenge tests:** This type of test must be performed under close supervision, preferably in an allergist's office or

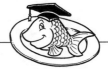

**Food for Thought**

For further information and a free newsletter on food allergies, send a self-addressed stamped envelope to:

The Food Allergy Network
10400 Eaton Place, Suite 107
Fairfax, VA 22030
800-929-4040

hospital, and it is considered the "gold standard" in food-allergy testing. Two capsules of dried food are prepared, one with the real McCoy and another with a nonreactive substance. Neither doctor nor patient knows which is which (a double-blind challenge). These challenges can rule out, as well as detect, allergies or intolerances to foods and other food substances such as additives.

## Treating a True Food Allergy

What's the treatment once you're diagnosed with a true food allergy? Avoid the offending food!

Although this list is not a substitute for consulting a registered dietitian, it can provide a pretty good idea of which food ingredients to avoid after you've been diagnosed with one of the following food allergies:

➤ **Cow's milk**—Check labels carefully and avoid all foods with the following ingredients: milk, yogurt, cheese, cottage cheese, custard, casein, whey, ghee, milk solids, curds, sodium caseinate, lactoglobulin, lactalbumin, milk chocolate, buttermilk, cream, sour cream, and butter.

➤ **Wheat**—Avoid all foods with the following ingredients: wheat, wheat germ, all-purpose flour, duram flour, cracker meal, couscous, bulgur, whole-wheat berries, cake flour, gluten flour, pastry flour, graham flour, semolina, bran, cereal or malt extract, modified food starch, farina, and graham.

➤ **Corn**—Avoid all foods with the following ingredients: fresh, canned, or frozen corn (regular and creamed), hominy, corn grits, maize, cornmeal, corn flour, corn sugar, baking powder, corn syrup, cornstarch, modified food starch, dextrin, malto-dextrins, dextrose, fructose, lactic acid, corn alcohol, vegetable gums, sorbitol, vinegar, and popcorn.

➤ **Soy**—Avoid all foods with the following ingredients: soy, lecithin, tofu, textured vegetable protein (TVP), tempeh, modified food starch, soy miso, soy sauce, teriyaki sauce, and soybean flour.

➤ **Nuts**—Folks who are allergic to peanuts and other types of nuts not only have to avoid the obvious plain nuts and nut butters, but also need to be on the lookout for "hidden" nuts tossed into baked goods, vegetarian dishes, candies, cereals, salads, and chicken stir-fry meals.

➤ **Eggs**—Avoid all foods that indicate the presence of an egg by listing any of the following ingredients: powdered or dry egg, egg white, dried egg

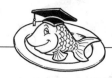

**Food for Thought**

Some people are diagnosed with allergies to food additives such as sulfites (food preservatives), tartrazine (food colorings), and MSG (flavor enhancer) and therefore must check ingredient labels with extreme care and ask a lot of questions when dining out.

yolk, egg substitute, eggnog, albumin, ovalbumin, ovomucin, ovomucoid, vitellin, ovovitellin, livetin, globulin, and ovoglobulin egg albumin.

➤ **Shellfish**—Avoid all shrimp, lobster, prawn, crab, crawfish, crayfish, clams, oysters, scallops, snails, octopus, squid, mussels, and geoducks.

Some people have such severe food allergies that they can even exhibit symptoms from the following:

➤ Kissing the lips of someone who has eaten the offending food

➤ Just smelling and inhaling the offending food while it cooks

➤ Coming into contact with utensils that have touched the offending food

# What's the Difference Between Allergy and Intolerance?

The difference lies in how your body handles the offending food. A food allergy affects the body's immune system; a food intolerance generally affects the body's metabolism. In other words, the body cannot properly digest a food or food substance, resulting in "intestinal chaos"—a.k.a. the gurgles.

## What's Lactose Intolerance All About?

If you can't stomach milk and you experience bloating, nausea, cramping, excessive gas, or a bad case of the runs after eating a dairy food, you are not alone. In fact, an estimated 30 to 50 million Americans suffer from some degree of lactose intolerance, which is the inability to digest the milk sugar *lactose*. In fact, I once had a client tell me he visited so many men's rooms while touring through Europe he was ready to write *The Complete Idiot's Guide to European Bathrooms.*

Why can't some people tolerate dairy foods? People who are lactose intolerant are unable to produce enough of the enzyme *lactase*, which is responsible for the digestion of lactose. Just imagine trying to tear down a skyscraper without a bulldozer; it's not gonna happen! Just like the bulldozer, *lactase* must break down, digest, and absorb lactose in the bloodstream. What's more, this type of intolerance affects people at different levels. Whereas one person might dash for the bathroom after just one sip of milk, others can tolerate small amounts of dairy without any problem.

**Food for Thought**

Don't confuse a lactose intolerance with a milk allergy. A lactose intolerance involves difficulty digesting the milk sugar lactose; a milk allergy involves an allergic reaction from the protein components in cow's milk. Folks who suffer from milk allergies cannot tolerate reduced-lactose products because the part of the milk they are allergic to (milk proteins) is still present.

Who generally tends to have a problem digesting milk?

➤ Up to 70 percent of the entire world's population does not produce enough of the enzyme lactase and therefore has some degree of lactose intolerance.

➤ In the United States alone, the following groups experience some or all symptoms of lactose intolerance:

More than 80 percent of Asian Americans

79 percent of Native Americans

75 percent of African Americans

51 percent of Hispanic Americans

21 percent of Caucasian Americans

➤ In rare cases, some people are born unable to produce the enzyme lactase due to a congenital defect.

➤ Following gastric surgery, people taking chronic antibiotics or anti-inflammatory drugs might also lose their ability (both short-term and long-term) to digest lactose.

➤ People might develop a temporary lactose intolerance during a bout of the flu, a stomach virus, or irritable bowel (spastic colon). During these instances, your doctor will probably tell you to avoid all milk and dairy because the enzyme lactase is easily destroyed with any stomach irritation. In these cases, when you recover, so does your ability to produce lactase.

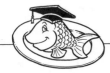

**Food for Thought**

For further information and a free brochure on lactose intolerance, call 800-LACTAID.

## Living with a Lactose Intolerance

The following tips are helpful for people who have difficulty digesting lactose. As mentioned earlier, the degree of lactose intolerance can vary from person to person; therefore, not everyone will be able to handle all of the suggestions. Give them each a shot, but be sure that you're in a comfortable place if some seem a bit risky. Keep in mind that lactose-containing foods are generally your best sources for the mineral calcium, so children and women with increased calcium requirements should load up on the non-dairy sources and speak with a registered dietitian about the possibility of calcium supplementation.

➤ Carefully look through the list of food ingredients and check for obvious and disguised lactose, including milk, cheese, cream, margarine, sour cream, milk solids, milk chocolate, whey, curds, malted milk, and skim-milk solids. Remember that people with severe lactose problems might not be able to tolerate even the small amounts in pancakes, biscuits, cookies, cakes, instant potatoes, salad dressings, sauces, gravies, lunch meats, soups, powdered coffee creamers, and whipped toppings.

➤ Be aware that a lot of over-the-counter medications have added lactose. Speak with your pharmacist if you're not completely sure.

➤ Although most lactose-intolerant people can't gulp down a straight glass of milk, some can tolerate smaller amounts of dairy combined with other foods. For instance, try a bowl of cereal with fruit and milk, or a slice of pizza with a lot of veggies (easy on the cheese), or a ham sandwich with one slice of cheese.

➤ Some people with lactose intolerance can tolerate yogurt because the bacteria in the yogurt actually metabolizes the milk sugar lactose for you.

➤ Also try cultured buttermilk and sweet acidophilis milk. Some folks find them easier to digest than regular milk.

➤ When real ice cream is a lethal poison, try a non-dairy substitute such as Toffuti or Rice Dream.

➤ Stock up on special lactose-reduced products, including Dairy Ease and Lactaid milk, cottage cheese, yogurts, cream cheese, and ice cream.

➤ Try the special tablets and drops that you can add to regular milk; they will almost completely break down the lactose after about 24 hours in the fridge.

➤ Also look for special lactase enzyme pills in your pharmacy that you can swallow *before* eating or drinking a dairy product. This comes in handy when you think you might encounter a difficult situation.

➤ In severe cases, even the lactose-reduced products might not be tolerated. But don't cheat your body of calcium just because you can't stomach the dairy. Buy calcium-fortified juice, calcium-fortified soymilk, and any other calcium-fortified food products you can get. Note: Definitely speak with your physician or a registered dietitian about calcium supplementation.

**Food for Thought**

Despite the widespread notion that chocolate, sugar, dairy products, and other fatty foods are responsible for pimples, most dermatologists today rarely identify an underlying relationship between acne and diet.

# Celiac Disease: Life Without Wheat, Rye, Barley, and Oats

Another food-related condition (less common than lactose intolerance) is *gluten-sensitive enteropathy*, better known as *celiac disease* or *gluten intolerance*. Celiac disease is a chronic disorder found in genetically susceptible individuals who exhibit severe intestinal distress after eating anything made with *gluten*, a protein found in wheat, rye, barley, and oats. People with this condition must follow a lifelong diet, avoiding all offending foods, or suffer the potential for malnourishment from chronic diarrhea and nutrient malabsorption.

### Nutri-Speak

**Gluten Intolerance** is an intestinal disorder that involves Gluten—a protein component of many grains. Gluten is broken down into two parts; gliadin and glutenin. Gliadin is the portion that can be toxic to the small intestines and may result in malabsorption of vital nutrients.

### Food for Thought

For further info on celiac disease, write to
   Celiac Disease Foundation
   13251 Ventura Blvd., Suite 3
   Studio City, CA 91604–1838
   818-990-2354

For further reading on life without gluten or wheat, order
   *Against the Grain*
   Jax Peters Lowell
   Henry Holt and Company, Inc.
   800-488-5233

As you can imagine, life on this diet is no picnic: A bowl of pasta, a bagel, cereal, crackers, or even a slice of bread can send a celiac's intestines into a sumo-wrestling match. Obviously, with the tremendous amount of food restrictions, members of the Gluten-Free Club should consult with a knowledgeable nutritionist. What's more, become best friends with your local health-food store: It's celiac-friendly and will generally carry the specialty items you need.

# Irritable Bowel Syndrome

Although not completely understood, irritable bowel syndrome (IBS) seems to be more common these days than the sniffles. With symptoms ranging from excessive gas, cramping, bloating, and intermittent bouts of constipation and diarrhea, IBS (also called a spastic colon) usually has nothing to do with food allergies or intolerances. It's more likely a functional problem with the muscular movement of your intestines. In fact, it's generally diagnosed when the serious gastrointestinal ailments are ruled out. Some doctors say that people can even bring it on with anxiety or nerves.

Dietary treatments that can help alleviate the symptoms include eating slowly, increasing fiber gradually, reducing might also want to keep a food log for a week or two to see whether any particular foods exacerbate the symptoms. (Some common culprits include alcohol, tobacco, caffeine, fatty foods, beans, sorbitol, spicy foods, and cruciferous veggies such as cauliflower, cabbage, and broccoli.) Also, see whether there's a correlation between your work schedule and the days you're feeling bad; some people find that the symptoms improve on the weekends when they're relaxing.

You can also try alternative remedies such as taking enteric-coated capsules of peppermint oil three times a day between meals (skip this one if you have heartburn), or explore yoga, meditation, or hypnosis to lessen stress and anxiety, which can sometimes wind up in your gut. Also, for women who notice IBS flare-ups around the time of menstruation, take evening primrose oil or black cohosh.

# For the Caffeine-Sensitive

Some people are extremely sensitive to caffeine; they become dizzy, shaky, and sometimes nauseous. Here's a list of some beverages and foods to watch:

| Food/Beverage | Caffeine (in Milligrams) |
|---|---|
| *Coffee (5 oz Cup)* | |
| Drip | 110–150 |
| Percolated | 40–170 |
| Decaffeinated | 2–5 |
| Freeze-dried instant | 40–108 |
| Decaffeinated | 2–3 |
| *Tea (Bags or Loose, 5 oz)* | |
| 1-minute brew | 9–33 |
| 3-minute brew | 20–46 |
| 5-minute brew | 20–50 |
| Iced tea (12 oz) | 22–36 |
| *Chocolate Items* | |
| Hot cocoa (5 oz) | 2–15 |
| Dry cocoa (1 oz) | 6 |
| Chocolate milk | 8 |
| Milk chocolate (1 oz) | 15 |
| Bakers chocolate (1 oz) | 25 |
| *Soft Drinks (12 oz)* | |
| Diet and regular | 35–60 |
| Caffeine–free | 0 |

If you think you may be suffering from a food sensitivity or intolerance—check it out. Keep a detailed food log for one week and include everything you eat and drink—you may even want to include the times of day that you are eating and drinking. Pay close attention to your body's reaction and see if you can find any correlation to a single food (like peppers, oranges, beans) or an entire food group (like milk, yogurt and cheese). Also, you can meet with a registered dietitian who can help you determine the foods that are aggravating your system.

## The Least You Need to Know

➤ A food allergy is when your body misinterprets a harmless food as an intruder and produces antibodies to fight off the foreign substance.

➤ A food allergy affects the immune system, whereas a food intolerance generally affects only the digestive system.

➤ Lactose intolerance is the inability to produce enough of the enzyme *lactase,* which is responsible for digesting the milk sugar lactose. Symptoms include bloating, cramping, gas, diarrhea, and nausea.

➤ Celiac disease is a condition that causes severe malabsorption after ingesting the protein gluten, which is found in wheat, rye, oats, and barley.

➤ Irritable bowel syndrome is a functional problem with the muscular movement of the intestines, resulting in intermittent bouts of constipation, diarrhea, bloating, and gas.

# Herbal Remedies

Herbal remedies were once considered taboo, something only used by witch doctors. Now, botanical supplements are moving into the mainstream, and even traditional M.D.s are taking the alternative route.

Although extensive research on herbal medicine has been done, you should always be wary of what you're taking. Do your homework, know your manufacturers, and read the bottles carefully; some of the herbal remedies out there have not been proven to be safe and effective, and it isn't easy to track problems related to herbal products. If you're looking for an alternative way to relieve a particular ailment, go ahead and get down with the herbal vibe. Just tell your physician what you're taking, especially if you're on other medication. Also, be safe and don't combine several remedies at the same time (which could lead to serious side effects)—and never use them when you're pregnant or planning to become pregnant.

This chapter provides the lowdown on popular herbs that have been shown to do some pretty impressive things. Read on to see if one of them might be right for you.

## Judging the Quality of Herbal Products

It can be quite overwhelming to choose a particular herb—all those bottles tend to look alike in the health food store, vitamin shop, pharmacy, and grocery store. And although herbs have properties that can affect our bodies internal functions, there are no regulations on herbal supplements within the United States to date. In fact, this lack of regulation means that different manufacturers use different measures of active ingredients per dose, and some may be unreliable. The following list provides brand manufacturers that you can trust—and probably produce many or all of the herbal supplements discussed in the chapter.

- ➤ Nature's Way
- ➤ Nature's Sunshine
- ➤ Gaia (primarily tinctures)
- ➤ Frontier
- ➤ Indian Botanicals

If you are seriously interested in the herbal world, find an herb-friendly health professional. You can call the American Herbalists Guild at 435-722-8434 for a list of professional practitioners.

### Q & A

**Are all herbs safe since they are natural?**

Most herbs can be quite safe if taken as directed under most circumstances. However, because herbs can potentially have medicinal abilities—you should never take them lightly. Read labels closely, follow dosage directions, and discontinue if you experience any uncomfortable side effects like throat irritations, upset stomach, diarrhea and headaches. Also, some people may even experience an allergic reaction to a particular herb.

# For Female Health

Over the centuries, many herbal products have been created for the special needs and health concerns of women. This section will cover Valerian Root, Black Cohosh, and Evening Primrose Oil.

## Valerian Root (Valeriana Officinalis)

**Use:** Three decades of extensive research has shown that valerian root is like a minor tranquilizer. It is known as a sleeping aid, and it might be useful for insomnia, mild anxiety and restlessness, lowering blood pressure, and reducing symptoms of menstruation and menopause. To date, it has not been proven to be habit forming.

**Dosage:** Tea, *tincture*, or an extract; it can also be added to bath water for external application. Relatively large amounts are required for effectiveness, typically about 50 to 100 drops or 1 tsp of dried root for tea. Take one hour before bed and repeat the dose 2–3 times if needed. Beware: It has a horrible odor, so you might want to invest in the tablet or capsule version (150–300 mg, 300–500 mg to aid in anxiety). It's not safe for long-term use, and it has no effect with alcohol but might intensify the effect of sedatives.

## Black Cohosh

**Use:** Some women take this for PMS and meno-pausal symptoms, but nothing has been clinically verified in humans. (However, it is big in Europe.) It suppresses the leutinizing hormone and therefore helps control hormone surges that cause discomforting menopausal symptoms. Relieving physical symptoms can lead to improving the emotional symptoms. In other words, some women get entirely depressed because they feel so physically lousy. Improve the hot flushes, bloating, etc, and the depression can sometimes improve.

**Dosage:** Tincture, 10–60 drops. As tea, 1–2 grams Note: Do not use with estrogen-positive cancers; long-term usage is not recommended.

## Evening Primrose Oil

**Use:** It is a natural source of an unusual fatty acid called gamma-linolenic acid (GLA), which occurs in only a few other plants such as borage oil and black currant. It modifies the synthesis of a group of hormones called *prostaglandins*, which are believed to be involved in a variety of PMS symptoms and are the target of anti-inflammatory drugs such as Advil or Motrin. In layman's terms: You can use this to help heal hard-core PMS symptoms in addition to arthritis pains and autoimmune diseases. It's also a great anti-inflammatory—and it promotes healthy growth of hair, skin, and nails.

**Dosage:** The recommendation is one 500 mg capsule twice daily; it takes 6–8 weeks before you see results.

# For Male Health

Like women, men can also benefit from herbs that target their special needs. Although men do not

### Nutri-Speak

**Tincture** is a liquid extract that that utilizes a combination of ethyl alcohol and water as the solvent. The advantages of using tinctures are that they have an increased shelf life and do not have to be refrigerated. The disadvantages are that they contain alcohol which is a problem for people who abstain and for children—and they do not taste pleasant.

### Nutri-Speak

**Prostaglandins** are hormonelike compounds that were first discovered in the prostate gland (*prosto-glandins*). Abnormal secretions of these compounds are thought to contribute to PMS (Premenstrual Syndrome).

**Premenstrual Syndrome** is a cluster of symptoms, including both physical and emotional pain, that some women experience before and during the onset of menstruation.

commonly buy and take herbs as often as women—they are becoming more popular. Here are two herbs that cover important male issues—Saw Palmetto and Yohimbe.

## Saw Palmetto

**Use:** This herb is used for BPH (*benign prostatic hyperplasia*). It reduces the size of the prostate in BPH and has a diuretic property. It might also stimulate the appetite and enhance the sex drive.

**Dosage:** 160 mg twice daily. There are long-term contradictions and drug interactions, so consult with a physician before using. Note: You must use a condom while engaging in intercourse because the semen might cause fetal damage.

## Yohimbe

**Use:** This aphrodisiac dilates blood vessels of the skin and mucus membranes (including those of the sexual organs). It is a monoamine oxidase inhibitor, which means that you should strictly avoid nasal decongestants, foods containing tyramine (such as liver, cheese, and red wine), and certain diet aids containing phenylpropanolamine. The drug should not be taken by anyone suffering from hypotension (low blood pressure), hypertension (high blood pressure), diabetes, or heart, liver, or kidney diseases. Effectiveness of this herb/drug has not yet been proven, and in the U.S., it's declared unsafe and is unavailable. If you really want to make it a part of your daily intake, you might need to trek to Germany; it's available in every sex shop!

**Dosage:** Usually administered in 5.4 mg doses, it is available as a prescription drug in many combinations with other so-called sexual stimulants such as strychnine, thyroid, and methyltestosterone.

# For Depression, Sleeping, and Aging

Are you feeling restless, tense, depressed, or having trouble sleeping at night? Or, maybe you simply want to defy some of the signs of aging. Read on—this section examines six herbs that may be worth a try: Gingko Biloba, DHEA, St. John's Wort, Kava-Kava, Asian Ginseng, and Chamomile.

## Gingko Biloba

**Use:** Derived from the gingko tree and originating in China 200 million years ago, it has been used for centuries as a digestive aid. Tests have shown that it thins the blood and therefore increases circulation in the brain and extremities, making it good for enhancing the memory and easing symptoms of age-related cognitive decline and early-stage dementia. One recent study showed that it slowed the progression of Alzheimer's disease in 27 percent of participants.

**Dosage:** Large doses are required, which explains why a concentrate is used rather than the herb itself. The typical dosage is 120–160 mg, but beware: Large doses might cause restlessness, diarrhea, nausea, and vomiting. Do not take this with other blood thinners (it can intensify the action and cause serious problems), and look for the standardized leaf extract, containing 24 percent flavone and 6 percent terpenes. (It is available as tincture, capsule, or tablets.)

# DHEA

**Use:** DHEA is the most abundant hormone produced by the adrenal glands; in the body, it is converted to testosterone and estrogen. Hormone production declines with age in both men and women (10 percent every 10 years after your mid-20s), so this supplement helps to maintain normal sex hormone levels, as well as inhibit damaging forms of stress and increase the production of antioxidant enzymes in the liver.

**Dosage:** If you are under 40, you might not need it, and it should not be used when pregnant or nursing or if you have had prior ovarian, adrenal, or thyroid tumors. Side effects that can occur with doses over 50 mg per day include acne, irritability, fatigue, and hirsutism in women (abnormal coarse hair growth usually on the facial area).

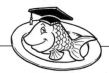

**Food for Thought**

A few drops of Lavender oil in the bath, can help you to relax. In fact, some say that after massaging your body with the lavender-bath water, you are more apt to have a sound sleep.

# St. John's Wort

**Use:** This herb might treat mild to moderate depression and seasonal affective disorder. Hypericin and pseudohypericin are the active ingredients, which aid in serotonin re-uptake inhibition in the brain. Although this might be one of the most popular and widely used herbs, its action as an antidepressant is not yet fully understood. Therefore, it is not a miracle drug or something that should be used lightly.

**Dosage:** It's based on the hypericin concentration in the extract. The minimal daily dosage recommended is 0.1 mg. Recommended dose is 300 mg of dried leaf and flower extract standardized to .3 percent hypericin three times per day; 40–80 drops of tincture three times per day; 1–2 cups of tea in the a.m. and p.m. made with 1–2 heaping tsp of dried herb per cup. It might take several weeks to kick in. Do not use with prescription antidepressants. Note: Might cause photosensitivity in those with particularly fair skin.

# Kava-Kava

**Use:** This herb addresses anxiety, tension, restlessness, stress, and insomnia. The relaxing properties of kava are related to kavalactones, the primary active ingredient. High-quality kava contains 5.5–8.3 percent of these compounds, which create changes in the brain activity that are similar to the effects of anti-anxiety drugs without their sedative or hypnotic effect.

**Dosage:** 140–210 mg divided over 2–3 doses. (Look for standardized extracts of 70 percent lactones.) Long-term consumption might turn the skin and nails yellow temporarily; if this occurs, stop taking immediately until the condition clears. This should not be taken with drugs that act on the central nervous system, such as alcohol, benzodiazepines, antidepressants, and barbiturates. Rare side effects include mild gastrointestinal disturbances.

## Asian Ginseng (a.k.a. Korean or Chinese)

**Use:** For supporting health—it alleviates fatigue or stress, enhances cognitive function and physical endurance, and aids in resistance to disease. It is widely used by athletes because of its ability to improve aerobic capacity and recovery time following exertion, but it does contain panaxosides, which have been shown to exert a hypoglycemic effect.

**Dosage:** 100 mg 1–2 times per day, usually used over a 2–3 week period, followed by 1–2 weeks of "rest" before resuming. In rare cases, it can cause over-stimulation, hence insomnia, and it is not recommended during pregnancy and lactation or for those with high blood pressure. Long-term use might cause menstrual abnormalities and breast tenderness in women.

## Chamomile

**Use:** This is known as a "cure-all," like Grandma's chicken soup. It's a cornerstone of European and American herbal medicine that has been used to treat irritable bowel syndrome, infant colic, mouth sores, anxiety, insomnia, menstrual cramps, and digestive problems.

**Dosage:** Because much of the value of the plant lies in its volatile oil, it is unfortunate that even a strong tea, properly prepared in a covered vessel and steeped for a long time, contains only about 10–15 percent of the oil originally present in the plant material. Whole extracts of the drug or preparations containing high quantities of the oil are more effective but are generally not marketed in the U.S. Boiling water is poured over a heaping tablespoon of dried flowers and strained after 10–15 minutes. You can drink it 3–4 times daily between meals. It might cause an allergic reaction in those with allergies to similar plants such as ragweed.

# Heart Disease

Heart disease remains to be a leading cause of death in both men and women. The following section provides information on two herbs that may help to fight heart disease; Garlic and Hawthorne.

## Garlic

**Use:** Garlic contains allicin, which lowers both cholesterol levels and blood pressure. There is evidence that garlic inhibits platelet aggregation, although it should not be used instead of stronger anti-clotting medication. It also has an overall positive effect on the cardiovascular system, and, according to some researchers, garlic stimulates the immune system, hence preventing cancer by hindering the growth of malignant cells.

**Dosage:** For therapeutic purposes, chew one fresh clove daily. (For *breath* purposes, you might want to follow it up with an Altoid, one of those "curiously strong mints!") There are also enteric-coated garlic-powder supplements, but note that the supplement should provide at least 5,000 mg allicin daily. Consumption of large quantities (five or more cloves daily) can result in heartburn, flatulence, and related gastrointestinal problems.

## Hawthorne

**Use:** Hawthorne is taken for cardiovascular ailments, including high blood pressure, hardening of the arteries, angina, and, potentially, early stages of congestive heart failure. It is not for acute attacks because the action is slow. This herb dilates the blood vessels, especially the coronary vessels, reducing peripheral resistance and thus lowering the blood pressure. It has a direct effect on the heart itself, which is especially noticeable in cases of heart damage.

**Dosage:** 160 mg of dried leaves and flowers (higher doses should only be used under strict M.D. supervision) or 20–40 drops of tincture 3 times daily.

# Liver Disease

The liver is one of the major organs that is impacted by alcohol and pharmaceutical drugs. This section reviews Milk Thistle—an impressive herb that has been shown to protect and regenerate the liver.

## Milk Thistle

**Use:** Milk thistle is taken for chronic inflammatory liver disease, such as cirrhosis and hepatitis, as well as more acute conditions such as toxic liver damage. It protects healthy liver cells or cells that are not yet damaged from the entry of toxic substances.

**Dosage:** Insoluble in water, it is ineffective if taken as a tea. (Studies show that less than 10 percent of the active ingredient is available in this form.) Use seed extracts standardized to at least 70 percent silymarin (the antihepatotoxic principle). The suggested daily dose provides 200 mg of concentrated extract 3 times daily in the treatment of liver disease, representing 140 mg of silymarin per capsule (in total, 420 mg daily). You can use one 200 mg dose as part of a cleansing/detoxification program. It might have mild laxative effects in some people.

# Respiratory Ailments

One of the top selling herbs in the United States, Echinacea has become an everyday household name. From fighting colds to ear infections, this section will run through everything you'll need to know.

# Echinacea

**Use:** Echinacea is popular for the prevention and treatment of the common cold and flu and adjunctive treatment in recent infections (middle ear, respiratory tract, urinary tract, and vaginal candidiasis). It is also an immunity booster. The myth that it's more effective with goldenseal is not true.

**Dosage:** 15–30 drops of tincture up to 5 times a day at the onset of cold symptoms and continued for least 10–14 days after. This varies, however, with the potency of the product—so read the bottle that you buy. Teas are not recommended because some of the active ingredients are not soluble in water. If you use it to prevent a cold, take echinacea three times daily for six to eight weeks. A "rest" period is recommended after eight weeks because its effects might diminish if used longer. Caution: Do not take echinacea if you have an autoimmune disease (MS or HIV).

# Arthritis

Arthritis involves the painful inflammation of joints—and can be caused by various conditions. If you are suffering from a form of arthritis, you may want to try one of these two supplements; Boswella and Glucosamine Chondroiten. Of course, before you pop any pill check with your physician—especially if you are already taking other medication.

## Boswella

**Use:** This is intended for the treatment of rheumatoid arthritis and osteoarthritis. It is a non-steroidal, anti-inflammatory agent that improves mobility and decreases joint pain and stiffness. At this point, it is still unclear whether long-term effects will reduce joint destruction.

**Dosage:** 150 mg, 3 times per day, lasting 8–12 weeks.

## Glucosamine and Chondroiten

Although this supplement is *not* herbal, it's still considered alternative and is definitely worth mentioning within this chapter.

**Use:** The combination of the two (glucosamine and chondroiten) is shown to slow and eventually eliminate osteoarthritis in many patients. In fact, it's estimated that up to 40 percent of osteoarthritis sufferers might see marked improvement after taking this supplement for approximately 2 months.

Glucosamine stimulates the production of collagen, which is the protein portion of a fibrous substance that holds the joints together in addition to being the main shock-absorbing substance that acts as a cushion between our joints. Hence, glucosamine helps the body repair damaged cartilage and eases the pain of osteoathritis.

Chondroiten sulfates act as "liquid magnets," helping to attract the fluid to the cartilage, which acts as a buffer. Chondroiten might also protect existing cartilage from premature breakdown by inhibiting certain enzymes that can destroy the cartilage.

**Dosage:** 1,500 mg per day of glucosamine and 1,200 mg per day of chondroiten. Note: The initial dosage should be adjusted according to your weigh, and you should speak with your physician about adjusting the dose when you are ready for a maintenance level.

# Migraines

Migraines are characterized by severe head pain, plus one or more of a range of symptoms including nausea, vomiting, and sensitivity to light. A migraine attack can last up to 72 hours and leave a person completely immobile. This section provides information on Feverfew—an herb that may help to alleviate these debilitating headaches.

## Feverfew

**Use:** This herb inhibits platelet aggregation and also helps prevent the vessels from constricting. The result is a reduction in severity, duration, and frequency of migraines and an improvement in blood-vessel tone.

**Dosage:** 125 mg of dried authentic feverfew leaf, containing a minimum of 0.2 percent of panthenolide, taken over a period of 4 to 6 weeks. The most common side effect is mouth ulceration, predominantly found in those who chew the leaves. (This should not be used by children.)

# Cancer

The incidence of cancer is quite low in the Asian countries. Therefore, scientists constantly conduct research to investigate, which of their cultural practices may help ward off this horrific illness. This section will provide you with some exciting news about Green Tea—and then you can read more in Chapter 18, "Diet and Cancer."

## Chinese Green Tea

**Use:** Green tea presents cancer-fighting properties that inhibit the interaction of tumor promoters, hormones, and growth factors with their receptors, which sort of seals off the tumor, preventing it from growing.

**Dosage:** The more tea you drink, the better it will be. It's nontoxic, but watch out for the caffeine.

# More Herbal Remedies Worth Mentioning

Yes, there are even more herbs to talk about. Find out how Ginger can settle your stomach, Bilberry can help your eyes, Rosemary can get your blood pumping, Peppermint can aid in indigestion, and Aloe can heal your wounds.

# Ginger

**Use:** Ginger might relieve motion sickness, nausea from morning sickness, and indigestion or an upset stomach. It has an overall calming effect on the digestive system because it increases the secretion of digestive juices, including saliva, neutralizing stomach acids, and toxins.

**Dosage:** Take capsules containing 500 mg of the powdered herb; the total daily dosage should not exceed 1 gram. It can also be consumed in the form of a tea of as candied ginger. Take 1,000 mg 30 minutes before traveling for motion sickness; 2 cups of tea using 1 tsp of fresh root or $1^1/_2$ tsp of powdered root per cup; or two 1-inch squares of candied ginger.

# Bilberry

**Use:** Taking bilberry addresses retinopathy, prevention of senile cataracts and macular degeneration, peripheral vascular disease, varicose veins, and hemorrhoids. It promotes the formation of normal connective tissue and protects from damage secondary to inflammation.

**Dosage:** Extract standardized to 25 percent anthocyanoside content is recommended at a daily dose of 480–600 mg in 2–3 divided doses, which may be reduced to a maintenance dose of 240 mg per day. The lower dose can be used by those interested in the prevention of eye or circulation disorders.

# Rosemary

**Use:** It'll spice up more than just that roast chicken—your entire circulatory system! Recommended for its tonic, astringent, and diaphoretic effects (it increases perspiration), rosemary is said to aid in digestion and can be made into a hair tonic that will prevent baldness. It is also great for those with low blood pressure and can be used to stimulate menstruation.

**Dosage:** Infused in tea, wine, a spirit, or a bath. Large quantities of the oil are needed for therapeutic purposes, and it's not safe when taken internally. (It can irritate the stomach, intestines, and kidneys.)

# Peppermint

**Use:** Peppermint has served as treatment for indigestion, flatulence, colic, and even menstrual cramping. Methol, the active ingredient, can aid in digestion because it reduces tonus of the lower esophageal sphincter and facilitates belching for relief.

**Dosage:** Taken in tea prepared from the leaves. Drink several cups for relief.

# Aloe

Aloe has two products that are completely different in terms of usage and chemical composition.

Aloe vera gel or mucilage is a thin, clear jelly-like substance that is used externally to treat wounds and sunburn. Although there is controversy about whether aloe gel retains its properties in preparation, fluid from a fresh leaf has shown to promote attachment and growth of normal human cells. This type of aloe is recommended as an external wound healer.

Aloe latex or juice is quite different. In fact, it acts as a laxative and is clearly not recommended.

# ...And Stay Away from These!

The following herbs might appear in over-the-counter products. Read labels and stay away; they have been shown to be dangerous!

# Ephedra/Ma Huang

**Use:** This herb has been taken to relieve constriction and congestion associated with bronchial asthma. It is also used as a nasal decongestant, to treat certain allergies, and to promote weight loss.

The real story is that it increases both systolic and diastolic blood pressure as well as the heart rate, which causes palpitations, nervousness, headaches, insomnia, and dizziness. It can be harmful and life-threatening—especially for those who suffer from heart conditions, hypertension, diabetes, and thyroid disease.

# Don Quai

**Use:** Some women have taken this herb to treat gynecological complaints, such as irregular periods and menopausal symptoms.

The real story is that excess dosage can negatively effect blood pressure, heart rhythm, and respiration.

Using herbs can be a convenient way to alleviate everything from headaches to upset stomachs. Use this chapter as a reference guide, and look things up when you are searching for a cure to a particular ache or ailment. Once again, I cannot stress the importance of checking things out with your physician—especially if you are taking medication and/or have a serious illness.

## The Least You Need to Know

➤ In the last decade, herbal remedies have become popular treatments for a variety of ailments. If you want to get into herbal culture, do it slowly and monitor yourself as you go along.

➤ Never indulge in herbal remedies when you're pregnant, planning on becoming pregnant, or lactating.

➤ Always consult with a physician before using herbs, especially if you're already taking other prescription drugs.

➤ Do some research: Know your manufacturers, be aware of what you're taking, read the bottles, and follow the instructions carefully. Adverse reactions are not uncommon.

➤ Avoid Don Quai and Ephedra (Ma Huang); they can affect blood pressure and heart rate in a negative manner.

# Part 5
# Pregnancy and Parenting

*Let the cravings begin! Being pregnant is both exciting and overwhelming, and the importance of good nutrition for mothers-to-be has been stressed over and over again. What's more, today most health experts also encourage exercise, which can help keep moms feeling more fit and mobile during their nine months of growing girth. Read on; in this section, I provide a lot of essential information that will help to manage your and your child's health.*

*This section is also dedicated to the younger folks. As a mother and nutritionist, I understand that sometimes it can be quite a challenge to get your kids to eat healthy. If we could only mold carrots and bananas into log shapes and pop a "Snickers" wrapper on top, life would be so much simpler. In this section, I'll offer creative suggestions for sneaking veggies into meals, making lower-fat after-school snack ideas, and provide tips to encourage more physical activity. Then, I'll address the college crowd and map out the best bites in the campus dining hall, along with the real deal on vending machines, late night munchies, and alcohol and partying and, of course, how to avoid those notorious "freshman 15" pounds that creep up on a lot of college students.*

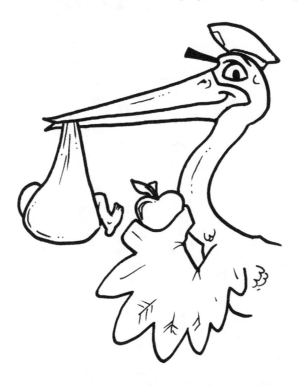

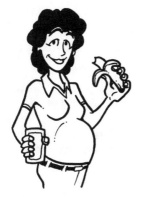

# Eating Your Way Through Pregnancy

Yippee, you're pregnant—congratulations on your exciting news! This chapter provides all the info you'll need to properly nourish yourself *and* your growing baby.

## Are You Really Eating for Two?

Has anyone ever said, "Go ahead and pack it in; you're eating for two"? Well, that's both true and false. *True* because your food selections will directly affect your growing baby. In other words, eat plenty of quality foods, loaded with nutrients, and you'll shower that growing bambino with all the right ingredients—and if you eat junk, your baby gets junk!

On the other hand, this statement is also *false* because you're clearly *not* eating for two adults. In fact, your growing baby is only a fraction of your size—so it's not the time to win a gold medal in the food Olympics.

## Increased Calories and Protein

It's true that you do require more calories. In fact, over the course of your pregnancy, you'll need to consume about an extra 70,000 calories. Obviously, this caloric increase is spread out over nine months: It ends up approximately 150 extra calories a day during the first trimester (the first three months) and around 300 extra calories a day during the second and third trimesters (the last six months).

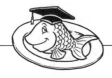

**Food for Thought**

You don't need to gain that much weight during the first trimester of your pregnancy. In fact, aim for a total of 2–5 pounds.

You'll also need an additional 10 grams of protein within those extra daily calories. Your daily dose goes from 50 to 60 grams when you're pregnant, for the development of your precious fetus. Getting this increased protein is *not* typically a problem. Most women already overshoot their needs, and consuming extra dairy and larger servings of lean meat, fish, poultry, eggs, and legumes will ensure that you get enough. For a more detailed description on how much protein you'll need, see the section "Adjusting Your Eating Plan," later in this chapter.

## A Weighty Issue: How Many Pounds Should You Gain?

It always seems like the first thing everyone asks when you return from your doctor's office is "How much weight did you gain?" None of their business! Understand that all women are different—and the rate and speed will vary from person to person. Some gain a lot in the second trimester, and then it drastically slows down in the third— whereas others have a nice, even gain throughout. Here's what's recommended for most healthy women:

| Pre-Pregnancy Weight | Suggested Gain | Weekly Gain in Second and Third Trimester |
| --- | --- | --- |
| Underweight Below 90% of desirable weight | 28–40 pounds | >1 pound |
| Normal weight (see range in Chapter 26) | 25–35 pounds | .8–1 pound |
| Moderately overweight More than 120–135% of desirable weight | 15–25 pounds | .7 pounds |
| Very overweight More than 135% of desirable weight | 15–20 pounds | .5 pounds |

Keep in mind that "desirable" weights fall within a range. You can see where you stand "pre-pregnancy" by comparing your weight in pounds with the height/weight chart in Chapter 26, "Come On, Knock It Off." Also, understand that there are special circumstances where some women will *need* to gain more, some less. For instance, women carrying twins will need to gain about 35–45 pounds, and although women with triplets almost *never* carry full term, (they typically deliver around 33 weeks) if they did, they would need to gain in the vicinity of 50–70 pounds—*and hire three full-time nannies and a massage therapist.* Rap with your doctor and listen to his or her advice on this weighty issue.

## Q & A

**Where does the extra weight go?**

Baby: 7–8 pounds
Placenta 1–2 pounds
Amniotic fluid: 1$\frac{1}{2}$–2 pounds
Uterine tissue: 2 pounds
Breast tissue: 1–2 pounds
Fluid volume: 6–10 pounds
Fat: 6+ pounds
*Total: 25–35 pounds*

# Adjusting Your Eating Plan

Let's ensure that you're gaining weight with the proper foods. Remember those five friendly food groups that have haunted you since page 1? *They're baa-ack.* Although individual requirements vary depending on calorie needs, the following chart gives some guidance in determining the basics of your diet:

| Food Group | Daily Servings | Sample Servings |
| --- | --- | --- |
| Breads/grains | 6+ | 1 slice bread, or $\frac{1}{2}$ small bagel, or 1 serving cereal, or $\frac{1}{2}$ cup cooked rice or pasta |
| Fruits | 3+ | 1 medium fruit, or 1 cup berries or melon, or $\frac{1}{2}$ cup fruit juice |
| Vegetables | 3+ | 1 cup raw leafy veggies, or $\frac{1}{2}$ cup cooked veggies |
| Milk/yogurt/cheese | 3–4 | 1 cup milk, or 1 cup yogurt, or $\frac{3}{4}$ cup cottage cheese, or 1 $\frac{1}{2}$ ounces of hard cheese |
| Meat/poultry/fish | 2–3 | 2–3 ounces lean meat, or 2 eggs (limit 2 per week), or $\frac{2}{3}$ cup of tofu, or 2–3 ounces of fish or poultry |
| Fluids | 8+ | 8 ounces of water, seltzer, and other beverages |
| Fats/sweets | Moderation | Try your best to keep these foods to a minimum. |

# Why All the Hype on Calcium?

Although calcium is needed throughout life, it is particularly important during pregnancy. (At last, you finally learn why everyone pesters you to drink your milk.) Your daily requirements remain at 1,000 milligrams—but some experts recommend up to 1,500 milligrams. That's approximately 3–4 servings of dairy (for example, 1 cup of milk + 1 cup pudding + 1 cup fruit yogurt + 1½ ounces of hard cheese).

## Q & A

**Won't the prenatal vitamins cover all the calcium my baby will need?**

Definitely not! Prenatal supplements supply about 200–250 milligrams per pill; that's not even one serving from the dairy group.

As you learned in Chapter 8, "Mighty Minerals: Calcium and Iron," calcium is responsible for strong bones and teeth, for the proper functioning of blood vessels, nerves, and muscles, as well as maintaining healthy connective tissue. During pregnancy, calcium is especially critical because you have to worry about your own bones *and* your growing baby's bones, tissues, and teeth as well. In fact, your baby counts on *your* calcium for normal development, therefore, when you skimp on the calcium-rich foods (and don't take supplementation), the calcium in your bones will be supplied to meet the increased demands of the growing fetus. In other words, you'll be placing yourself at a much greater risk for osteoporosis. See Chapter 8 for the calcium content of various foods, both dairy and nondairy.

### Overrated—Undercooked

Don't think, "Hey, I'm pregnant; I can eat *whatever* and *whenever* I want!" With pregnancy comes increased caloric and nutrient requirements, but you can meet these needs without putting on 20 pounds of flub. Don't deprive yourself of cravings; that's one of the fun things about pregnancy. (Cap'n Crunch was one of mine.) Just don't go overboard. Extra weight gained during your pregnancy is extra weight you'll be wearing *after* the baby is born.

## Hiking Up the Iron

Ever wonder why the prenatal vitamins are loaded with iron? It's because during pregnancy, your body requires about double the amount of this mineral than usual. In fact, you go from normally needing 15 milligrams to requiring a daily dose of 30 milligrams when you're expecting.

Why do pregnant women require more iron? Remember, iron is found in your blood and is responsible for carrying and delivering oxygen to every cell in your body. Pregnant women have an *expanded* blood volume, so it makes sense that more blood requires more iron. Also, you have to supply oxygen to both your cells *and* the cells of your growing baby. Once again, this greater demand for oxygen requires greater amounts of iron.

Because nursing your baby *also* requires an increase in a variety of nutrients, nursing women will also benefit from following the same general eating guidelines discussed in this chapter. Take a look:

|  | **Before** | **Pregnant** | **Lactating** |
| --- | --- | --- | --- |
| Calories | Varies | +300 | +500 |
| Protein (g) | 50 | 60 | 65 for first six months<br>62 for second six months |
| Calcium (mg) | 1,000 | 1,000 | 1,000 |
| Folic Acid (mg) | 400 | 600 | 500 |
| Iron (mg) | 15 | 30 | 15 |

*These requirements are for healthy women 19–50 years of age.*

Just because the prenatal vitamins are brimming with the stuff, don't think you can slack off in the food department. Understand that prenatal supplements (providing around 30–60 milligrams) are merely "just in case"—you still need to eat a lot of iron-rich foods. On the eating plan, you require 2–3 servings of protein foods each day. This will help satisfy your body's extra demand for *both* protein and iron because the best absorbable iron is found in the foods within this group. For further tips on boosting your iron, flip back to Chapter 8:

➤ **Best sources of heme iron:** Animal foods such as liver, beef, pork, lamb, veal, chicken, turkey, and eggs.

➤ **Good sources of nonheme iron:** Non-animal foods such as enriched breads and cereals, beans, dried fruits, seeds, nuts, broccoli, spinach, collard greens, broccoli, barley, chickpeas, and blackstrap molasses.

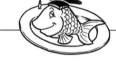

**Food for Thought**

Pregnant women with lactose intolerance should eat plenty of *nondairy* calcium-fortified foods, along with the special lactose-reduced products. Also, speak with your physician about calcium supplementation. (For further information on lactose intolerance, see Chapter 20, "Food Allergies and Other Ailments.")

# Blast Your Baby with Vitamins!

During pregnancy you want to provide your growing baby with plenty of nutrients—including the antioxidants: vitamin C and beta carotene. Read on and learn which fruits and vegetables supply the biggest bang for your buck.

➤ **Fruits rich in vitamin C:** Orange, grapefruit, mango, strawberries, papaya, raspberries, tangerine, kiwi, cantaloupe, guava, lemon, orange juice, grapefruit juice, and other vitamin C fortified juices.

➤ **Vegetables rich in vitamin C:** Broccoli, tomato, sweet potato, pepper, kale, cabbage, brussels sprouts, rutabaga, cauliflower, and spinach.

➤ **Fruits rich in beta carotene:** Apricot, cantaloupe, papaya, mango, prunes, peach, nectarine, tangerine, watermelon, and guava.

➤ **Vegetables rich in beta carotene:** Broccoli, brussels sprouts, carrots, collard greens, escarole, dark green lettuce, spinach, sweet potato, kale, butternut squash, chicory, red pepper, and tomato juice.

# Keep on Drinkin', Sippin', Gulpin', and Guzzlin'!

Proper hydration is another vital component for a healthy pregnancy. Did you know that the average female is about 55–65 percent water, and the average newborn is about 85 percent water? During this nine-month period of bodily change, shift, and growth (to put it mildly), your fluid demands skyrocket for the following reasons:

➤ You need to maintain your *expanded* blood supply and fluid volume. You see, through the blood and lymphatic system, water helps deliver oxygen and other nutrients all over your body.

➤ Like always, fluids are needed to help wash down your food and assist in nutrient absorption.

➤ Extra fluids, along with fiber, can help to alleviate some of the bothersome plumbing problems (alias "mom-to-be" constipation).

➤ Fluid provides a cushion for the developing fetus and also helps lubricate your joints.

➤ Lastly, fluid is needed for the normal functioning of *every* cell in your body.

"Favorable fluids" you should be guzzling down include water, club soda, bottled water, vegetable juice, seltzer, fruit juice, and low-fat milk.

Liquids you should steer clear of are alcohol, coffee, tea, soft drinks, diet cola (and other artificially sweetened drinks), and questionable herbal teas.

Also realize that in some instances, you might need even *more* than the already increased amount: for example, if you're perspiring in hot weather, or when you're exercising, or if you have any type of fever, vomiting, or diarrhea. (Obviously, in the last case, contact your doctor immediately.)

# Foods to Forget!

The following is a suggested list of foods to *avoid* until after the baby is born:

➤ **Raw foods:** Because these foods can increase your risk for bacterial infection, avoid anything raw, including sushi and other seafood, beef tartar, undercooked poultry, raw or unpasteurized milk, soft cooked and poached eggs, or raw egg that's possibly found in eggnog, cookie dough, caesar salads, and milkshakes.

➤ **Nitrates, nitrites, and nitrosamines:** These are possible cancer-causing chemicals and are found in hot dogs, bacon, bologna, and other processed cold cuts.

➤ **Alcohol:** Because alcohol can damage the developing fetus (fetal alcohol syndrome), avoid all beer, wine, and liquor.

➤ **Caffeine:** Although there is insufficient evidence to conclude that caffeine adversely affects reproduction in humans, it does pass through the placenta and into the baby's body. Therefore, it is smart to avoid coffee, tea, and other highly caffeinated beverages—but speak with your personal physician.

➤ **Herbal teas:** Some herbal teas can have medicinal properties. Check out anything questionable with your nutritionist or physician before assuming that it's okay to drink.

➤ **MSG:** Monosodium glutamate can cause uncomfortable side effects for the pregnant mom, including headaches, dizziness, and nausea.

➤ **Artificial sweeteners:** This is a tough judgment call. Although some health professionals claim artificial sweeteners are perfectly safe during pregnancy, others say you should completely avoid them. In my opinion, why play around with your baby's health? You can live without them for nine months.

## Q & A

**What is gestational diabetes?**

Gestational diabetes is the onset of high blood sugar (or carbohydrate intolerance) that is generally detected around the 28th week of pregnancy. Because this condition is caused by the placenta putting out large doses of anti-insulin hormones, as soon as the placenta is removed (during the baby's delivery), the condition disappears in almost all cases. Women diagnosed with gestational diabetes have very specific dietary concerns and should work with a qualified nutritionist (registered dietitian) on appropriate meal planning.

# The Many Trials and Tribulations of Having a Baby

When embarking on the road to motherly bliss, some women glow and others, shall I say, turn green. I was one of the unlucky green women. Although agonizing and uncomfortable (to put it *mildly*), these lousy side effects, including constipation, nausea, water retention, and heartburn, are merely normal pregnancy occurrences and most certainly worth the beautiful end product.

**Food for Thought**

Getting enough of the vitamin folic acid can *drastically* reduce the risk for babies born with neural tube defects such as spina bifida. So fill up on the green leafy veggies and get precautionary backup from a prenatal vitamin that supplies folic acid.

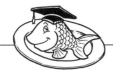

**Food for Thought**

Sometimes, the increased iron can cause constipation, diarrhea, dark-colored stools, and abdominal discomfort. Don't be alarmed; it's just par for the course. Be sure to increase your fiber and fluids and move around as much as possible.

## The "Uh-Oh, Better Get Drano" Feeling

Most pregnant women experience the constipation blues at one time or another during the nine-month haul. Why does food tend to stop dead in its tracks before reaching its final destination anyway? Unfortunately, there are a bunch of explanations:

➤ Hormonal changes

➤ The increased pressure on your intestinal tract as your baby grows

➤ All of the extra iron in your prenatal supplements

➤ Not enough fiber in your diet

➤ Not drinking enough fluids

➤ Plain old lack of exercise

Yes, it's true that the first three circumstances are completely uncontrollable, but let's focus on the last three: fiber, fluid, and exercise, which are quite controllable and can *dramatically* decrease your plumbing problems.

First, increase your dietary fiber by eating more fresh fruit, veggies, and whole grain foods. Better yet, flip back to the fiber chapter (Chapter 6, "In and Out with Fiber") and read the tips for boosting your daily intake. Next, drink a ton of fluids. Stay tuned for Chapter 23, "Exercising Your Way Through Pregnancy," which provides exercise guidelines during pregnancy.

## Ugh! That Nagging Nausea

Commonly known as "morning sickness," the awful nausea and vomiting can occur at *any* time of the day, so don't be misled. One bit of reassuring news: Although horridly unpleasant, it's *normal* and thought to simply be a side effect from the hormonal changes that take place during pregnancy. If you're on a first-name basis with your toilet, hang in there; the nausea usually disappears by week 14.

Here are some tips to help reduce the nausea:

➤ Nibble on carbohydrate-rich foods throughout the day. They are easy to digest and will provide your body with some energy (calories). For example, bagels, pretzels, crackers, cereal, and rice cakes are all primo snacks.

➤ If you tend to be nauseated in the early morning, keep some of the preceding carbs by your bed. Pop something into your mouth *before* getting up; this will start the digestive process and get rid of excess stomach acid.

➤ Most women find cold foods easier to tolerate than hot foods; however, everyone is unique. What makes one woman sick might be soothing to another. In other words, listen to your own body and go ahead with whatever works best for you.

➤ Avoid any sharp cooking odors, and open the windows for some fresh air.

➤ When you just can't take solid foods, suck on an ice pop or frozen fruit bars or sip on lemonade and fruit juice.

➤ Avoid high-fat foods because they sit longer in your stomach and can exacerbate the nausea.

➤ Sometimes, iron supplements can intensify nausea. If you are taking iron pills, take them with a snack or two hours after a meal with some ginger ale. If the nausea persists, you might also want to speak with your doctor about possibly holding off on the iron until you feel better.

➤ Do *not* take prenatal vitamins on an empty stomach; take them with a meal or snack.

*Contact your doctor immediately if you have persistent vomiting, are losing weight, or are too nauseated to take in fluids.*

## What's All the Swelling About?

Edema is the uncomfortable swelling, or retention of water, that occurs primarily in your feet, ankles, and hands during pregnancy. As long as there's no increase in blood pressure or protein in the urine, edema is normal and unfortunately tends to get worse in the last trimester. However, there is no need to panic; most of this bothersome fluid will be lost during and shortly after your baby's delivery.

Make yourself more comfortable from the effects of edema:

➤ Lie down with your feet elevated on a pillow.

➤ Remove all of your tight rings.

➤ Wear loose, comfortable shoes.

➤ Ease up on the salty stuff such as sauerkraut, pickles, soy sauce, salty pretzels, and chips.

➤ *Never* restrict your fluid intake; always continue to drink plenty of fluids.

## Oh, My Aching Heart

Contrary to the name, *heartburn* is actually a burning sensation in your lower esophagus that is usually accompanied by a sour taste. Although this dreadful feeling can happen at any time during your pregnancy, it's most common toward the last few months, when your baby is rapidly growing and exerting pressure on your stomach and uterus. What's more, during pregnancy, the valve between your stomach and esophagus can become relaxed, making it easy for the food to occasionally reverse directions.

Some simple remedies to ease heartburn:

➤ Relax and eat your food slowly.

➤ Instead of eating a lot at one sitting, eat several smaller meals throughout the day.

➤ Limit fluids *with* meals, but increase fluids *between* meals.

➤ Chew gum or suck candy. Of course, your dentist will hate me, but it can help to neutralize the acid.

➤ Never lie flat after you have eaten. In fact, keep your head elevated when you sleep with the help of extra pillows and by placing a couple of books underneath the mattress to help tilt it slightly upward.

➤ Avoid wearing tight clothing. Stick with items that are loose and comfortable.

➤ Stand up and walk around. This can help encourage your gastric juices to flow in the right direction.

➤ Keep a log and track some foods that might be triggering your heartburn. Some common culprits include regular and decaf coffee, colas, spicy foods, greasy fried foods, chocolate, citrus fruits and juices, and tomato-based products.

➤ Do not take any antacids without your doctor's approval.

## Five-Day Pregnancy Meal Plan

Here's a five-day meal plan to get you started on your healthy eating track. You'll notice the adjustments for the first trimester at the bottom of each menu; this is because your body requires fewer calories during the first three months and more during the last six months.

## Menu 1

Breakfast
1 cup whole-grain cereal topped with
1 cup 1% low-fat milk & 1 Tbs of chopped nuts
$^1/_2$ cantaloupe (or 1 cup of berries)
8 ounces grapefruit juice

Lunch
Turkey/cheese sandwich (2 oz turkey, 1$^1/_2$ oz cheese, with roasted peppers on 2 slices whole-wheat bread)
1 cup vegetable soup
Glass of seltzer water with 4 ounces cranberry juice

Snack
Yogurt/fruit shake (blend 1 cup low-fat frozen yogurt, 1 banana, and $^1/_2$–1 cup strawberries or blueberries)

Dinner
Tossed salad with 2 Tbs dressing
5 ounces grilled chicken breast, cut into chunks and stir-fried with 1 cup of assorted veggies (with 1 Tbs olive oil and 1 tsp of low-sodium soy sauce)
1 cup of brown rice
Seltzer or water with fresh lemon

Snack
1 cup 1% low-fat milk
4 graham crackers topped with 1 Tbs of peanut butter

Nutrition Information:

| | |
|---|---|
| Calories: 2,544 | Iron: 25 mg |
| Fat: 26% (74 grams) | Calcium: 1,645 mg |
| Carbohydrate: 53% | Folic acid: 465 mcg |
| Fiber: 38 grams | B6: 4.7 mg |
| Protein: 21% | Zinc: 18 mg |

For the first trimester, skip the midnight snack of milk, graham crackers, and peanut butter, and you'll have the following nutrition information:

| | |
|---|---|
| Calories: 2,288 | Iron: 24 mg |
| Fat: 24% (62 grams) | Calcium: 1,335 mg |
| Carbohydrate: 54% | Folic acid: 438 mcg |
| Protein: 22% | B6: 4.5 mg |
| Fiber: 37 grams | Zinc: 16 mg |

## Menu 2

<u>Breakfast</u>
1 cup oatmeal with $^1/_4$ cup raisins
Whole-wheat pita bread
2 tsp reduced-fat margarine and 1 Tbs jam
1 cup 1% low-fat milk

<u>Lunch</u>
Open-faced tuna melt (recipe in Chapter 11, "Now You're Cooking")
Carrot sticks with 2 Tbs of low-fat dressing
8 ounces of orange juice
Apple

<u>Snack</u>
1 cup low-fat fruit yogurt
2 oatmeal raisin cookies
Seltzer with lemon

<u>Dinner</u>
4 ounces broiled beef sirloin
$1^1/_2$ cups linguini with $^1/_2$ cup marinara sauce
1 cup steamed spinach with garlic and 1 tsp olive oil
1 cup fruit salad with 1 Tbs of chopped walnuts
Water or seltzer

<u>Snack</u>
Frozen yogurt pop
6 mini flavored rice cakes

<u>Nutrition Information</u>:

| | |
|---|---|
| Calories: 2,517 | Iron: 20 mg |
| Fat: 24% (67 grams) | Calcium: 1,772 mg |
| Carbohydrate: 55% | Folic acid: 406 mcg |
| Fiber: 34 grams | B6: 2.5 mg |
| Protein: 21% | Zinc: 19 mg |

For the first trimester, skip the night-time snack of frozen yogurt and rice cakes, and you'll have the following nutrition information:

| | |
|---|---|
| Calories: 2,342 | Iron: 20 mg |
| Fat: 24% (63 grams) | Calcium: 1,667 mg |
| Carbohydrate: 54% | Folic acid: 402 mcg |
| Fiber: 34 grams | B6: 2.4 mg |
| Protein: 22% | Zinc: 19 mg |

## Menu 3

<u>Breakfast</u>
2 whole-grain waffles
1 Tbs margarine
1 cup strawberries (or small banana)
1 cup low-fat fruit yogurt
1 cup 1% low-fat milk

<u>Lunch</u>
Egg white-veggie omelet (recipe in Chapter 11)
Toasted bagel with 2 Tbs of cream cheese and 1 Tbs jam
1 serving canned peaches in light syrup
Seltzer water or club soda

<u>Snack</u>
Granola bar
1 cup frozen seedless grapes
8 ounces orange juice

<u>Dinner</u>
Tossed salad with 2 Tbs dressing
4–5 ounces of grilled fish
1 ½ cup of couscous
Steamed carrots
Frozen fruit bar
Water or seltzer with lemon

<u>Snack</u>
1 slice of whole-grain toast
1½ ounces of low-fat cheese

<u>Nutrition Information:</u>

| | |
|---|---|
| Calories: 2,554 | Iron: 15 mg |
| Fat: 25% (70 grams) | Calcium: 1,827 mg |
| Carbohydrate: 55% | Folic acid: 457 mcg |
| Fiber: 30 grams | B6: 2.1 mg |
| Protein: 20% | Zinc: 10 mg |

For the first trimester, skip the night-time snack of whole-grain toast and cheese, and you'll have the following nutrition information:

| | |
|---|---|
| Calories: 2,322 | Iron: 13 mg |
| Fat: 24% (63 grams) | Calcium: 1,363 mg |
| Carbohydrate: 57% | Folic acid: 435 mcg |
| Fiber: 27 grams | B6: 2.0 mg |
| Protein: 19% | Zinc: 8 mg |

## Menu 4

Breakfast
French toast a la mode (recipe in Chapter 11)
8 ounces grapefruit juice

Lunch
Chef salad with lettuce, tomato, carrots, and 1 ounce roast beef
2 ounces turkey breast
$1^1/_2$ ounce Swiss cheese
2 Tbs vinaigrette dressing
Whole-grain roll
$^1/_2$ cup dried apricots mixed with 2 Tbs of almonds
Club soda

Snack
1 cup frozen yogurt topped with granola
Nectarine

Dinner
$1^1/_2$ cups cooked pasta with 3 ounces shrimp, 1 cup cooked broccoli (or peapods and carrots),
$^1/_2$ cup marinara sauce
1 cup fresh strawberries with 3 Tbs whipped cream
Club soda with lemon

Snack
Slice of angel food cake
1 cup low-fat milk

Nutrition Information:

| | |
|---|---|
| Calories: 2,550 | Iron: 23 mg |
| Fat: 25% (71 grams) | Calcium: 1,764 mg |
| Carbohydrate: 55% | Folic acid: 446 mcg |
| Fiber: 32 grams | B6: 2.3 mg |
| Protein: 20% | Zinc: 14 mg |

For the first trimester, skip the night-time snack of angel food cake and milk plus the granola on the frozen yogurt at midday, and you'll have the following nutrition information:

| | |
|---|---|
| Calories: 2,232 | Iron: 21 mg |
| Fat: 25% (61 grams) | Calcium: 1,400 mg |
| Carbohydrate: 55% | Folic acid: 406 mcg |
| Protein: 20% | B6: 2.0 mg |
| Fiber: 29 grams | Zinc: 12 mg |

## Menu 5

Breakfast
1 cup whole-grain cereal
1 cup 1% low-fat milk
1 cup raspberries
1 slice raisin bread with 1 Tbs of peanut butter
8 ounces orange juice (calcium-fortified)

Lunch
1¹/₂ cup rice and 1 cup black beans
1 cup fresh fruit salad topped with 2 Tbs of granola and 1 Tbs of chopped walnuts
Club soda

Snack
Yogurt/fruit shake
1 chocolate chip cookie

Dinner
Seasoned swordfish steaks (5 ounces)
1 cup steamed kale with 1 tsp olive oil and garlic
Baked sweet potato with 2 tsp of margarine
Baked apple with cinnamon
Water

Snack
1 cup of frozen seedless grapes or a frozen fruit bar
1 cup 1% low-fat milk

Nutrition Information:

| | |
|---|---|
| Calories: 2,485 | Iron: 26 mg |
| Fat: 25% (69 grams) | Calcium: 1,443 mg |
| Carbohydrate: 58% | Folic acid: 642 mcg |
| Fiber: 53 grams | B6: 3.4 mg |
| Protein: 17% | Zinc: 16 mg |

For the first trimester, skip the night-time snack of milk and grapes *plus* the chocolate chip cookie at midday, and you'll have the following nutrition information:

| | |
|---|---|
| Calories: 2,246 | Iron: 26 mg |
| Fat: 25% (62 grams) | Calcium: 1,100 mg |
| Carbohydrate: 58% | Folic acid: 625 mcg |
| Fiber: 51 grams | B6: 3.2 mg |
| Protein: 17% | Zinc: 15 mg |

Eating a balanced and varied diet will provide you and your baby with the 40 or so nutrients important for good health. Pay extra attention to folate, iron, calcium and protein—and take good care of yourself by monitoring your weight gain and being physically active. Pregnancy is one of the most exciting times in a woman's life, so enjoy!

---

### The Least You Need to Know

➤ You'll need about an extra 70,000 calories during the entire nine-month haul! That's about 150 extra calories each day during the first trimester and around 300 extra calories each day during the second and third trimesters.

➤ Adequate protein, calcium, iron, folic acid, and a variety of other nutrients are required throughout your pregnancy to cover the increased demands of the growing fetus.

➤ Healthy, normal weight women should aim for a 25–35 pound weight gain.

➤ Although nausea, constipation, water retention, and heartburn can be quite unpleasant, rest assured they are generally normal side effects of pregnancy.

---

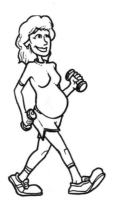

# Chapter 23

# Exercising Your Way Through Pregnancy

> **In This Chapter**
>
> ➤ The pros of exercising through pregnancy
>
> ➤ How much and how hard
>
> ➤ Important tips for safety
>
> ➤ Appropriate exercise programs

Way back in the olden days (you know, when our parents had us) pregnancy was a time for rest—not exercise. *You're pregnant? Relax, put your feet up, and have a few bon bons.* Today, we know better. In fact, research shows that pregnant women who regularly exercise have fewer aches and pains, better self esteem, more stamina, strength, and energy, and perhaps less fear of the delivery room.

Naturally, pregnancy is not the time to beat the world record in the high jump or place in the New York City marathon, but you can certainly continue with a modified version of your regular exercise regimen. You can even begin a prenatal exercise program if you're a newcomer to the world of fitness. Compare delivering a baby to participating in an Olympic event: The nine-month pregnancy is your chance to train for the big day.

## Most Doctors Give the Green Light for Exercise

Most obstetricians today are keen on the idea of pregnant women exercising their way to the delivery room—within the limits of common sense, of course. However, because certain medical instances rule out exercise, and nobody knows you medically better than your obstetrician, never begin exercising without first discussing it with your personal physician.

## Q & A

**Can you start exercising for the first time when you're pregnant—even if you're totally out of shape?**

Yes! In fact, studies report that beginners can safely reap the benefits from exercise as long as they take it easy, appropriately warm up and cool down, keep their heart rates within a safe range, and have appropriate supervision for at least the first few sessions. Naturally, fitness novices must get the okay from their docs before jumping in.

## *What Do the Experts Say?*

This is a summary of the appropriate guidelines and recommendations from the American College of Obstetricians and Gynecologists (ACOG) on exercise during pregnancy and postpartum.

For healthy pregnant women who have no additional risk factors, ACOG recommends the following:

1. During pregnancy, women can continue to exercise and derive health benefits even from mild to moderate exercise routines. Regular exercise—at least three times per week—is preferable to intermittent activity.

2. Avoid exercise in the supine position (lying on your back) after the first trimester. This position can decrease the cardiac output (blood flow) to the uterus. Also, avoid prolonged periods of motionless standing.

3. Pregnant women have less oxygen available for aerobic activity and therefore should not expect to be able to do what they did pre-pregnancy. Pay close attention to your body, and modify your exercise intensity according to how you feel. Always stop exercising when you feel fatigued and *never* push your body to exhaustion.

   Although some women might be able to continue with their regular weight-bearing exercises at the same intensity as they did pre-pregnancy, non–weight-bearing exercises such as swimming and biking might be easier to do and present less risk of injury.

4. Your changing size, shape, and weight can make certain exercises difficult. Avoid activities that can throw off your balance and possibly cause you to fall. Further, avoid any exercise with the potential for even mild abdominal trauma.

5. Pregnancy requires an additional 300 calories a day. Thus, women who exercise during pregnancy should be particularly careful to eat an adequate diet.

6. Pregnant women who exercise in the first trimester should stay cool by drinking plenty of water, wear appropriate clothing, and avoid very humid or hot environments.

7. Resume your pre-pregnancy exercise routines gradually after giving birth. Many of the physical changes that take place during pregnancy persist for four to six weeks.

**Food for Thought**

Pick up *Fit Pregnancy* magazine and get the latest scoop on keeping fit while you're expecting. From the folks over at *Shape* magazine, it hits the newsstands three to four times each year.

You should not exercise during pregnancy if you have any of the following conditions:

➤ Pregnancy-induced hypertension (high blood pressure)

➤ Preterm rupture of membranes

➤ Preterm labor during the prior or current pregnancy

➤ Incompetent cervix/cerclage (a surgical procedure to close the cervix to keep the fetus intact in utero)

➤ Persistent second or third trimester bleeding

➤ Intrauterine growth retardation

**Q & A**

**Do fit women have easier deliveries than unfit women?**

I hate to say it, but probably not. An easy delivery has more to do with genetics, the positioning of the baby, and a lot of luck. I've heard of "super fit" women who had labors from hell, and I've heard of sedentary women who popped out babies with just four pushes. Go figure.

However, one thing is for sure: Fit moms can better handle prolonged, agonizing labor and bounce back with a quicker recuperation period than unfit moms.

In addition, women with certain other medical or obstetric conditions, including chronic hypertension or active thyroid, cardiac, vascular, or pulmonary disease, should be evaluated carefully in order to determine whether an exercise program is appropriate.

# Warming Up, Cooling Down, and All the Stuff in the Middle

Pregnant or not, the ABCs of exercise remain the same. Be sure to begin each session with an appropriate warm-up—some light aerobic activity that will rev up your system and prepare your body for the exercise to follow. Next, continue with a low- to moderate-intensity aerobic segment and pay close attention to your body's cues. During pregnancy, work at a comfortable pace, stop when you feel fatigued, and never push yourself to exhaustion. Lastly, always end your aerobic session with a proper cooldown; gradually slow down the pace to bring your heart rate back to a resting level. See Chapter 14, "Getting Physical," for further details on exercise programs.

**Food for Thought**

The mysterious art of yoga involves breathing, relaxation, stretching, and body awareness. Therefore, yoga can play a magical role in making you feel terrific during and after your pregnancy.

## Stretch Your Bod—Carefully

Regular, consistent stretching can help to maintain your flexibility and prevent some of the muscle tightness that typically sneaks up on you during the last trimester. As always, stretching must precede some type of warm-up activity to increase your circulation and internal body temperature. Also, be sure to ease into each stretch gradually and hold for 10–30 seconds; never bounce! During pregnancy, the object is to stretch nice and easy. Don't ever push a stretch past the point of your pain-free range of motion.

## Keep a Check on the Intensity

As of 1994, the American College of Obstetricians and Gynecologists (ACOG) lifted the rule that limited pregnant exercisers to a heart rate of 140 beats per minute or less. Today, there are no limitations on heart rate: You can monitor your own intensity as long as you exercise common sense. Keep in mind, you should *always* be able to comfortably carry on a conversation to ensure you are working in a safe aerobic range, and never push through fatigue, cramping, or any other discomfort. (Review the section on checking your heart rate in Chapter 14.)

Understand that being pregnant means you will typically fatigue more easily. Therefore, be cautious in the gym and modify your pre-pregnancy routine by decreasing both workout intensity and length. Also, don't expect to keep up with those nonpregnant jocks; find some less competitive opponents.

### Q & A

**What should I expect during the first, second, and third trimesters?**

During the first trimester, size is not the issue; your raging hormones are! Because some women feel incredibly tired and queasy, listen to your body and do whatever activity you can manage until you feel better.

During the second trimester, most women bounce back and feel like themselves again. If you feel up to it, this is a terrific time to incorporate regular exercise into your weekly schedule.

During the last trimester, your growing waistline and weight might affect your stamina, agility, and balance. Think about switching to gentler activities that won't strain your joints and muscles (for instance, swimming and walking).

## "Energize" Without All the Slamming and Jamming!

When it comes to selecting the type of exercise, every woman is different. One woman might be perfectly okay with modifying her usual sport (for instance, a runner might continue to jog at a slower pace), but other women are uncomfortable with the jarring and jolting on the joints—especially in the last trimester, when weight begins to climb. Think about switching to gentler activities, such as walking instead of running, swimming instead of high-impact aerobics, or pedaling on a stationary bike.

### *Take a Walk with Your Baby*

Some of the great things about walking include that there's no crashing impact, you can select your own pace and distance, you get quality "think time" (a precious commodity after the baby arrives), and you can do it just about anywhere. For some fresh air, go for a trek around the neighborhood or hit a scenic trail. If the weather doesn't suit you, try a treadmill, or wander about your local shopping mall. Anything goes; just remember these key points:

➤ You need to keep a strong, upright posture; lead with your chest.

**Food for Thought**

Don't wait to get thirsty: Keep a water bottle close by and drink before, during, and after your workouts to ensure that you and your baby are adequately hydrated.

➤ Rhythmically move your arms forward and back from the shoulders. Do not swing them higher than your chest or across your midline.

**Overrated—Undercooked**

Reduce your risk for injury by avoiding activities that require a lot of balance and coordination because as your body shifts, so does your center of gravity due to your enlarged belly, breasts, and uterus. Back off from things that might land you on the ground: skiing, horseback riding, biking, and skating. Avoid sports that involve sharp, jerky movements such as swinging a tennis racket, volleyball, bowling, and so on.

➤ Do not walk outdoors when the ground is icy. Remember, your balance is not as keen as it used to be.

➤ Don't try to conquer steep hills that can send your heart rate soaring or place a lot of stress on your back.

➤ Do not walk in steamy, hot, or humid weather.

➤ Keep your body and baby well hydrated. Drink before, during, and after your walk.

➤ Eat a snack before you start your walk to prevent a drop in your blood-sugar.

➤ Wear comfortable shoes with good support. Some women's feet swell during pregnancy, so you might need shoes or sneaks at least a half size bigger.

➤ Wear appropriate clothing. On cold days, wear layers that can be shed and tied around your waist as you heat up.

# Sign Up for a Prenatal Exercise Class

Prenatal exercise classes are specially designed for expectant moms and take into consideration your shifting center of gravity, reduced stamina, and ever-changing bod. Generally, these specialty classes focus on thorough warm-ups, cool-downs, aerobic workouts, and stretching. In some instances, they might also include strength training and yoga. All exercises are carefully choreographed to keep you energized, but in a comfortable and appropriate fashion. Furthermore, you won't feel self-conscious because everyone in the class is in the same boat—give or take a few inches (or yards) around the waist. In other words, it's highly unlikely that the woman standing next to you will be wearing a thong leotard (*and if she is, more power to her*). It's also a nice place to bond, swap pregnancy war stories, and meet other women who are soon to have kids the same age as your own.

You can typically find out what's available in your area by checking with the local health clubs, hospitals, birthing centers, or even your obstetrician's office.

## Q & A

**What the heck are Kegals?**

Kegals are exercises to strengthen the muscles within the pelvic floor (sort of deep inside, between your vagina and belly button). To figure out where these muscles are, stop and start your urine flow when your sitting on the toilet. Once you find them, regularly strengthen your pelvic-floor muscles with tightening and relaxing exercises. Pull upward and inward toward the body's midline, hold for about 5–10 seconds, and then relax. Repeat them for as many times as you can, as often as you are willing. Kegal exercises can be done sitting, standing, or lying down and can drastically help to increase genital circulation, strengthen and maintain the pelvic floor muscles, and prevent incontinence after the baby is born.

# Yes, "Moms-to-Be" Can Lift Weights

Being pregnant doesn't necessarily mean passing up the weight room. In fact, some light weight training might cut back on some of the back and shoulder pain associated with enlarged breasts, extra weight, and a growing uterus. It might also reduce the leg cramps and neck strain that some women experience toward the last trimester. Personally, my favorite benefit from prenatal lifting is that your muscles will be primed for the "baby *aftermath.*" That is, you'll be ready to lug around your pocketbook, diaper bag, and stroller on one arm, while carrying your baby on the other. To this day, I still amaze my sister Debra with the amount of equipment I can juggle with just two arms!

If you're experienced with weights, you can continue with a modified version of your regular routine. (Adjust the amount of weight and number of reps to how you feel.) However, if you are a novice with the dumbbells and machines, this is definitely not the time to lift anything unsupervised. You can ask a qualified trainer who is experienced with pregnant women to show you the ropes.

Some things to consider:

➤ Regroup your weight-training goals. Instead of focusing on intense workouts that will increase strength and define your muscles, relax, take it easy, and simply concentrate on strength maintenance.

➤ Because you might become less agile and coordinated due to the extra weight you are carrying, consider sticking with the machines. They offer much more support and require less balance than the free weights.

**253**

➤ Be aware that some machines require inappropriate positioning, and as your belly expands in front, you literally might not be able to fit on some of the machines comfortably. (Ah, isn't pregnancy fun?) But don't let that halt the workout: Ask a trainer to show you some safe (perhaps nonmachine) exercises. Or simply forget about that exercise until you're back to your post-pregnancy routine.

➤ The amount of weight you should lift depends on your strength pre-pregnancy and how you feel during your pregnancy. Lift what feels slightly challenging during the last few reps, not an amount that really pushes your limit.

➤ Pay close attention to your form and concentrate on smooth and steady breathing.

➤ Don't be discouraged if you have to cut back on the weights as you get further into your pregnancy. In fact, expect to cut back. Remember, you're pregnant—not Wonder Woman. Women typically get more tired and have less agility and balance toward the end of the nine-month term.

➤ If at any point you feel nauseous, dizzy, overly fatigued, or any other uncomfortable sensation (cramping, knotting, tingling), stop exercising immediately and speak with your doctor before continuing.

### Q & A

**Can I lie on my back and do sit-ups?**

Yes, but only during the first trimester. After the fourth month, you risk pinching off the inferior vena cava, an important large vein that carries blood back to the heart. During pregnancy, the weight of your growing uterus might compress this vein and cause you to feel faint. Instead of stomach exercises on your back, ask a trainer to show you how to work your abdominals on your side or standing up.

## Bouncing Back After the Baby Arrives

Generally, five to six weeks after delivering your bundle of joy, your doctor will give you the okay to resume all exercise—which is easier said than done. Between the sleep deprivation and feeling like your body's been through a war, merely scheduling in the time and getting the motivation is a feat in itself. Take a deep breath and round up some energy because exercise can do wonders for both your mind and body. Start slow, go at your own pace, and gradually ease back into your pre-pregnancy routine.

## The Least You Need to Know

➤ Women who regularly exercise during pregnancy tend to have fewer aches and pains, better self esteem, and more stamina, strength, and energy.

➤ Because some medical instances rule out exercise, always get the okay from your doctor before beginning an exercise program.

➤ Because pregnancy generally reduces your stamina, speed, and agility, expect to modify your pre-pregnancy routines by decreasing your workout intensity and length. Also, always keep your heart rate within a comfortable working range and never push your body to exhaustion.

➤ Most pregnant women prefer gentler activities that do not strain the joints such as swimming, walking, and stationary bikes—especially during the last trimester when your girth and weight start to climb.

➤ Drink plenty of water before, during, and after exercise to ensure that you and your baby are well-hydrated.

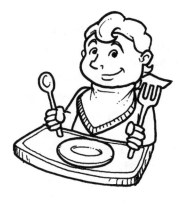

# Feeding the Younger Folks

Being a kid these days is a pretty demanding job. Between homework, after-school activities, sports, being popular, and keeping up with fashion, it's especially important that the younger folks learn to keep their bodies fit and healthy so that they're better-equipped to take on the world.

As a mother, as well as a nutritionist, I understand that nobody knows your children better than you. Therefore, this chapter is not about telling you what you should and shouldn't feed your kids but merely offers suggestions and guidelines to help you in this endeavor. Read on to learn how to encourage your kids to eat nutritious foods and get plenty of physical activity. Bear in mind that healthy kids grow up to be healthy adults.

# Your Very First Food Decision: Breast Milk or Formula?

Most pediatricians and nutritionists across the board agree that breast milk is the food of choice for growing babies. First, nursing is a beautiful mother-baby bonding experience, and it's economically savvy. In other words, it's cheap! But most importantly, breast milk has the capability to protect your baby from several infections because it is believed to carry immunities (protective substances) from mother to infant. *Colostrum*, the yellowish pre-milk substance secreted in the first few days after delivery, might carry even more antibodies—plus it's loaded with protein and zinc.

For all you women who choose not to nurse, or aren't able to nurse, don't lose any sleep. Companies today make sophisticated baby formulas that closely mimic the components in human milk. What's more, babies that are formula-fed can receive just as much "snuggling time" and form close bonds with mom as babies that are breast-fed. Whatever you decide (the bottle or the breast), rest assured all kids have a shot at Harvard University and the Olympic soccer team!

# When and How to Start Solids

Although you might choose to nurse past six months, at this point your growing baby will need more calories and iron than breast milk or formulas alone can supply. Generally, pediatricians recommend beginning solid foods between four and six months. Here are some strategies for getting started:

➤ A general rule of thumb is to introduce only one new food at a time (over three to five days) to rule out food allergies and intolerances. If your baby tolerates a food, and you don't notice any adverse reactions (skin rashes, wheezing, diarrhea, stomach aches), you can graduate on to the next food item.

As your baby moves up in age and food variety, keep a watchful eye on highly allergic items such as wheat, egg white, nut butters, and cow's milk. In fact, avoid giving egg whites, regular dairy, and peanut butter until after the first year.

➤ Rice cereal is usually recommended for the first food introduction because it is the least allergenic. Follow the directions on the box (usually 3–5 tablespoons of dry cereal is mixed with breast milk, formula, or water). Although it might seem bland to you, don't add anything else (sugar, salt, honey). Your baby will find it perfectly fine, and it's really the texture that you want him or her to get used to.

➤ After cereal has passed the test, try some pureed fruit and pureed veggies. (I recommend that you start with the veggies.) Watch how your baby starts to master the art of pushing the food back into the mouth with the tongue; what a genius! You can also give your baby unsweetened 100 percent fruit juice at this point, but be sure to dilute it to half-strength with water.

➤ By age 6 to 10 months, your baby's digestive system is maturing and it's time to introduce all sorts of mashed concoctions. Try strained meats, chicken, turkey, egg yolks (continue to avoid egg whites), and mashed lentils and beans.

➤ By 12 months, you can go ahead and substitute regular cow's milk for formula, with your pediatrician's okay. Encourage at least three full cups of milk per day, but not so much that your child will be too full for the solid foods that supply the necessary calories and iron. You can also go ahead and add cheese and plain yogurts.

➤ Go at your own pace, and listen to what your pediatrician has to say about the growth and development of your little one—clearly the best indication of your baby's nutritional status.

**Food for Thought**

It's a good idea to start with vegetables *before* fruit. After introducing the sweetness of fruit, some infants are not so willing to eat the vegetables.

Popular first-year foods:

➤ Rice cereals

➤ Squash

➤ Green beans

➤ Yogurt, plain

➤ Peaches

➤ Chicken

➤ Turkey

➤ Barley cereals

➤ Sweet potato

➤ Peas

➤ Applesauce

➤ Plums

➤ Beef

➤ Oat cereals

➤ Carrots

➤ Avocado

➤ Bananas

➤ Pears

➤ Lamb

# The Wrong Stuff

Watch out for certain foods. During the first year, avoid foods that are difficult to chew and could cause choking such as nuts, popcorn, hard candy, and raw carrots. Also avoid foods that have tough outer skins, such as grapes and hot dogs, and foods that are thick and sticky, such as peanut butter.

Honey should definitely be avoided in children under one year of age because it can cause infant botulism. Honey is sometimes contaminated with spores of clostridium botulinum, and in an infant's intestine, these spores can grow and produce a toxin that can make a baby sick and—in extreme cases—cause death. Adults need not worry because "friendly" bacteria present in their intestines prevents these spores from growing.

Be extra cautious when introducing foods that tend to be highly allergenic, such as egg whites, wheat, corn, nuts, seafood, citrus fruits, cow's milk, chocolate, cocoa, seafood, pork, berries, soy, and tomatoes.

# The Right Stuff for Growing Kids

These are the basic guidelines for children three years and older. Keep in mind that this chart represents the minimum requirements. Obviously, active kids who participate in after-school sports (or kids who just plain run around a lot) will need more food than the average couch potato. Also, expect the portions sizes to vary; younger children generally eat much smaller portions than older kids.

| Food Group | Suggested Servings/Day | Key Nutrients |
|---|---|---|
| Bread and grain group | 6+ | Carbohydrates, B-vitamins, iron |
| Vegetable group | 3+ | Vitamin C, vitamin A, folic acid, magnesium, fiber |
| Fruit group | 2+ | Vitamin C, vitamin A, potassium, fiber |
| Milk, yogurt, and cheese group | 3+ | Calcium, riboflavin, protein |
| Meat, poultry, dried beans, eggs, and nuts group | 2 | Protein, B-vitamins, iron, zinc |

## Q & A

*Should I worry if my kids aren't getting enough food?*

Probably not. Children generally eat when they are hungry and stop when they are full. You might, however, want to pay attention to daily food choices among various food groups. If certain foods are consistently left out, brainstorm on ways to work them into the day.

## Be a Healthy Role Model

Monkey see, monkey do! As your children grow, they observe and copy everything you do—eating habits included. Remember, actions speak much louder than words, so start munching on those fruits and vegetables.

## Cook with Your Kids, Not for Them!

Introduce your kids to healthy eating and the kitchen! I've found that children are more interested and willing to eat unfamiliar foods when they participate in the preparation. Try some of the following suggestions:

➤ Select a few nights each week and involve your kids with dinner planning and preparation. Designate different jobs for each child.

➤ You might prefer to single out one child at a time. For instance, Tuesday night might be the night you and your son whip up a creative dinner concoction for the family. Thursday night might be a special night for just you and your daughter to plan the evening spread.

➤ How about an entire "theme night?" For example, one night might be Japanese. Make chicken teriyaki over rice; you can set up a table on the floor, sit on pillows, and use chopsticks instead of forks. Or make it Greek night and serve Greek salads while wearing togas.

Healthy after-school snacks include

➤ Fresh fruit

➤ Veggies and low-fat dip

➤ Yogurt and granola

➤ Fig bars and low-fat milk

➤ Fruit cocktail in light syrup

➤ Bananas and apple slices with peanut butter

➤ Carrots and celery with salsa

➤ Whole-wheat toast with apple butter

➤ Trail mix (nuts and raisins)

➤ Dried fruit

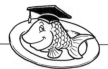

**Food for Thought**

Until the age of 24 years, kids are laying down the foundation for a lifetime of strong, healthy bones, so discourage all of the sugary beverages and encourage them to drink milk and calcium-fortified juice.

**Food for Thought**

Make mealtime fun for your younger kids: Set a place at the dinner table for a special doll or stuffed animal.

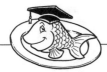

### Food for Thought

Typically, the more color on your plate, the more vitamin content. For example, a plate of noodles with broccoli, tomato sauce, and parmesan cheese will have a lot more color and vitamin content than a plate of plain noodles with butter.

➤ Cereal with fruit and low-fat milk

➤ English muffin pizzas

➤ Frozen fruit bars

➤ Frozen yogurt pops

➤ Banana-Berry Frosty (see recipe)

➤ Peanut Butter Yogurt Milkshake (see recipe)

➤ Animal crackers and graham crackers

➤ Pretzels and fruit juice

➤ Vegetable soup and pita bread

➤ Flavored rice cakes

➤ Jazzed-Up Popcorn (see recipe)

## Fun and Easy Recipes

Here are a few recipes that will help your kids enjoy cooking.

### Breakfast Berry Crepes

*Serves four*

Nonstick vegetable spray

$1/2$ cup blueberries

2 cups whole-grain flour

$1/2$ cup raspberries

1 egg, beaten

$1/2$ sliced strawberries

$2^1/2$ cups low-fat milk

Place flour in a bowl and add egg plus 2 cups of milk (save $1/2$ cup). Beat with a wire whisk until all lumps are gone and the mixture is completely smooth. Gradually add the remaining $1/2$ cup of milk to make a thin batter. Use nonstick cooking spray on hot skillet (medium-high temperature), and pour enough batter in the pan to make a large circle. Sprinkle the desired amount of fruit on top and press down into the crepe. Cook for approximately 2–3 more minutes and then flip the crepe and cook the other side. Carefully lift onto a plate and roll it all the way up.

*From the kitchen of Andrea Mendonca*

## Jazzed-Up Popcorn

Make air-popped popcorn, spray on some nonstick cooking spray, and then jazz it up with one of the following ingredients:

Parmesan cheese

Chili powder and garlic

Ground cinnamon

Low-sodium soy sauce

## Tuna Salad Cones

*Serves four*

Open a can of water-packed tuna and drain off liquid. Mash up tuna and mix in grated carrots, chopped tomatoes, and some shredded low-fat cheddar cheese (optional). Lightly mix with low-fat mayonnaise or Italian salad dressing, and scoop into flat-bottomed ice cream cones (not the sugar kind). Serve for lunch or at a party; your kids will love them!

*From the kitchen of Lisa, Jason, and Harley Bauer*

## Banana-Berry Frosty

*Serves Two*

1 cup low-fat milk

2 tsp vanilla

$1/_2$ cup of fresh strawberries

3–4 ice cubes

$1/_2$ banana

Place all the ingredients into the blender and mix until smooth and fluffy.

*From the kitchen of Jesse and Cole Bauer*

### Peanut Butter Yogurt Milkshake

*Serves Two*

4 big scoops of vanilla Frozen Yogurt

1–2 Tbs peanut butter

1 cup low-fat milk

Mix all the ingredients in the blender until thick and smooth.

*From the kitchen of Haley and Mike Simon*

### Food for Thought

Unfortunately enough, recent studies report that 21 percent of American kids 12 to 19 are obese.

For further reading, look for

*The Can-Do Eating Plan for Overweight Kids and Teens,* Michelle Daum, M.S., R.D. Avon Books, 1997 800-223-0690

# What About Sweets?

Clearly, some foods are healthier than others, but there's room in every meal plan for all foods, even the junky stuff. Develop a positive attitude about food by emphasizing healthy choices and limiting—but not eliminating— the not-so-healthy cakes, cookies, and candy. In fact, forbidding your kids to eat certain foods doesn't work; it only makes the high-fat stuff that much more enticing.

Place a limit of 1–2 dessert-like foods each day—and keep the serving sizes relatively small (2 cookies, small slice of cake, 1 scoop of ice cream). You can also serve healthier dessert alternatives such as chocolate fondue (orange segments, banana slices, and berries dipped in chocolate syrup) or an Angel food cake topped with strawberries. Both can satisfy a sweet craving with a lot less fat and sugar.

### Q & A

How can you get your finicky child to eat healthier?

Education is an important tool. Children as young as two years old can begin to understand the importance of certain food groups. Make it simple and fun by incorporating games, taste tests, and color drawings. A great idea is to hang a sticker chart on the fridge and reward your child each time he or she tastes a new food at a meal—or eats a vegetable at dinner. Don't get hung up on the portion sizes; remember, kids have small capacities and the idea is to create a willingness toward new food (not a clean plate award).

What about your teenagers? As your kids grow up, you tend to have much less control over what they eat. Continue to encourage healthy food choices and certainly downplay the unhealthy stuff—but be careful not to create an obsessive environment of "bad food/good food." It can backfire into a serious eating disorder.

# The Sneaky Gourmet: 15 Ways to Disguise Vegetables

Your kid won't go near vegetables? See if you can sneak in a few here and there with some of these suggestions:

1. Add a mixed vegetable medley to your meatloaf recipe.

2. Scatter cooked vegetables throughout pasta and then cover with marinara sauce.

3. Grate carrots into tuna or chicken salad and stuff in a pita pocket.

4. Make homemade pizza. Toss on sliced mushrooms and chopped broccoli *before* spreading on the cheese.

5. Make vegetable lasagna. You can stick with a single vegetable such as spinach (see the Spinach Lasagna recipe in Chapter 19, "Going Vegetarian") or mix in a variety of chopped, cooked vegetables such as zucchini, cauliflower, broccoli, carrots, mushrooms, green beans, and so on.

6. Add cooked peas, corn, and carrots to mashed potatoes.

7. Serve vegetable soup with crackers.

8. Puree cooked squash and carrots, and then add small amounts into your ground beef or ground turkey. Shape into hamburgers or turkey-burgers and cook on the grill.

9. Top a baked potato with chopped broccoli and low-fat melted cheese.

10. Make low-fat zucchini and carrot muffins.

11. Serve "make-your-own tacos" and have different stations set up with lean ground beef (or ground turkey), sliced tomatoes, shredded lettuce, and carrots.

12. Make chicken-vegetable kabobs. Alternate chunks of grilled chicken, peppers, tomatoes, onions, zucchini, and mushrooms on metal skewers. Set up a variety of dips that your kids can have fun experimenting with, such as barbecue sauce, honey mustard sauce, sweet and sour sauce, and low-fat salad dressings. Of course, maybe you'll get lucky and your kids will simply like the original marinade.

13. Finely chop cooked broccoli and thoroughly mix into your rice.

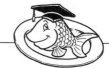

**Food for Thought**

Research has shown that vitamin C and Omega 3 fats (fats found in oily fish) can reduce asthmatic symptoms in children.

14. Turn your kids on to wok cooking and have them assist with washing and cutting up the vegetables. Try chicken-vegetable stir-fry, beef-vegetable stir-fry, or seafood-vegetable stir-fry. Pour them all over rice or linguini and hand out the chopsticks.

15. Make a spinach dip with low-fat plain yogurt, low-fat sour cream, and pureed cooked spinach. Have them dip carrots, celery, peppers, and zucchini slices. If they don't want to dip with raw veggies, give them some crackers; at least they'll get the spinach from the dip.

**Food for Thought**

Have your kids log their exercise for a week so that they understand the importance of regular physical activity and feel proud about the accomplishment.

Monday: Rode my bike for 1 hour
Tuesday: Dance class for 45 minutes
Wednesday: Walked the dog 20 minutes

# Turn Off That Tube!

Too much television generally means too much sitting around. Put a two-hour limit on TV watching and encourage your kids to get up and move. Teach them about the importance of exercise and have them do something physical for at least 30 minutes every day. Have them walk the dog, jump rope, skate, throw a ball around, swim, play tag, play basketball, sign up for an after-school class, or join a sports team.

## The Least You Need to Know

➤ Most health experts recommend breast milk over formula because breast milk is believed to pass protective substances from mother to baby.

➤ Typically between four and six months, your pediatrician will give you the okay to start your baby on solids. Stick with one food at a time to rule out food allergies.

➤ All growing kids should eat a daily total of at least 6 servings of breads and grains, 2 servings of fruit, 3 servings of veggies, 3 servings of dairy, and 2 servings of meat, poultry, dried beans, fish, eggs, or nuts. Expect younger kids to eat much smaller serving sizes than older children.

➤ Let kids be kids and occasionally eat junk food. Understand that an obsessive environment of denial can backfire.

➤ Put a two-hour limit on television watching and encourage your kids to become physically active.

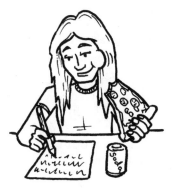

# Chapter 25

# Eating Through the College Years

---

## In This Chapter

➤ The pros of eating breakfast

➤ Healthy meals in the campus dining hall

➤ The "freshman 15"

➤ All about alcohol and partying

➤ Test your nutrition I.Q.

---

This chapter isn't aimed at parents; it's aimed at you young adults who are venturing off to college and experiencing—maybe for the first time—what it really means to take care of yourself. Are you up to it? Let's find out: Does this routine sound familiar?

The day begins with no breakfast; "Who has time?" With an English class at 8 A.M., you're lucky if you can get dressed, brush your teeth, and run out the door. Breakfast is just *not* a priority.

By lunchtime, you're delirious with hunger and ready to collapse. Food card in hand (no money needed and all the food you can eat: *what a concept!*), you're off to the campus dining hall. Lunch consists of a cheeseburger, french fries, and a cola, topped off with chocolate cake or a donut. (Gotta keep up that strength, you know—two more grueling classes ahead.)

By 6 P.M., you stumble back into the dining hall, exhausted from your chaotic day. You load your tray with anything that looks appealing: fried chicken and mashed potatoes, burritos and sour cream, or pepperoni pizza, of course, washed down with another cola. Hey, because it's all free, why not grab a few cookies and a soft-serve ice cream cone before heading back to the dorm?

It's time to face the music: You're a nutrition nightmare!

# Mistake #1: No Time for Breakfast

You might be amazed to learn that mom was right: Eating breakfast is important. Unfortunately, many college students skip this essential meal.

Remember, when you wake up from a good night's sleep, your body has been fasting for at least eight hours. (Unless there was a late-night party, in which case we're talking about two hours.) As I've mentioned earlier in the book, "break-fast" in the morning helps kick your system into gear by supplying food energy to your body. Without food, you're tired, sluggish, and probably fighting to stay awake during morning classes. Fueling your body with a healthy breakfast can keep you alert and focused during your morning schedule.

## *Skipping Breakfast to "Save Calories?" I Don't Think So!*

By the way, for all you students who skip breakfast to "save calories," think again. The majority of breakfast skippers wind up so ravenous by lunchtime and dinner that they overcompensate and pig out.

Here's an example of how not eating breakfast can become a diet disaster: Nancy, a student at University of Michigan, skipped breakfast regularly to lose weight. She would then find herself so famished by lunchtime that she would inevitably over-eat—and, of course, sabotage her diet in the process. I recommended that she experiment with a healthy breakfast for two weeks to see whether eating in the morning would help control her midday munchies. Sure enough, she felt more energetic and alert during her morning routine and ate *substantially* less at lunch, enabling her to lose three pounds.

**Food for Thought**

The campus dining hall is loaded with *both* healthy and not so healthy foods. Balance out your meals and select a variety of nutritious foods *most* of the time, and you can certainly sneak in some of the "not so healthy stuff" every once in a while. The key is to keep fat intake down (less than 30 percent of calories should come from fat) while eating a variety of foods from all of the food groups.

# Mistake #2: Too Many High-Fat Food Choices

For many young people, going off to college is their first time away from home. It's not easy having to constantly fend for yourself when you're used to the luxury of Mom's home cooking. Oh, the memories of a stocked fridge, fresh fruit, and hot meals on the table every night.

Hey, being on your own is no reason to slouch off in the food department. Most of the foods mentioned in the "college scenario from hell" are loaded with fat, sugar, and salt, which can lead to a host of problems, including weight gain and even serious illnesses. Furthermore, these foods lack vitamins, minerals, and other essential nutrients that your body needs to function properly.

You say it's impossible to eat right at school? There's actually a lot of good food in your campus dining hall. Read on and learn to choose foods that will make you look and feel your best all the time.

# Making the Grade in the Campus Dining Hall

The following is a collection of food stations commonly found in university dining halls. Find the stations that your school offers, and learn to ace the test with nutritious choices at breakfast, lunch, and dinner.

## Cereal Bars

There is nothing quicker and more satisfying than a bowl of cereal in the morning. Enjoy both the hot and cold varieties; they're high in carbohydrates, chock-full of nutrients, and generally very low in fat.

**Choose more often:** First, choose high-fiber cereals such as All-Bran, Raisin Bran, Bran Flakes, Bran Chex, or any others with the word "bran" in the name. Fiber not only relieves constipation, but also protects against certain cancers. Pour on plenty of low-fat milk or yogurt to boost your daily calcium, and don't forget to toss in a lot of fresh fruit (bananas, peaches, blueberries, strawberries, apples, raisins, raspberries, pineapple—whatever) for extra vitamin content and added sweetness. Don't stop at the cold cereals: Warm up those cold winter mornings with a hearty bowl of hot oatmeal or cream of wheat.

**Choose less often:** Forget about those sugary cereals. They might be delicious, but some brands actually pack more sugar into one serving than a piece of cake. If high-sugar cereal is a must, mix it with a healthier cereal to reduce the sugar. For example, mix half a bowl of Frosted Flakes with half a bowl of Bran Flakes. After a while, you might even prefer the healthier cereal. Avoid pouring on "whole fat" milk. It is loaded with artery-clogging saturated fat. Switch first to 2% milk and then 1%. Hey, if you're extra determined, go for the skim (no fat at all).

## Salad Bars

The word "salad" usually brings to mind an array of lettuce, tomatoes, cucumbers, carrots, onions, broccoli, peppers, and so on. All of these salad ingredients offer vitamins, minerals, fiber, and—the best news of all—very few calories. Unfortunately, salad bars also offer a variety of high-fat side items that can turn your health-conscious plate into a catastrophe. Read on, and pass your next trip to the salad bar with flying colors.

**Choose more often:** Pile your plate with a lot of colorful raw vegetables. Jazz up your salad with protein and turn it into a meal. Throw on some chickpeas, beans, eggs, low-fat cheeses, sliced turkey or roast beef, or plain tuna. Stick with a "light" or low-fat dressing, or use plenty of balsamic vinegar with a touch of oil. If regular dressing is a must, opt for vinaigrettes, or go easy on the higher fat selections (1–2 tablespoons).

**Choose less often:** Don't pile your plate with mayonnaise-laden side dishes such as macaroni salad, cole slaw, potato salad, and carrot-raisin salad. If your waistline can't afford extra fat calories, beware of other high-fat side items such as oily pasta salads, cheese, olives, avocado, bacon bits, sunflower seeds, nuts, croutons, and creamy salad dressings.

## Hot Stations

Ready to load your tray with whatever looks most delicious? Decisions, decisions, decisions! First, figure out which entree and side dish fit into your fat budget. Make savvy choices by understanding the healthier methods of meal preparation. Naturally, an occasional trek on the dark-side is okay, but generally stick with the foods on the *Choose More Often* list.

**Choose more often:** Look for entrees and side items that are grilled, baked, steamed, broiled, blackened, lightly stir-fried, mesquite-grilled, poached, and lightly marinated. Choose dishes made with teriyaki, soy sauce, barbecue sauce, tomato sauce, marinara sauce, honey mustard sauce, white wine sauce, or broth:

➤ Eat plenty of skinless chicken and turkey and all types of seafood. Even an occasional portion of lean, red meat (2–3 times per week) can fit into a healthy eating plan. When selecting a soup, opt for non-creamy versions such as vegetable-barley, chicken-noodle, lentil-bean combos, tomato-rice, minestrone, Manhattan clam chowder (the red, not the white), and garden-vegetable. Stick with nonfried side dishes, such as steamed or sautèed vegetables,; corn-on-the-cob; mashed, baked, or roasted potatoes; rice; couscous; and pastas in light oil or red sauce.

➤ Be imaginative, and mix together several items that are offered to create your own original meal. For example, scoop rice into vegetable soups, mix vegetables into pastas, spread yogurt on a baked potato. The sky's the limit.

**Choose less often:** Don't chow down on all of those fried favorites: fried chicken, fried fish, fried eggs, pan-fried burgers, french fries, onion rings, fried potato skins, hash browns, vegetable tempura, and so on. Also stay away from entrees that are loaded with whole-milk cheese such as lasagna, baked ziti, cheesy burritos, chicken/veal/eggplant parmesan, grilled cheese sandwiches, macaroni and cheese, calzones, and cheesy pizza (especially with pepperoni and sausage). Let's not forget those artery-clogging rich pasta sauces such as fettucini alfredo (heart attack on a plate).

Avoid creamy soups such as cream of broccoli, cream of mushroom, French onion soup (with cheese), New England clam chowder, and lobster bisque. Also beware of chicken skins and higher fat meats such as hot dogs, bacon, sausage, pepperoni, chicken wings, buffalo wings, and ribs. Limit the amount of eggs you eat for breakfast to twice per week. Although the whites are pure protein, the yolks contain too much cholesterol.

# Refrigerator Items

A meal doesn't have to be hot—and there are a lot of healthy options hidden in the refrigerator section of your dining hall. From sandwiches to prepared salads and yogurts, as long as you make smart choices, a "cold" meal can be nutritious and satisfying.

**Choose more often:** Stick with lower-fat sandwiches such as turkey breast, grilled chicken, lean roast beef, and ham. Add some extra fiber by throwing on some veggies and choosing whole wheat bread over white bread. Stick with mustard, ketchup, or light salad dressing as a spread. Get into low-fat yogurts; they're loaded with calcium and protein and tend to be low in calories. Prepared salads with chicken, turkey, roast beef, ham, and moderate amounts of cheese are also smart alternatives; just go easy on the dressing.

**Choose less often:** Don't make it a habit to gobble down sandwiches loaded with globs of mayonnaise such as tuna salad, chicken salad, egg salad, and seafood salad. Avoid pre-prepared sandwiches that contain high-fat meats such as salami, bologna, pepperoni, and bacon. Furthermore, limit the salads and sandwiches that come with a lot of extra cheese and oil.

# Beverages

Feel like a tall, cold glass of cola? *No!* With all the beverages at your fingertips, why not select something healthier? The following guidelines provide you with the best bets for quenching your thirst.

**Choose more often:** Drink water, water, and more water. Plain old water might sound boring, but it happens to be the "superhero" of all beverages. Not only is water the best way to quench your thirst and hydrate your body, but it also helps to move things along. (I think you get the picture). Mix club soda, seltzer, mineral water, or sparkling water with fresh lemon, lime, orange, or even some fruit juice for flavor.

If $H_2O$ doesn't thrill you, at least select a drink that offers you some nutrition rather than pure sugar. For example, natural fruit juices contain several vitamins such as A, C, potassium, magnesium, and other B-vitamins, depending on the type of juice. Low-fat milk and chocolate milk are also smart alternatives because they both provide calcium and protein.

**Choose less often:** Don't guzzle down all of those sugary drinks (soda, fruit punch, sugary iced teas). These are pure sugar, no nutrition. Diet beverages are not such a bargain either; with all those artificial sweeteners, who needs them? Go easy on coffees and teas as well. With all that caffeine, you'll be jittery, irritable, and bouncing off the walls.

# Potato Bars

Take advantage of this no-fat complex carbohydrate and *mangia*. Not only are baked potatoes low in calories (about 150 for a medium potato), but also they are loaded with potassium, vitamin C, and a decent amount of fiber if you eat the skin. Don't glob on the butter and sour cream (too much fat); instead, try some of these healthier alternatives:

**Choose more often:** Try a baked potato topped with

> Broccoli and marinara sauce
> Cottage cheese
> Vegetarian chili
> Tossed salad and light vinaigrette
> Salsa, ketchup, or barbecue sauce
> Dijon mustard
> Low-fat yogurt (plain and flavored)
> Cooked veggies and parmesan cheese
> Stir-fried vegetables with soy sauce
> One pat of butter or margarine

**Choose less often:** You already know what I'm gonna say about this one. Lay off the mounds of butter and sour cream!

## Desserts

The perfect ending to a meal—or maybe not.

**Choose more often:** Select fresh fruit, frozen yogurt, Jell-O, angel-food cake, low-fat cookies, sorbet, frozen fruit bars, applesauce, and baked apples. If you feel like going all out, share a decadent dessert with a friend.

**Choose less often:** Don't make it a habit to top off each meal with a high-fat dessert such as chocolate cake, cookies, ice cream sundaes, strawberry shortcake, puddings, custards, and apple pie a la mode.

# Breakfast Ideas in the Campus Dining Hall

- ❏ Low-fat milk, toast with jam, and an orange
- ❏ Bowl of cereal, low-fat milk, banana, and orange juice
- ❏ Yogurt with cereal and raisins and a glass of milk or juice
- ❏ Bagel with a thin layer of cream cheese and tomato slices, glass of milk, and an apple
- ❏ Oatmeal with sliced peaches and a glass of grapefruit juice
- ❏ Pancakes with strawberries, bananas, or other fruit (and go "light" on the butter and syrup) with a glass of milk or hot tea with lemon
- ❏ Waffle topped with peaches and yogurt and a glass of grapefruit juice
- ❏ Scrambled eggs, bagel with jam, and a glass of orange juice

❏ Vegetable omelet, fresh fruit salad, and a glass of milk

❏ Poached eggs on a English muffin, light hot cocoa, and sliced melon

## Lunch Ideas in the Campus Dining Hall

❏ Turkey breast sandwich on whole-wheat bread, carrot sticks, and frozen yogurt with granola

❏ Bowl of lentil soup, a baked potato topped with broccoli and marinara sauce, and an orange

❏ Vegetable pizza and fresh fruit salad

❏ Hamburger on a bun, side salad, and an apple

❏ Grilled chicken sandwich with lettuce, tomato, two cookies, and low-fat milk

❏ Grilled vegetables with cheese in a pita pocket and fruit salad

❏ Chicken noodle soup, low-fat yogurt, and a frozen fruit bar

❏ Large tossed salad with beans and chickpeas, pita bread, and a low-fat fruit yogurt topped off with a pear

❏ Salad with turkey breast, roll, and angel food cake topped with strawberries

❏ Baked potato with broccoli and cheese, side salad, and fresh pineapple slices

❏ Roast beef or ham sandwich, cup of tomato soup, and some grapes

❏ Peanut butter and jelly sandwich, bowl of vegetable soup, and an apple

## Dinner Ideas in the Campus Dining Hall

❏ Veggie burger on a bun, salad, and fresh fruit

❏ Chicken burrito with salsa, a side of vegetables, and an orange

❏ Grilled chicken breast, mashed potatoes, and carrots with two cookies and a light hot cocoa

❏ Vegetable pizza, side salad, and fresh fruit

❏ Pasta with vegetables and tomato sauce, sprinkled with parmesan cheese, and some Jell-O

❏ Broiled fish with sautéed vegetables over rice and a frozen yogurt cone with sprinkles

❏ Vegetarian chili, a large salad, and some angel food cake

❏ Chicken kebab, veggies over rice, and a frozen yogurt-banana split

❏ Large salad with beans, a bowl of minestrone soup, and fruit ices

❏ Lightly stir-fried shrimp and vegetables over linguini with sliced peaches for dessert

❏ Chicken fajitas with salsa and a frozen fruit bar

# The Infamous "Freshman 15"

College is the time to gain knowledge—not weight. Why do so many freshman girls (and some guys) put on the pounds during their first year of school?

You can partially blame it on a decline in your RMR. The *resting metabolic rate*, also known as *basal metabolic rate*, is the number of calories that you burn when your body is not active. Most little kids have super high RMRs; they can eat a ton and not gain any weight. As you age and enter adulthood, your RMR usually slows down and you can't burn calories so effortlessly anymore. (At least that's true for the majority of us. Some people maintain wicked high metabolisms forever and ever. Lucky devils.)

The undeniable reason for the increased weight (better known as the notorious "freshman 15" pounds of flub) is poor eating habits and lack of exercise. Let's take a look at some common culprits.

> **Nutri-Speak**
>
> **Resting Metabolic Rate** is also known as *basal metabolic rate*, it's the number of calories that you burn when your body is not active (or at rest).

## Late-Night Munchies and Ordering In

Many college students make a habit of skipping meals, only to find themselves ravenous late at night. Does this sound familiar: "Hello, Domino's, I'd like to order a large supreme pizza." Your body needs fuel *throughout* the day, not at the end of your day (such as when you eat that family-size bag of Doritos at 2 A.M.). Keep in mind: Calories eaten during the day are much more likely to be burned than calories eaten just before bedtime because you burn more calories while active than while lying around. Take advantage of the campus dining hall during regular mealtimes, and avoid the unnecessary eating late at night.

## Vending Machines

Stop! Don't push that button before you inspect the goods. Tragically enough, the majority of tempting treats that scream "Eat me" from behind the glass windows are loaded with fat. For example, a bag of M&Ms has 10 grams of fat, a Snickers bar has 14 grams of fat, two jumbo chocolate-chip cookies have 18 grams of fat, and those "only sold in vending machines" cheese and crackers contain 11 grams of fat. Remember, the object of a healthy eating plan is to take in less than 30 percent of your total calories from fat, and one of the vending machine losers can really dent your day.

As for the times that you absolutely can't pass by without sticking your change into the slot, shoot for the healthier alternatives: for instance, pretzels, fig bars, low-fat granola bars, and wheat crackers. If your sweet tooth won't let up, occasionally satisfy the junk-food urge with hard candies, licorice, jelly beans, gummy bears, and other gooey-chewies. They don't provide anything in the way of nutrition (straight sugar), but at least they are generally low in fat (sort of the best of the worst).

## Getting Sloppy in the Dining Hall

Piling your tray with unhealthy, high-fat foods during mealtimes can also make you a candidate for weight gain. No more excuses, it's time for some major damage control. Reread the section "Making the Grade in the Campus Dining Hall."

## Lack of Exercise

Another common weight-gain culprit is inactivity. The name of the game is balance; calories in equals calories out. In other words, eating a lot of garbage and sitting around on your butt all day (whether studying or watching soap operas) will put on the pounds, simply because you're taking in more calories than you're burning off. All types of exercises burn calories, walking, jumping rope, aerobic classes, stair climbing; it doesn't necessarily have to be something intense.

## Alcohol and Partying

It's true, some studies suggest that an occasional drink can actually benefit your health. Come on, who are we kidding? That's not the kind of drinking most college kids are into. It's more like *party all night and drink 'til you drop*. Maybe I can convince you to ease up on the booze by first providing the caloric facts. Alcohol is loaded with calories. More specifically, it is loaded "nutrient-less" calories (seven per gram, to be exact). Just another possible reason for weight gain.

| Alcoholic Beverage | Serving Size (Fluid Ounces) | Approximate Calories |
|---|---|---|
| Beer | 12 | 150 |
| Light beer | 12 | 100 |
| Bloody Mary | 5 | 115 |
| Gin and tonic | 7.5 | 170 |
| Daiquiri | 4.5 | 250 |
| Piña Colada | 4.5 | 260 |
| Screwdriver | 7 | 175 |
| Tequila Sunrise | 5.5 | 190 |
| Tom Collins | 7.5 | 120 |
| Gin/rum/vodka/whiskey 100 proof | 1.5 (1 shot) | 125 |
| Gin/rum/vodka/whiskey 80 proof | 1.5 (1 shot) | 100 |
| Wine, red and white | 5 | 105 |
| Champagne | 5 | 133 |
| Martini | 2.5 | 155 |

Incidentally, alcohol can also lead to late-night eating. One of my clients, Lisa, reminisces of a pizza place located right next to the popular off-campus bar. Every

Thursday, Friday, and Saturday night, the place would be mobbed with semi-drunk kids pigging out on pizza, all claiming "Purple Pizza" (the name of the place) had the best pizza in the entire world. Ironically enough, one day Lisa stopped in and had a slice for lunch without her usual alcohol buzz. Not even edible!

Whether you munch out with a group of friends, or devour your roommate's Pop-Tart stash, alcohol can certainly cloud your thinking and instigate a late-night eating orgy.

Another reason to lay off the booze: "Oh, my aching head." You can literally lose an entire day between the headaches, nausea, fatigue, and other lousy symptoms that occur from drinking one too many.

For the *occasional* times you drink, follow these guidelines:

➤ Make sure you have food in your stomach before you drink. Food can act as a buffer and delay the absorption of alcohol into the bloodstream.

➤ Know your limit. Everyone has his own capacity for alcohol, and it's important to know when to stop. Bear in mind that you will not impress a potential crush if you are stumbling (or vomiting) all over yourself at a party.

➤ Ask the bartender to dilute your drinks with extra fruit juice, seltzer water, or club soda. Also, order wine spritzers (half wine, half seltzer).

➤ Alternate every other drink at a party with plain water, fruit juice, or any other non-alcoholic beverage. This way, you're never empty-handed.

➤ Better yet, stick with non-alcoholic drinks and avoid alcohol altogether.

# Pop Quiz: Test Your Nutrition I.Q.

Take the following quiz and test your nutritional smarts:

1. **Circle the two beverages that are the best bets in the campus dining hall:**
   a. Sweetened iced teas
   b. Water
   c. Orange juice
   d. Soda

2. **Which of the following sandwiches has the most fat?**
   a. Tuna salad sandwich
   b. Roast beef sandwich
   c. Turkey breast sandwich
   d. Grilled chicken sandwich

3. **Eating breakfast can help you control your weight.**
   a. True
   b. False

4. **A low-fat topping for a baked potato is**
   a. Sour cream
   b. Butter
   c. Margarine
   d. Marinara sauce

5. **Choose the breakfast cereal that offers the most fiber:**
   a. Cap'n Crunch
   b. Raisin Bran
   c. Rice Krispies
   d. Frosted Flakes

6. **Which type of potato has the most fat?**
   a. Baked potato
   b. Roasted potato
   c. French-fried potato
   d. Mashed potato

7. **Circle the following high-fat salad bar items:**
   a. Olives
   b. Beans
   c. Bacon bits
   d. Chickpeas

8. **Which is the healthier soup?**
   a. Cream of broccoli
   b. Vegetable barley

9. **It is perfectly okay to eat lean red meat once in a while.**
   a. True
   b. False

10. **Some of the healthiest desserts in the dining hall include**
    a. Applesauce
    b. Frozen yogurt
    c. Angel food cake
    d. All of the above

Answers:

| | |
|---|---|
| 1. b and c | 6. c |
| 2. a | 7. a and c |
| 3. True | 8. b |
| 4. d | 9. True |
| 5. b | 10. d |

---

### The Least You Need to Know

➤ Take responsibility for yourself and select well-balanced, healthy meals in the campus dining hall.

➤ Don't forget to start your day with a nutritious breakfast. Eating breakfast helps regulate your appetite the rest of the day so you won't overeat at lunch and dinner.

➤ Avoid those dreaded "freshman 15" pounds by dodging vending machines, stopping late-night ordering, making low-fat selections in the campus dining hall, and getting off the couch to exercise.

➤ Alcohol contains a lot of "empty calories," and excessive drinking might result in weight gain.

# Part 6
# Weight Management 101

*Weight control seems to be a full-time job for some people; they're on and off every diet on the planet. I have a friend, Joan, who once told me her biggest fear of death is that they will print her weight in the obituary! Needless to say, she's alive and well and on another crazy diet.*

*It's finally time to stop going up and down like a yo-yo and stick with a sensible plan of attack. Whether you want to lose weight, gain weight, or most importantly, stop obsessing, this final section covers it all, so read on. I provide weight-loss programs to help knock off (and keep off) those extra unwanted pounds, along with calorie-cramming strategies to help you skinny folks beef up your bods. I also take a look at life-threatening eating disorders and where to find help when food and exercise go beyond health and get way out of control.*

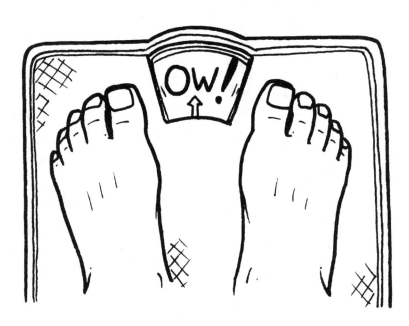

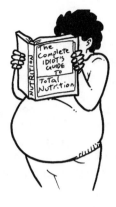

# Chapter 26

# Come On, Knock It Off

---

### In This Chapter

➤ Why crash dieting *doesn't* work

➤ Identifying your ideal body weight

➤ Lose weight on a well-balanced program

➤ Understanding the language of "bubbles"

➤ Maintaining your weight after you've lost

---

Let's take a walk down memory lane. We've had the Scarsdale Diet, the Grapefruit Diet, the Banana-Cottage Cheese Diet, the Cabbage Soup Diet, the High-Protein Diet, and even the "Lose 10 Pounds in a Week Eating Rice & Mashed Potatoes" Diet (obviously developed by a constipated psychopath).

Unfortunately, crash dieting is an American sport that just won't go away. They're sort of like trick candles on a birthday cake: Every time you blow one out, another one pops up to taunt you. But with all these blubber-blasting gimmicks, our national waistline continues to bulge! In fact, most people who lose weight on these crazy programs wind up gaining it all back—plus some extra pounds to boot. What's more, the fad diets usually leave you deprived and irritable.

# What's the Best Diet Anyway?

If you're looking for a quick fix, this chapter is *not* going to help you. The bottom line is that people should lose weight eating the very same healthy foods that they will continue to eat *after* they have lost the weight—that is, a lot of complex carbs coming from whole grains, fruits, and vegetables, low-fat dairy, and lean sources of protein foods. Makes perfect sense, right? To lose weight *forever,* you must work on changing your eating behavior forever. Read through and try my bubble plan. You've got nothing to lose except some unwanted pounds—and perhaps a lifetime of professional dieting.

### Food for Thought

For your personal nutrition profile, visit my Web site at www.joyof-nutrition.com. Simply fill out your food for a typical day (plus your height, weight, and age), and I'll show how you measure up to your daily requirements for vitamins, minerals, calories, carbohydrate, protein, fat, sugar, fiber, and much more.

## What Should You Weigh?

First, figure out a realistic weight to strive for. Here's a quick way to estimate your healthy weight range:

➤ **For men:** Start with 106 pounds for 5 feet, and then add 6 pounds for every inch over 5 feet (or subtract 6 pounds for every inch under 5 feet).

Then, calculate the weight range for your frame by subtracting or adding 10 percent of the sum to your number.

*Example:* A man standing 5'10" will calculate 106 + 60 = 166 pounds. If he is small-framed, he *subtracts* 10% of that from 166 pounds to get 150 pounds. If he is large-framed, he *adds* 10% to 166 to get 182 pounds. Therefore, a man who is 5'10" has a healthy weight range between 150 and 182 pounds.

➤ **For women:** Start with 100 pounds for 5 feet, and then add 5 pounds for every inch over 5 feet (or subtract 5 pounds for every inch under 5 feet). Then, calculate your weight range by subtracting and adding 10 percent of that sum to your number.

*Example:* A woman standing 5'5" will calculate 100 + 25 = 125 pounds. If she is small-framed, she *subtracts* 10% of that from 125 pounds to get 112.5 pounds. If she is large-framed, she *adds* 10% to 125 to get 137.5 pounds. Therefore, a woman who is 5'5" has a healthy weight range between 112.5 and 137.5 pounds.

Here's another quick way to get a visual of your weight range. Simply use it as a guideline because the numbers seem to slightly vary from chart to chart.

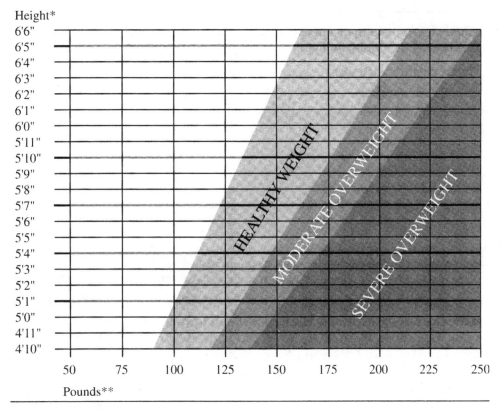

Height*

Pounds**

*Without shoes.
**Without clothes. The higher weights apply to people with more muscle and bone, such as many men.

Source: *Report of the Dietary Guidelines Advisory Committee on the Dietary Guidelines for Americans, 1995,* pages 23-24.

# Testing Your Body Fat: Getting Pinched, Dunked, and Zapped

Although your weight indicates the sum total of *all* your body parts, it doesn't take into consideration your body composition (the amount of body fat versus lean body mass), which is important to know because muscle weighs more than fat. In fact, some people might appear a bit high on the weight chart *but* have very little body fat, indicating that the weight is coming from muscle mass and *not* blubber mass. (Of course, *you* know whether that extra weight is solid muscle or just...extra weight.)

To get a more accurate idea about where you stand in terms of fat, check out your body fat percentage by getting pinched, dunked, or zapped—especially if you regularly work out. Compare your results with the normative ranges in the following chart:

| Percent Body Fat for Women | | |
| --- | --- | --- |
| *Age* | *Good* | *Excellent* |
| 20–29 | 20.6–22.7 | 17.1–19.8 |
| 30–39 | 21.6–24.0 | 18.0–20.8 |
| 40–49 | 24.9–27.3 | 21.3–24.9 |
| 50–59 | 28.5–30.8 | 25.0–27.4 |
| 60– | 29.3–31.8 | 25.1–28.5 |
| **Percent Body Fat for Men** | | |
| 20–29 | 14.1–16.8 | 9.4–12.9 |
| 30–39 | 17.5–19.7 | 13.9–16.6 |
| 40–49 | 19.6–21.8 | 16.3–18.8 |
| 50–59 | 21.3–23.4 | 17.9–20.6 |
| 60– | 22.0–24.3 | 18.4–21.1 |

## Skin-Fold Calipers

Getting "pinched" involves what are called *calipers*, a contraption that looks like a handgun with salad tongs. A tester positions the gun on certain parts of your body and grabs your fat so that it is pulled away from your muscle and bone. (Sounds painful, but it's not.) After gathering a few different measurements, typically from the back of your arm, your thigh, your abdomen, your shoulder, and your hip, the tester will plug each number into a formula to calibrate your overall body fat percentage.

**Food for Thought**

Take a trained athlete and a couch potato of the same height and weight: The athlete looks healthier and leaner and most likely wears a smaller clothing size than the couch spud. This is because muscle weighs more than fat, even though it takes up less space.

Although the calipers are quick, simple, and convenient, the test results can sometimes be skewed if a tester pinches some muscle along with the fat *or* does not pinch enough of the fat. You will also need to have this type of test performed *before* a workout; during exercise, your skin slightly swells, which can make you appear fatter than you are.

## Underwater Weighing

Getting "dunked" is actually the most accurate of the classic methods of body-fat testing. Basically, you sit on a scale in a small pool of warm water. Next, you blow *all* the air out of your lungs and dunk underneath until you are completely submerged for about five seconds. Your underwater weight will then register on a digital scale; a tester plugs that number into a formula to determine the percent of body fat.

## Bio-Electrical Impedance

Getting "zapped" requires you to lie on your back with one electrode attached to your hand and another to your foot. A signal is then sent from one electrode to the other. The faster the signal travels, the more muscle you have. On the other hand, the slower the signal moves, the more fat you have because fat impedes or blocks the signal.

# How Many Calories Should You Eat for Weight Loss and Weight Maintenance?

Counting the calories in each morsel of food that you eat is *not* the way to go. But you can get a general idea of how many total calories you should eat each day, to either maintain *or* lose weight, with the following formula:

1. First find your BMR (basal metabolic rate: the amount of calories needed to perform your normal bodily functions at rest).

   BMR = your current weight × 10

2. Next, multiply your BMR × an activity factor.

   BMR × 0.30 (for average daily activities)

3. Last, add your BMR to your activity factor.

Here's an example of a 130-pound woman:

   130 pounds × 10 = BMR of 1,300 calories

   1,300 calories × .30 = 390 activity factor

   1,300 + 390 = 1,690 calories per day

People who participate in regular physical activity more than three times a week will need to raise the activity factor to .40–.60.

**Food for Thought**

If you decide to work with a nutritionist, remember: You want a food partner, not a food dictator! Find a qualified registered dietitian (R.D.) who will move at your pace and make you feel completely comfortable. For a registered dietitian in your area, call the American Dietetic Association at 800-366-1655.

The example shows that an average 130-pound woman can maintain her weight on 1,690 calories per day. Now, let's say she wants to lose a few pounds. To lose weight, she needs to create a negative balance by reducing the amount of daily calories and increasing her exercise to burn even more calories. For instance, she needs to get on a 1,400 calorie food plan, plus work out aerobically 4–5 days per week. She'd have no problem shedding some weight safely and efficiently.

Plug your own stats into the formula, and figure out what it will take calorically to melt away those unwanted pounds. Understand that no one should ever eat less than 1,200 calories per day; you will slow down your metabolism and set yourself up to gain all the weight back. Even if you are very petite, and the math works out to be less than 1,200—stick with 1,200 calories and jack up your exercise.

# The "Bubble Game" and Your Personal Weight-Loss Plan

Now that you've done the math, roll up your sleeves and get ready to learn about bubbles. On the following pages you'll be provided with several plans that use bubbles to represent servings sizes (○ ○ ○). Each bubble plan is designed to provide a specific caloric level—1,200 cals, 1,400 cals, 1,600 cals, or 1,800 cals. You'll select one of the balanced weight-loss plans experiment and create an in-between plan of your own. Make it into a game and simply follow the bubble sheets by focusing on the number of total daily servings from each of the five food groups. Notice that all the calculations have been done for you, so there's no need to count a single calorie. In fact, calorie counting from here on in is off limits.

**Food for Thought**

People are different and lose weight at different speeds on different plans. For instance, you and your friend might do the math and come up with the same 1,400-calorie weight-loss plan, but she might lose 1–2 pounds each week, and you might only lose half a pound each week. In this case, assume that you have a slower metabolism and need to step up your exercise and use the lower 1,200-calorie plan.

## *Understanding the Bubbles*

A bubble is simply a serving size; therefore, the number of bubbles in each food group is the total number of servings in your plan for each day. For example, if you are following the 1,200-calorie plan, you have two fruit bubbles and three grain/bread bubbles, which represents two servings of fruit and three servings of grain. Browse the various items under each food category, and learn exactly what counts as one serving so that you know how to plan your foods for the day.

It's *not* necessary to weigh or measure; an eyeball guess-timation will work just fine. Here's how to guesstimate your serving sizes, and remember, this is only a general list; there are a gazillion other foods that can fit perfectly into each category, so go ahead and plug in your favorites.

### *One Grain/Bread Bubble = Approximately 80 Calories*

- ○ 1 medium slice of *any* type of bread
- ○ ¹/₂ small bagel or English muffin
- ○ Small pita bread (or ¹/₂ large)
- ○ 1 serving cereal (hot or cold)
- ○ ¹/₂ cup cooked pasta, rice, barley, or couscous
- ○ *Small* baked potato or sweet potato (size of your fist)
- ○ ¹/₂ cup peas or corn
- ○ 1 ounce (small bag) pretzels
- ○ Low-fat granola bar
- ○ 2 fig cookies

Note: Some vegetables are included in this group because they are very starchy.

Here are some common grains and how they can count:

➤ Pasta entree = four grain bubbles

➤ Side of pasta or rice = two grain bubbles

➤ Large baked potato = two grain bubbles

➤ Large, hot pretzel = three grain bubbles

➤ Potato knish = three grain bubbles

➤ Large New York bagel = three to four grain bubbles

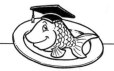

**Food for Thought**

A sensible weight-loss plan should shed pounds slowly but steadily—approximately one to two pounds per week.

### One Vegetable Bubble = Approximately 25 Calories

Most vegetables are unlimited; just make sure to eat your *minimal* quota!

❍ 1 cup raw vegetables

❍ ¹/₂ cup cooked vegetables

❍ 1 cup vegetable juice

The only exceptions are the starchy potatoes, peas, and corn, which get counted as grains.

### One Fruit Bubble = Approximately 60–90 Calories

❍ Any medium piece of fruit (apple, small banana, pear, and so on)

❍ ¹/₂ small cantaloupe

❍ Large wedge of watermelon or honey dew

❍ 1 cup fresh fruit salad or berries

❍ Small glass fruit juice (about ¹/₂ cup)

❍ Large scoop of fruit sorbet

❍ Noncreamy frozen fruit bar

❍ Small handful of dried fruit

### One Milk Bubble = Approximately 90–150 Calories

❍ 1 cup low-fat milk (skim or 1%)

❍ 1 8-ounce container of nonfat (flavored) yogurt

❍ Small low-fat frozen yogurt

❍ 2–3 slices of low-fat hard cheese (or 1¹/₂ ounces)

❍ ³/₄ cup (big scoop) low-fat cottage cheese

❍ 1 cup low-fat pudding

❍ Skim milk cappuccino, café latté, or hot cocoa

❍ 3–4 Tbs parmesan cheese

### 1 Milk Plus 1 Fat = Approximately 150–200 Calories

○ 1 cup whole milk

○ Regular cheese on anything

○ One scoop real ice cream

○ Regular hot chocolate, cappuccino, or café latté

○ 1 cup chocolate pudding

○ *Anything* else made with whole milk

### One Protein Bubble = Approximately 225 Calories per 3 Ounces

○ Approximately 3 ounces of lean meat, poultry, or fish (the size of a deck of cards), unless otherwise indicated

○ Chicken breast (3 ounces)

○ Turkey breast (3 ounces)

○ Lean red meats (3 ounces)

○ Turkey burger or veggie burger (3 ounces)

○ All seafood and fish (3 ounces)

○ Tofu (6 ounces)

○ Egg whites (approximately 4)

○ Whole eggs (2)—but eat occasionally

○ Beans (¹/₂–1 cup cooked)

### One Fat Bubble = Approximately 45 Calories

○ Any time you *think* something is prepared with fat: for example, sautéed vegetables—a sauce on your fish—fried chicken cutlet, etc.

○ Any time you use 1 tsp butter, oil, margarine, or mayonnaise

○ 1 Tbs cream cheese, peanut butter, or salad dressing

○ 2 Tbs of sour cream

For reduced-calorie spreads, double the serving size; you do *not* need to count fat-free spreads at all.

### "Free Foods" That Don't Count as Anything!

○ Mustard

○ Cocktail sauce

○ Ketchup

○ Salsa

○ Soy sauce*

○ Tomato sauce

○ Teriyaki sauce*

○ Bouillon*

○ Worcestershire sauce

○ Sugar

○ All spices and seasonings

○ Sugar substitutes

○ Jams and jellies

○ Hard candies (3 per day)

○ Pancake syrup (a circle only)

○ Chewing gum (1 pack per day)

○ Fat-free salad dressings and spreads (in moderation)

○ Coffee/tea

○ Horseradish

○ Sugar-free beverages

*These foods are extremely high in salt; when they're available, choose the low-sodium versions.*

## Tracking Your Food on the Daily Bubble Sheets

Make 20 or more copies of the food plan on the following pages that's right for you, and chart your daily food intake for the first few weeks, just to get the hang of it. After eating each meal or snack, check off the appropriate bubbles at the bottom. This will help you to keep an eye on exactly how much food you've eaten and how much is left for the rest of the day.

## Approximately
## 1,200 Calorie Food Plan

Breakfast


Lunch


Snack


Dinner


Snack


---

Grains and breads: ○ ○ ○

Vegetables: ○ ○ ○

Fruits: ○ ○

Milks: ○ ○

Protein foods: ○ ○

Fats: ○ ○

Water: ○ ○ ○ ○ ○ ○ ○ ○

**Sample Day of
1,200 Calorie Food Plan**

<u>Breakfast</u>
1 serving of dry cereal
1 cup skim milk
1 banana

<u>Lunch</u>
Large salad with 3 ounces grilled chicken with 1 Tbs of dressing (or 2 Tbs of low-fat Italian salad dressing)
Small pita bread

<u>Snack</u>
Low-fat frozen yogurt

<u>Dinner</u>
Lean steak, 3 ounces
A lots of steamed broccoli
Small baked potato with 1 tsp of margarine
1 cup fresh strawberries

Grains and breads: ☑ ☑ ☑

Vegetables: ☑ ☑ ☑

Fruit: ☑ ☑

Milk: ☑ ☑

Protein foods: ☑ ☑

Fat: ☑ ☑

Water: ☑ ☑ ☑ ☑ ☑ ☑ ☑ ☑

### *Approximately*
### *1,400 Calorie Food Plan*

Breakfast

Lunch

Snack

Dinner

Snack

---

Grains and breads: ○ ○ ○ ○

Vegetables: ○ ○ ○

Fruits: ○ ○ ○

Milks: ○ ○

Protein foods: ○ ○

Fats: ○ ○

Water: ○ ○ ○ ○ ○ ○ ○ ○

## Sample Day of
## 1,400 Food Calorie Plan

Breakfast
Toasted English muffin with 1 Tbs cream cheese
1 cup low-fat milk plus 1 cup blueberries in a blender with ice

Lunch
3 ounces turkey breast on a plain tortilla wrap
Lettuce, tomato slices, and mustard
An apple

Snack
A pear

Dinner
Tossed green salad with 1 ounce of grated low-fat cheese and fat-free dressing
4 ounces grilled fish in lemon
Medium baked potato with 2 Tbs sour cream
Steamed spinach

---

Grains and breads: ☑☑☑☑

Vegetables: ☑☑☑

Fruits: ☑☑☑

Milks: ☑☑

Protein foods: ☑☑

Fats: ☑☑☑

Water: ☑☑☑☑☑☑☑☑

## Approximately
## 1,600 Calorie Food Plan

Breakfast

Lunch

Snack

Dinner

Snack

---

Grains and breads: ○ ○ ○ ○ ○ ○

Vegetables: ○ ○ ○

Fruits: ○ ○ ○

Milks: ○ ○

Protein foods: ○ ○

Fats: ○ ○ ○

Water: ○ ○ ○ ○ ○ ○ ○

### Sample Day of
### 1,600 Calorie Food Plan

<u>Breakfast</u>
Bowl of oatmeal with some skim milk
Container of nonfat flavored yogurt
Small glass orange juice

<u>Lunch</u>
Hamburger on bun
Side salad with 1 Tbs dressing
Fresh fruit salad

<u>Snack</u>
Frozen fruit bar

<u>Dinner</u>
Stir-fry chicken and a lot of veggies (use only 1–2 tsp oil and soy sauce)
1 cup brown rice
Small frozen yogurt

Grains and breads: ☑ ☑ ☑ ☑ ☑ ☑

Vegetables: ☑ ☑ ☑

Fruits: ☑ ☑ ☑

Milk: ☑ ☑

Protein foods: ☑ ☑

Fats: ☑ ☑ ☑

Water: ☑ ☑ ☑ ☑ ☑ ☑ ☑ ☑

### Approximately
### 1,800 Calorie Food Plan

Breakfast


Lunch


Snack


Dinner


Snack

---

Grains and breads: ○ ○ ○ ○ ○ ○ ○

Vegetables: ○ ○ ○ ○ ○ ○

Fruits: ○ ○ ○ ○

Milk: ○ ○ ○

Protein foods: ○ ○

Fats: ○ ○ ○

Water: ○ ○ ○ ○ ○ ○ ○

## Sample Day of
## 1,800 Calorie Food Plan

Breakfast
Egg-white omelet with veggies (use 1 whole egg plus 2 egg whites and nonstick cooking spray)
2 slices whole-wheat toast with 2 tsp reduced-fat margarine
Sliced bananas and strawberries, $\frac{1}{2}$ cup
1 cup of skim milk

Lunch
1 slice vegetable cheese pizza
Tossed salad with low-fat dressing

Snack
Peach
2 fig cookies

Dinner
Grilled swordfish (3–4 ounces),
Marinate in lemon and 1 tsp olive oil
$1\frac{1}{2}$ cups pasta with marinara sauce
Grated low-fat mozzarella cheese ($1\frac{1}{2}$ oz)
Cooked carrots and green beans
A baked apple

Grains and breads: ☑ ☑ ☑ ☑ ☑ ☑ ☑

Vegetables: ☑ ☑ ☑ ☑ ☑ ☑

Fruits: ☑ ☑ ☑ ☑

Milk: ☑ ☑ ☑

Protein foods: ☑ ☑

Fats: ☑ ☑ ☑

Water: ☑ ☑ ☑ ☑ ☑ ☑ ☑ ☑

# No More "I've Blown It" Syndrome; All Foods Are Allowed

Are you guilty of the "all-or-nothing" mentality? Do you place all your faves "off limits" when you diet, and then, the second you eat anything on the "bad list," you go whole hog and eat the house? *("I've already blown it—might as well polish off the rest of the chips and cookies. I'll start fresh on Monday.")*

Diets fail when you're deprived of your favorite foods—even if they aren't healthy. You *don't* gain weight from occasionally eating moderate amounts of high-fat foods. In fact, you *lose* weight because in the end, you don't feel deprived, and you're not tempted to bag your whole weight-loss program.

The following list shows you that almost *anything* can fit in: You just have to cross off the appropriate bubbles and account for the food item during that day. Try your best to stick with healthier choices most of the time, but go ahead and occasionally splurge on pizza, cookies, cake, or anything else that tempts your palate; I encourage it! Simply stay within your daily bubble limit by shifting other meals around to compensate, and you'll still lose weight.

**Food for Thought**

Did you know that six pieces of broken cookie equals an entire cookie that you could have enjoyed?

## Fat-Combo Foods

Fat-combo foods have fat built in. In other words, they are not straight oil, dressing or butter—but fat combos such as pizza, chocolate, and so on.

➤ Cookies (2 medium) = 1 grain, 1 fat

➤ Cake (medium slice, *any* type) = 2 grains, 2 fats

➤ Doughnut = 2 grains, 2 fats

➤ Large bakery cookie = 2 grains, 2 fats

➤ Scone (medium) = 2 grains, 2 fats

➤ Danish/pastry = 2 grains, 2 fats

➤ Bakery muffin (large) = 3 grains, 2 fats

➤ Potato chips (small bag) = 1 grain, 1 fat

➤ Corn chips (small bag) = 1 grain, 1 fat

➤ Chocolate bar (Kit-Kat, Snickers, and so on) = 1 grain, 3 fats

➤ Coleslaw ($^1/_2$ cup) = 1 vegetable, 1 fat

➤ Potato salad ($^1/_2$ cup) = 1 grain, 1 fat

➤ Real ice cream (2 scoops) = 2 milks, 2 fats

- ➤ French fries (about 20) = 2 grains, 2 fats
- ➤ Chinese lo mein (1 cup) = 2 grains, 2 fats
- ➤ Cornbread (medium piece) = 1 grain, 1 fat
- ➤ Cream soups (1 cup) = 1 grain, 1 fat, 1 vegetable
- ➤ Macaroni and cheese (1 cup) = 2 grains, 1 milk (or protein), 1 fat
- ➤ Pizza (1 medium slice) = 2 grains, 1 milk (or protein), 1 vegetable, 1 fat

*Notice that for macaroni and cheese and pizza, the cheese can either be counted as milk or protein.*

### Q & A

**Where do you carry your excess padding, on your belly or butt?**

Studies have shown that people carrying excess fat on the upper body and stomach suffer *more* health risks than people carrying fat on the hips and buttocks. Weight that is carried in the abdominal region is closer to the heart and the larger coronary arteries—versus weight on the hips. Therefore, it poses a greater risk for heart disease

# Setting Realistic Goals

Don't overwhelm yourself trying to lose a tremendous amount of weight. Instead, break it into smaller, more achievable short-term goals. For example, if you have your heart set on losing, say, 40 pounds, aim for 10 pounds at a time. Even with a mere eight pounds to lose, strive for knocking off two pounds at a time.

Also, understand that genetics play a key role in determining your body makeup, so don't dream about that "Barbie-doll body"; it's not gonna happen. Take a look at your mom, dad, and other relatives; biology isn't destiny, but heredity does play an integral part in shaping your shape.

The most important thing is to learn to love the body you have and keep your focus on ways to

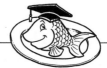

**Food for Thought**

Don't obsess over the scale; it can drive you nuts! Limit the times you weigh yourself to no more than once or twice a week. In fact, avoid hopping on the scale each time you hit the bathroom by packing it away in the closet between weigh-ins, *or* simply weigh yourself outside your home (at the gym, your doctor's office, and so on).

make it healthy. You might never be a size 6 or have bulging muscles, but you can learn to be happy with the body you have by taking care of it.

## Get Moving and Keep Moving

Following a healthy food plan is only half of the weight-loss equation: You've gotta move to lose! Numerous studies have shown that exercise helps promote weight loss *and* weight maintenance by revving up your metabolism (that is, burning more calories). What's more, exercise relieves stress and can even psych up your state of mind so that you're motivated to make smart food choices during the day.

## Maintaining Your Weight After You've Lost It

So you have reached your goal—now what? "Hooray!" on one hand, "Eek!" on the other! Maintaining your weight is actually harder than losing weight because there's no goal to strive for; you're already there. Hang tight and read the following tips. This time, your shapely physique is here to stay.

➤ The trick is to loosen the diet reins, but not too much. Continue with a *modified* version of your bubble plan (in your head only) because it's well balanced and encourages you to eat healthfully.

➤ Figure out a five-pound weight range with your present weight in the middle. For example, if your weight is 130 pounds, give yourself a range of 128–132 pounds. Continue to weigh in once every week or so, and if you go over the range, get back on the bubble sheets.

➤ Plan one meal "off" each week—in other words, a meal that doesn't fit or calculate into your plan (anything you'd like). If your weight continues to stay put, add a second meal off, or possibly a dessert. Experiment and see what your body can handle; everyone is different.

➤ You might prefer to simply add a few more grains to your plan (or a fruit and milk). See what your weekly weigh-ins reveal (or if your clothes seem to "shrink" or "grow") and never panic if you think you've gained. Just take away some of the additions the following week. Remember, the key to maintaining is to find out how much food your body can handle.

➤ Absolutely continue with your regular exercise program. Exercise allows you to eat more food because it burns mega calories and keeps you tight and toned because it zaps body fat and increases your lean body mass.

**The Least You Need to Know**

➤ Fad diets don't work. People should lose weight eating the very same healthy foods they will continue to eat after the weight is lost.

➤ Your weight on the scale is the sum total of all your body parts (fat mass and lean mass); therefore, it's also helpful to test your body-fat percentage because this identifies how much of your body is actually fat.

➤ Don't set your heart on a Barbie/Ken-doll body. Plan realistic weight-loss goals by understanding that genetics play a key role in body make-up.

➤ Learn to love the body you have, and focus on making it healthy, not necessarily perfect.

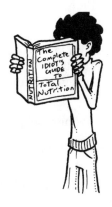

# Chapter 27

# Adding Some Padding

**In This Chapter**

➤ Strategies to help you gain weight

➤ High-calorie meals and snacks

➤ Refreshing shakes to boost your calories

Is your metabolism so speedy that you burn calories quicker than you can pack 'em in? Maybe you're one of those "uninterested in food" people, who look down at their watches and think, "Oops, I forgot to eat lunch." Whatever the reasons for your thin physique, fear not: With some attention and determination, you can start an upward trend on your bathroom scale.

## Is Being Underweight a Health Concern?

For some people being too thin can be a health concern—specifically for people that are underweight because they undereat. When your body does not receive adequate food energy (calories), it basically runs out of gas and leaves you feeling fatigued, irritable, and with decreased concentration. Further with an inadequate food intake you run the risk of developing vitamin and mineral deficiencies that may cause serious long-term problems (e.g., to little calcium and Vitamin D = bone loss).

On the other hand being underweight may *not* pose a health risk and merely be about improving appearance. Some people are born with fast metabolisms that burn calories quicker than they can eat them. In this case your caloric intake is most probably providing your daily requirements for nutrition, and you'll have to learn to eat more, more often, and calorically dense foods to try and defy your genetics.

To check if you are underweight, flip back to Chapter 26, "Knock It Off," and look at the height/weight charts provided (or follow the equation provided).

# Six Tips to Help You Pack in the Calories

Gaining weight requires devouring more calories than you burn. In fact, to gain one pound, you need an extra 3,500 calories coming from food. Naturally, that's not at one sitting, but by simply eating an extra 500 calories a day, you can gain a pound per week—because 500 calories × 7 = 3,500 calories.

Stick with the basic food principles and concentrate on the following tips:

➤ Eat larger portions at your three main meals; even consider adding an extra meal to your day.

➤ Snacks are important! Plan at least three snacks a day. Snack #1 can fit between breakfast and lunch; snack #2, between lunch and dinner; snack #3, before bedtime. Tote along some trail mix, dried fruits, crackers, sports bars, fig bars, and nuts, or keep them in your desk at work.

➤ Add calorically dense foods to your meals. For example, toss beans, seeds, nuts, peas, avocado, cheese, and dressings into salads. Add shrimp, fish, chunks of chicken, and a lot of parmesan cheese to pastas. Add crackers, rice, corn, noodles, and beans to your soups. Don't forget the bread basket; spread on the margarine and dig in!

➤ Guzzle tons of pure fruit juice or milk (preferably 1% or 2%) with and between your meals; it's a great way to painlessly add calories.

➤ Add powdered dry milk to your soups and casseroles.

➤ Try a calorically dense supplement, such as Ensure Plus, Sustacal, Boost, Carnation Instant Breakfast, and Nutriment. Just make sure you drink them between meals or with meals—not instead of meals—or you won't be getting extra calories at all.

➤ Consult a qualified exercise trainer about embarking on a weight-lifting program. It can help you build muscles and put on some pounds.

**Nutri-Speak**

**Calorically dense foods** provide a lot of calories and fat in a relatively small portion size. (Nuts, seeds, and avocado are examples.)

# Adding More of the Good Stuff

Although the idea is to increase your calories, you also want to keep your diet well-balanced and nutritious. The last thing you want to do is shovel in chocolate bars, donuts, cakes, cookies, and other "nutrient-less" stuff that will pad you with fat and supply zippo in the nutrition department. Instead, eat more of the good stuff and stick with foods that are calorically dense. Here are some examples:

| Basic, Healthy Meal | To Add Some Calories |
|---|---|
| Vegetable omelet | Add cheese and a bagel with margarine. |
| Salads | Add shredded cheese, avocado, olives, and plenty of dressing. |
| Pizza | Add extra cheese and vegetables. |
| Pasta | Add olive oil, olives, and parmesan cheese. |
| Chicken stir-fry | Add peanuts or cashews. |
| Burritos | Add guacamole or sour cream. |

Here are some high-calorie and nutritional snack ideas:

➤ Frozen-yogurt milkshake (anything goes)

➤ Bowl of cereal with fruit and low-fat milk

➤ Tortilla chips with salsa and guacamole

➤ Peanut butter and jelly on crackers

➤ Bran, corn, or blueberry muffins

➤ Peanut butter on apple slices or bananas

➤ Cheese and crackers

➤ Cereal mixed with yogurt

➤ Dried fruit and nut mixture

➤ Fruit bars and granola bars

## Shake It Up Baby

Shakes can be a refreshing, filling alternative to snacks and can add a significant amount of calories to your day. Try these ideas:

➤ Process in a blender: 4 ice cubes, $1/2$ cup orange juice, $1/2$ cup of melon chunks, 1 banana or $1/2$ cup strawberries, and wheat germ (optional). Add more or less juice and fruit to achieve the desired consistency.

➤ Mix Carnation Instant Breakfast or Ovaltine with 1 cup of low-fat milk; drink it with your breakfast or have it for a mid-morning or bedtime snack.

➤ Puree 10 oz silken tofu, $3/4$ cup apple juice, 1 banana, or $1/2$ cup blueberries in a blender and top with walnuts or almonds.

➤ For a thick smoothie, puree 1 cup yogurt, 2 tsp honey, 1 banana, and $3/4$ cup fruit juice. (Pineapple or orange juice works well.) Mix in wheat germ if desired.

Wanna Gain Some Weight? Try This Sample Menu:

## Sample Menu

Breakfast
Bran flakes (large bowl) with low-fat milk
2 handfuls of raisins
Large glass of orange juice
Bagel with margarine

Snack 1
8 oz low-fat milk with Carnation Instant Breakfast
Large blueberry muffin

Lunch
Chicken-salad sandwich on whole-wheat bread
Bowl of vegetable soup with crackers
Apple
Large glass of fruit juice

Snack 2
Peanut butter on crackers with low-fat milk
Dried fruit and nuts
Glass of juice

Dinner
Vegetable cheese pizza
A lot of Italian bread
Salad with olive oil and vinegar
Flavored fruit drink

Bedtime snack
Frozen yogurt cone with sprinkles

By following these tips and becoming consistent with larger meals and frequent snacks, you should be able to gain some weight. Remember to focus on more servings of the five major food groups—grains, fruits, vegetables, meats, other proteins foods, and dairy—and not try to gain weight by overdoing foods from the pyramids tip.

### The Least You Need to Know

➤ To gain weight, you must take in more calories than your body burns.

➤ Increase your daily calories by eating bigger portions with your meals and by snacking on calorically dense foods that also offer nutrition.

➤ Guzzle tons of fruit juice, make creative shakes, or drink the popular supplements that are on the market.

➤ Embark in a weight-lifting program. It can help beef up your muscles and your weight.

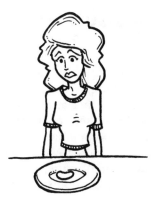

# Chapter 28

# Understanding Eating Disorders

---

## In This Chapter

➤ All about anorexia nervosa and bulimia

➤ What is compulsive overeating?

➤ Real-life stories from people with eating issues

➤ How to help a friend with an eating disorder

---

The ideal of beauty has become more and more slender—a bone-thin slender, in fact, that most people are not capable of achieving through healthy, normal eating. Surrounded by skinny-minnies on TV, movies, and magazines, it's no wonder that millions of Americans each year suffer from serious eating disorders. More than 90 percent of those afflicted with eating disorders are adolescents and young adult women, who are at a time in their lives when the quest for that "ideal bod" is overwhelming.

Many psychological theories about eating disorders have been proposed, and today, there are numerous comprehensive treatment centers to help people struggling with anorexia nervosa, bulimia, and compulsive overeating. As a society, we need to overcome this obsession with unreasonably low weights and learn to accept and love the healthy genetic shapes we were given. This chapter provides you with the basics on eating disorders so that you can better understand the world of dieting gone haywire—and perhaps help a friend, a relative, or even yourself.

*I would also like to extend a very special thanks to three of my clients, who have allowed me to share their struggles with food.*

# Anorexia Nervosa: the Relentless Pursuit of Thinness

Anorexia nervosa is a complex psychological disorder that literally involves self-starvation. People who suffer from this illness eat next to nothing, refuse to maintain a healthy body weight for their corresponding height, and frequently claim to "feel fat" even though they are obviously emaciated. Because anorexics are severely malnourished, they often experience symptoms of starvation: brittle nails and hair; dry skin; extreme sensitivity to the cold; anemia (low iron); lanugo (fine hair growth on body surface); loss of bone; swollen joints; and dangerously low blood pressure, heart rates, and potassium levels. If not caught and treated in time, victims of anorexia nervosa can literally "diet themselves to death."

The prevalence of anorexia nervosa is estimated at 0.1–0.6 percent of the general population, with 90 percent of the sufferers women and roughly 6 percent boys and young men. Although any personality can fall victim to this life-threatening illness, most anorexics tend to be perfectionists who keep their feelings bottled up inside, straight-A students, good athletes, and people who always do the right thing. For anorexics, restricting and controlling food becomes a way to cope with just about anything.

Here are some of the warning signs of anorexia nervosa:

➤ Abnormal loss of 15 percent (or more) of normal body weight with no medical reason for the loss. It can also be a failure to gain an expected amount of weight during a period of growth for younger children and adolescents.

➤ An intense fear of becoming fat or gaining weight, along with strict dieting and severe caloric restriction—despite a rail-thin appearance.

➤ In females, absence of at least three consecutive menstrual cycles otherwise expected to be normal.

➤ Always moving the diet "finish line." *("Just five more pounds and then I'll stop.")*

➤ Constant preoccupation with food. Anorexics will often cook and prepare food for others but refuse to eat anything themselves.

➤ Distorted body image. For example, claiming to "have fat hips" even though scales and mirrors show that they are severely emaciated.

➤ Strange eating rituals such as cutting food into tiny pieces, taking an unusually long time to eat a meal, and constantly preferring to eat alone.

➤ Obsessively over-exercising despite fatigue and weakness.

➤ Becoming socially withdrawn, isolated, and depressed.

**Nutri-Speak**

**Anorexia nervosa** means "appetite loss of nervous origins." **Bulimia** means "ox-like hunger."

### *"Weighting to Be Normal"*

*At 13 years of age and 172 pounds, I wasn't very involved in the world around me. Sure, I saw the fried chicken, mashed potatoes, cakes, and cookies, but boys, clothing, and beaches eluded me. Don't get me wrong, I wasn't miserable all the time; I just wasn't particularly happy. In fact, most of the time I was nothing; I was just FAT!*

*Like most perfectionists, I seemed to do everything to extremes. Initially, I ate to the fullest, and later, when my doctor told me I needed to lose weight, I dieted to the skinniest. 365 days later and 52 pounds lighter, the new Jane emerged. I had exercised and dieted my way to health. Burgers and taxis were out, low-fat foods and biking were in.*

*Not surprisingly, my doctor was ecstatic with my success, and my family was beaming with pride. My friends, on the other hand, were filled with that strange combination of jealousy and admiration, and finally for the first time in my life, guys noticed me. They whistled when I walked down the street and approached me at school. "Wow," I thought. "If I can get this much attention at 120 pounds, imagine how great life could be at 110."*

*At 100 pounds, I thought I had found bliss: I could count my ribs, pull down my pants without unbuttoning them, and most importantly, I could go an entire day on just a small fat-free frozen yogurt.*

*The months flew by, and my weight continued to plummet. Exhausted, freezing, and wearing size-0 clothing, I had propelled myself into a lonely abyss. Summer nights felt like the dead of winter, and the urge to sleep was unstoppable. I knew I was sick—everyone knew I was sick—and I was ultimately diagnosed with anorexia nervosa.*

*Although I rejected the notion of having a disease, I struggled both mentally and physically with solid foods and decreasing my amount of exercise. Gradually over the course of a year, I regained both my body and my life. I admit, low-fat foods and exercising are still entrenched in my life, but this time in a healthy manner, not as a destructive disaster. I must push myself to eat a risky meal (a "scary" meal with fat) every other day and allow myself to indulge in a dessert treat twice a week. Although I still obsess about my weight, it's no longer about losing; instead, it's about maintaining. I have been at my current healthy, thin weight of 112 pounds for the last year, and I guess you can say I have finally found an ideal way to exercise my "control." I "control" what I eat and how much I exercise, not in a freezing abyss, but in a hot, sweaty gym.*

*—Jane Stern, an 20-year-old recovered anorexic*

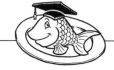

**Food for Thought**

For further reading, order *The Eating Disorder Catalog*, Gurze Books, 800-756-7533, www.gurze.com.

# Bulimia Nervosa

The eating disorder termed *bulimia* is at least two or three times more prevalent than anorexia nervosa. In fact, recent surveys report that about 1 percent of the general population and 4 percent of women aged 18–30 suffer from this troublesome disease. People with bulimia have repeated episodes of *binge eating*—rapidly consuming large quantities of food and then ridding their bodies of the excess calories by vomiting, abusing laxatives or diuretics, and/or exercising obsessively. In most cases, this binge/purge syndrome is an outlet for anxiety, frustration, depression, loneliness, boredom, or sadness. Because most bulimics are typically normal weight, they can keep this a secret and go undetected for years. Although some researchers think the problem is getting worse, others believe that people are just more willing to seek help, and therefore, it's noticed and treated more often.

Here are some of the warning signs of bulimia:

➤ Dissatisfaction with body shape and constant preoccupation with becoming thin.

➤ Recurrent mood swings and depression.

➤ Frequent episodes of rapidly consuming large amounts of food (binge eating), followed by attempts to purge (get rid of food) through self-induced vomiting, use of laxatives or diuretics, prolonged exercise, or by following severe low-calorie diets between binges.

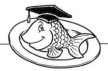

### Food for Thought

Many people aren't diagnosed with anorexia or bulimia but suffer from less serious "food issues" that nonetheless control and hinder their lives.

Remember you only have one life to live. Get help and live it to the fullest!

➤ Serious physical complications from chronic vomiting, including erosion of dental enamel from acidic vomit, scars on the hands from sticking fingers down the throat, swollen glands, sore throat, irritation of the esophagus, and poor digestion (heartburn, gas, diarrhea, constipation, bloating). The more serious physical dangers include severe dehydration, loss of potassium (because potassium controls the heart beat), and rupture of the esophagus.

➤ Awareness that eating pattern is abnormal.

➤ Fear of not being able to control eating voluntarily.

➤ Light-headedness and dizziness or fainting.

➤ Frequent weight fluctuations of 10 pounds in either direction from the constant bingeing and purging.

### *"My Vicious Cycle of Starving-Stuffing"*

*It all started when I was preparing to go off to college. My anxiety stemmed from separating from my family and manifested itself in a body-image and eating problem. Up until this time, I was a "normal" eater, eating when I was hungry, stopping when I was full, and occasionally overeating during special occasions. I ate chocolate bars, pizza, and movie popcorn without as much as a blink. What was it like then?*

*Suddenly, it was as if my body wasn't mine anymore. It became this "thing" separate from myself. I became hyper-aware and mentally obsessed with how to control my shape through obsessive exercise and restrictive eating patterns. Skipping two meals in a row and exercising two hours a day became normal to me. I used to stand in front of my dorm room mirror naked, poking and scrutinizing myself out loud. My self-esteem was so low that I actually needed someone to validate all of my insecurities. My overweight roommate would look on in disgust, reassuring me that I wasn't fat. A lot of people in my life got tired of reassuring me of this.*

*I did not allow myself to enjoy "forbidden foods" for a long time through college. I felt proud of this control but ironically continued with my dissatisfaction over my "chunky body" (which has always been very thin, so I'm told). But after a while of rigid restriction, my body rebelled and my disordered eating took on a new twist: a few days of restricting (sometimes as low as 500 calories a day) and then bam—I would "sabotage" all of my efforts by stuffing myself until I was uncomfortably full! Feeling disgusted, depressed, and ENORMOUS, I would get rid of the calories by making myself vomit, and then struggle back to my extremely low-cal, restrictive diet, and the vicious cycle continued. My weight could fluctuate 10 pounds depending upon the day of the week, but to the outside world, I still remained a "normal" little person.*

*I also developed strange idiosyncrasies. Certain colors had to be eaten together, and certain foods had to "match" each other, for no particular reason except that they made sense to me. I would also weigh myself up to 25 times each day. There was no room for error, spontaneity, or change.*

*Finally, coming to terms with the fact that this obsession with food and exercise was ruining my life, I started to see a psychotherapist. For the first time, I realized that my "food thing" was only a symptom of unlimited emotions that I had bottled up inside. I needed to work hard to break free from my extremist attitudes and my belief that being less than perfect was not worth being. (What is "perfect" anyway?)*

*Today, I allow myself to feel entitled to my words and actions and realize that a middle ground is healthier in relation to feeling, thinking, and eating. I've also worked with a nutritionist for the past year. She has taught me that restricting inevitably leads to bingeing, and I'm desperately trying to do away with black/white days (restricting or bingeing) and instead focus on the "gray."*

*I no longer let one M&M dictate my self-esteem, and I have learned that normal eating is flexible and always changing. It's okay to eat a big piece of cake on my birthday, chocolate when I have PMS, and movie popcorn once in a while. "Normal eating" means eating healthy most of the time, while allowing yourself to indulge when you feel like it. It's feeding yourself when you're hungry and sometimes when you're not—even just for the fun of it! It's feeding your mind as well as your body and realizing that weight fluctuations are normal. It is seeing life as more than what you put in your mouth and enjoying social situations for the conversation and laughter. It is learning to accept our bodies, our strengths, and our limitations as well. I admit, every day is a struggle right now, but at least I finally believe that I am worth it.*

—*A 27-year-old recovering bulimic*

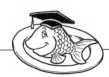

**Food for Thought**

Eating disorders can sometimes run in families. In fact, the rate of anorexia among sisters has been estimated at 2–10 percent.

# Compulsive Overeating

People who compulsively overeat repeatedly consume excessive amounts of food, sometimes to the point of abdominal discomfort. However, unlike bulimics, they do not get rid of the food with any of the methods mentioned earlier. In fact, most people with this type of eating disorder are overweight from the constant bingeing and have a long history of weight fluctuations.

Because compulsive overeaters feel out of control with their food (and often eat in secret), there seems to be a high incidence of depression, in addition to the serious medical complications that go hand in hand with being overweight.

### "Dieting My Way to Obesity"

*The cycle began when I was 11 or 12. I wore a size 7 and thought I looked fat. I dieted, starved, exercised, overate, and ended up a size 9. I did the size 7–9 dance several times until I finally graduated to the 9–11 routine. This continued until I ultimately reached size 13.*

*The turning point from "eating problem" to "life-threatening disorder" happened in my adult years after the break-up of a serious relationship. I just couldn't face the anxiety of the dating world again! It was also right after my grandmother passed away and my father had a heart attack. Starting a high-powered, senior-level job, my binges became out of control. Suddenly, walking home from work, I felt an urgent need to eat; I stopped at a grocery store, a deli, and a restaurant, buying chips, cakes, ice cream, and cookies. I reached my apartment and rushed into the kitchen, still wearing my heavy winter coat and hat, and started shoveling cake into my mouth. My hands were shaking and not able to get the cake in fast enough. I finished the entire cake, a pint of ice cream, and 20 Oreos before I was finally calm enough to take off my coat and order Chinese take-out.*

*This routine went on night after night for months. Within six months, I was up 85 pounds, and for the first time in my life, I topped 200 pounds on the scale. I was depressed, desperate, and terrified. I cried on and off all day long—in the shower, on the train, and in my office, frantically searching for help from diet centers, obesity researchers, and hospital programs. I frequently and seriously contemplated suicide. I was humiliated and weighed 250 pounds. I felt like a heroin addict, only I was addicted to food.*

*With the understanding, support, and guidance from trusting, caring, and knowledgeable practitioners, a psychiatrist, a nutritionist, group therapy, and anti-depression medication, I am presently working my way out of this perpetual hell. I now follow a non-deprivational approach—all foods in moderation. Believe me, it took a lot for me to be willing to try this because all I've ever known is either 750-calorie diets or 20,000-calorie binges. Today, I allow myself a chocolate bar if I really crave one, and if I need to overeat (not binge) because of a heavy, stressful workload—I give myself permission.*

*I presently weigh 185 pounds, eat normally, and, at 45, have a rebirth of hope.*

—*A 45-year-old compulsive overeater*

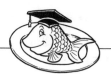

**Food for Thought**

Healing Connections is a nonprofit organization that strives to save lives through education, prevention, intervention, advocacy, and financial assistance for people suffering from anorexia and bulimia. They also provide educational workshops in schools and businesses. For more information, or to make a tax-deductible donation, contact Jennifer Kellman, 1461A First Avenue, Suite 303, New York, NY, 10021, or phone 212-585-3450.

# How to Help a Friend or Relative with an Eating Disorder

Combating an eating disorder is huge and generally involves a collaborative team of specialists, including a psychiatrist (or psychologist) to work through the psychological dynamics, a physician to monitor physical status, and a nutritionist (or dietitian) to reintroduce food as an ally—not an enemy. Here are some things you can do if you suspect a friend or family member has an eating disorder:

➤ Call your local hospital (or some of the treatment centers listed later in this chapter) and gather information on the various programs in your area. Ask about individual therapists, group therapy sessions, and nutritionists that specialize in food issues.

➤ In a very caring and gentle way, discuss your concerns with your friend or relative, and provide some of the professional resources and phone numbers that you've found. Be very supportive and patient; even offer to go along for any initial consults.

➤ If the person is a minor and refuses to get help, you might need to speak with a family member.

## Where to Go for Help

The following organizations can provide information, literature, and qualified referrals for the treatment of eating disorders:

**National Association of Anorexia Nervosa and Associated Disorders**
P.O. Box 7
Highland Park, IL 60035
847-831-3438

**American Anorexia Nervosa/Bulimia Association**
165 West 46th Street
New York, NY 10036
212-575-6200

**National Eating Disorder Organization**
**Laureate Eating Disorder Unit**
6655 South Yale Avenue
Tulsa, OK 74136
918-481-4044

Some of the comprehensive treatment centers available include

**Eating Disorders Clinic**
The New York State Psychiatric Institute
Columbia-Presbyterian Medical Center
722 West 168th Street
New York, NY 10032
212-960-5746

*Treatment is free for individuals who meet criteria for this research program.

**Eating Disorder Program**
The Cornell Medical Center—Westchester Division
21 Bloomingdale Road
White Plains, NY 10605
914-997-5875

**The Renfrew Center**
475 Spring Lane
Philadelphia, PA 19128
800-736-3739
215-482-5353

## The Least You Need to Know

➤ Anorexia nervosa is a life-threatening eating disorder that involves self-induced starvation and refusal to maintain a normal healthy weight.

➤ Bulimia nervosa is a serious eating disorder that involves repeated episodes of rapidly consuming large quantities of food and then ridding the body of the excess calories by self-induced vomiting, laxatives or diuretic abuse, and/or prolonged exercising.

➤ Compulsive overeating is repeatedly eating excessive amounts of food. Unlike bulimics, compulsive overeaters do not purge and therefore tend to be extremely overweight.

➤ Treating an eating disorder generally requires a collaborative approach from a psychiatrist or psychologist, a physician, and a nutritionist.

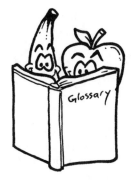

# Recipes for Your Health

## Jam in Popovers

*Serves eight*

1 cup flour                          1 egg

$^1/_4$ tsp salt                     Nonstick vegetable spray

1 cup 1% low-fat milk                1 tsp baking powder

1 Tbs canola oil                     Jam or preserves

Preheat oven to 425°. Use nonstick vegetable spray on muffin tin (or popover tin). Measure out all ingredients and pour into a blender. Blend well. Next, pour mixture into prepared muffin tray, filling each tin only $^1/_2$ to $^2/_3$ of the way. Bake 25–35 minutes until sides are rigid and top is puffed.

Each popover with an additional teaspoon of jam (optional) is the equivalent of one serving. Serve with plenty of fresh fruit.

<u>Nutrition Analysis</u>
Calories: 112
Total fat: 3 grams
Saturated fat: .5 grams
Dietary fiber: 0.5 grams
Protein: 3 grams
Sodium: 136 mg
Cholesterol: 28 mg

*From the kitchen of Meg Fein*

## Breakfast Berry Crepes

*Serves four*

2 cups whole-grain flour

$^1/_2$ cup blueberries

1 egg, beaten

$^1/_2$ cup raspberries

$2^1/_2$ cups low-fat milk

$^1/_2$ cup sliced strawberries

Nonstick vegetable spray

Place flour in a bowl and add egg plus 2 cups of milk. (Save $^1/_2$ cup.) Beat with a wire whisk until all lumps are gone and the mixture is completely smooth. Gradually add the remaining $^1/_2$ cup of milk to make a thin batter. Use nonstick cooking spray on hot skillet (medium-high temp), and pour enough batter in the pan just to make a large circle. Sprinkle desired amount of fruit on top and press down into the crepe. Cook for approx. 2–3 more minutes and then flip the crepe and cook the other side. Carefully lift onto a plate and roll it up.

Nutrition Analysis
Calories: 325
Total fat: 4 grams
Saturated fat: 1.6 grams
Dietary fiber: 5 grams

Protein: 15 grams
Sodium: 95 mg
Cholesterol: 59 mg

*From the kitchen of Andrea Mendonca and Jesse and Cole Bauer*

## Greek "Village" Salad

*Serves six*

4 large tomatoes, cut into chunks

1 large cucumber, peeled and sliced

2 green peppers, cut up into rings

1 large red onion, cut into rings

$^1/_2$ pound feta cheese, sliced and crumbled

Dried oregano, to taste

Black pepper to taste

$^1/_2$ cup *Olympia Dukakis's Light Greek Salad Dressing* (a personal favorite)

Place the cut tomatoes in a salad bowl with the peppers, onions, cucumber, and half of the crumbled feta cheese. Mix in the light Greek salad dressing and some black pepper to taste. On top, arrange the rest of the feta in neat slices and sprinkle with the oregano and a bit more dressing.

Nutrition Analysis
Calories: 180
Total fat: 13 grams
Saturated fat: 6 grams
Dietary fiber: 2 grams

Protein: 7 grams
Sodium: 509 mg
Cholesterol: 33 mg

*From the kitchen of Olympia Dukakis*

## Garden Tostada

*Serves four*

8 corn tortillas

$^1/_4$ cup nonfat mozzarella

$^1/_4$ cup nonfat sour cream

Salad

$^1/_2$ red bell pepper, chopped medium

$^1/_4$ cup chopped scallions

1 Anaheim chile pepper, seeded
  and chopped medium

4 Tbs prepared salsa

2 ripe tomatoes, chopped medium

2 Tbs vinegar

2 cups black beans, drained

3 cups shredded dark-green lettuce

Preheat oven to 375°. Place corn tortillas on cookie trays; do not overlap. Bake for 5 minutes and turn over. Bake for 10 more minutes or until curled and golden brown. Combine salad ingredients in large mixing bowl. To serve: Place 2 corn tortillas on each plate. Place salad mixture on top of each tortilla. Place 1 Tbs of nonfat mozzarella and 1 Tbs of sour cream over each tortilla.

### Nutrition Analysis
Calories: 300

Total fat: 2 grams

Saturated fat: 0 grams

Dietary fiber: 9 grams

Protein: 15 grams

Sodium: 200 mg

Cholesterol: 0 mg

*Copyright* Food for Health *newsletter, 1996. Reprinted with permission.*

## Curried Chicken and Rice

*Serves four*

1¹/₂ cups water

1 cup chicken broth

1 cup canned crushed tomatoes

¹/₄ cup dark, seedless raisins

1 tsp curry powder

¹/₂ tsp cumin

1¹/₄ cups uncooked basmati rice

12 oz. chicken breasts, boneless, skinless, cut into ¹/₂-inch cubes

2 cups broccoli florets

4 Tbs nonfat plain yogurt

In a large sauce pan, combine all ingredients *except for chicken, broccoli,* and *nonfat yogurt.* Bring to a boil, reduce to a simmer (turn stove to medium or medium-low), and cook covered for 8 minutes or until liquid is almost evaporated. Add chicken breast and broccoli florets and cook an additional 5 minutes or until chicken is done and rice is tender. It might be necessary to add more water. Serve with nonfat yogurt spooned over the top of each portion.

Nutrition Analysis

Calories: 370

Total fat: 1 grams

Saturated fat: 0 grams

Dietary fiber: 4 grams

Protein: 28 grams

Sodium: 230 mg

Cholesterol: 50 mg

## Eggplant Parmigiana

*Serves four*

1 large eggplant

1 cup nonfat plain yogurt

2 cups corn-flake crumbs

Olive oil cooking spray

Pinch cayenne pepper

1 cup grated nonfat mozzarella cheese

¹/₄ tsp garlic powder

16 oz. pasta sauce

Preheat oven to 350°. Slice eggplant lengthwise into ¹/₄-inch thick slices. (It is optimal to get 6 or 8 slices; that way, you have 1¹/₂ to 2 slices per person.) Combine corn-flake crumbs, cayenne pepper, and garlic powder in large mixing bowl. Coat eggplant slices with yogurt on both sides and then press both sides into corn-flake crumb mixture.

Set coated eggplant on cookie tray sprayed with olive oil cooking spray, and spray top of eggplant lightly with olive oil spray. Bake for 15 minutes or until crisp and golden brown. Top with grated nonfat mozzarella and bake an additional 3–5 minutes until cheese melts. Serve each portion over ¹/₄ cup hot pasta sauce.

Nutrition Analysis

Calories: 160

Total fat: 0 grams

Saturated fat: 0 grams

Dietary fiber: 4 grams

Protein: 11 grams

Sodium: 500 mg

Cholesterol: 5 mg

## Chicken Teriyaki over Linguine

*Serves four*

**Pasta**
8 oz. dried linguine noodles

**Sauce**

Vegetable oil cooking spray

12 oz. chicken breast strips (skinless)

1 Tbs low-sodium soy sauce

2 Tbs orange juice

1 1/4 cups water

3 cups fresh mixed stir-fry vegetables

1 cup snow peas

1/2 cup sliced green onion (scallions)

1 Tbs cornstarch

Cook linguine in 2 quarts of rapidly boiling water. Follow package directions for cooking times. Pasta is done when tender but slightly firm in center. Drain in colander.

Make the sauce: Heat a large 12-inch nonstick skillet and spray with vegetable oil cooking spray. Cook chicken strips just until done, approximately 5–7 minutes; set chicken aside. In the same skillet, add the soy sauce, orange juice, and 1 cup water. Bring to a simmer. Add all the vegetables and cook until tender, approximately 6 minutes. Dilute the cornstarch in 1/4 cup water and stir into the vegetable mixture. Broth should form a light glaze. Add chicken and serve over pasta.

Nutrition Analysis

Calories: 220

Total fat: 1 grams

Saturated fat: 0 grams

Dietary fiber: 9 grams

Protein: 25 grams

Sodium: 260 mg

Cholesterol: 50 mg

*Copyright* Food for Health *newsletter, 1996. Reprinted with permission.*

## Asparagus with Dijon Sauce

*Serves four*

$^3/_4$ pound fresh asparagus spears

$^1/_4$ cup reduced-sodium chicken broth

2 tsp Dijon mustard or tarragon Dijon mustard

1 Tbs grated Romano or Asiago cheese

Break woody ends off asparagus and place in skillet. Pour broth over asparagus and then cover and steam over medium heat until crisp-tender (about 4 minutes). Remove asparagus to warm serving plate with slotted spatula and keep warm. Add mustard to skillet; increase heat to high and bring to a boil, stirring constantly. Pour over asparagus and sprinkle with cheese.

*Microwave Method*

Break woody ends off asparagus and place in 2-quart rectangular microwave-safe dish. Pour broth over asparagus; cover with vented plastic wrap and cook on high power 3 to 4 minutes or until crisp-tender. Pour off liquid into 1-cup glass measure. Keep asparagus covered. Whisk mustard into juices. Cook uncovered at high power until boiling, about 30 seconds. Pour over asparagus; sprinkle with cheese.

Nutrition Analysis
Calories: 20
Total fat: 0.7 grams
Saturated fat: 0.4 grams
Dietary Fiber: 1.4 grams

Protein: 3 grams
Sodium: 51 mg
Cholesterol: 1 mg

*Copyright 1995, The American Dietetic Association. "Skim the Fat: A Practical and Up-to-Date Food Guide." Used with permission.*

## Traditional Tapioca

*Serves four*

2 Tbs quick-cooking tapioca

3 Tbs sugar

1/8 tsp salt

1 egg, beaten

2 cups skim milk

$^1/_2$ tsp vanilla

Mix all ingredients (except vanilla) in a saucepan. Let stand 5 minutes. Bring to a full boil, stirring constantly. Remove from heat. Stir in vanilla. Stir again after 20 minutes. Chill.

Nutrition Analysis
Calories: 115
Total fat: 1.5 grams
Saturated fat: 0.5 grams
Dietary Fiber: 0 grams

Protein: 1.4 grams
Sodium: 172 grams
Cholesterol: 55 mg

*Copyright 1995, The American Dietetic Association. "Skim the Fat: A Practical and Up-to-Date Food Guide." Used with permission.*

## Cinnamon Apple Phyllo Rolls

*Serves six*

1 box of phyllo dough, room temperature
(you need 3 strips)

3–4 medium-sized apples (cleaned, peeled, seeded,
coarsely chopped, and rinsed in water and lemon juice)

1 Tbs margarine

$^1/_4$ cup sugar

$^1/_4$ cup brown sugar

$^1/_2$ tsp cinnamon

$^1/_4$ tsp cloves (optional)

$^1/_2$ tsp vanilla

Nonstick vegetable spray

Melt margarine in a skillet and add apples, sugar, spices, and vanilla, stirring often. Cook until tender. Remove from heat and let it cool to room temperature. Preheat oven to 400°. Take 3 sheets of phyllo dough and cut them into $^1/_2$- or $^1/_3$-sheet strips. Lightly spray over each group of strips with nonstick vegetable spray, spoon apple mixture onto the strips, and roll up. Place them on a cookie sheet seam-side down, and again lightly gloss the outer phyllo with non-stick cooking spray. Bake 20–30 minutes, until lightly browned.

### Nutrition Analysis

Calories: 274

Total fat: 4 grams

Saturated fat: .5 grams

Dietary fiber: 2 grams

Protein: 2 grams

Sodium: 175 mg

Cholesterol: 0 mg

*From the kitchen of Meg Fein*

## Caribbean Rice Salad

*Serves four*

**Rice**

1$^1/_2$ cups white long-grain rice

2$^1/_4$ cups water

**Dressing**

2 Tbs cider vinegar

2 Tbs orange juice

4 Tbs nonfat Italian salad dressing

**Salad**

1 15$^1/_4$ oz. can black beans, drained and rinsed

1 orange, peeled, diced into $^1/_2$-inch cubes, and seeds removed

1 mango, peeled, chopped into $^1/_2$-inch cubes, and pit removed

1 fresh tomato, diced into $^1/_2$-inch cubes

$^1/_2$ jalapeño pepper, minced fine, seeds and veins removed,

$^1/_2$ red bell pepper, sliced into thin strips and seeds removed

$^1/_4$ cup sliced green onions

6 cups shredded dark-green lettuce

Prepare long-grain rice according to package directions. If you are in a hurry, use instant rice instead. Allow to cool to room temperature. (This process can be hurried by putting the cooked rice in your freezer in a shallow pan.)

Combine dressing ingredients together and toss with salad ingredients; toss with rice and serve. You can use additional orange segments and pepper strips for garnish if you want. Divide entire tossed salad between 4 plates and serve.

<u>Nutrition Analysis</u>

Calories: 340

Total fat: 1 grams

Saturated fat: 0 grams

Dietary fiber: 8 grams

Protein: 11 grams

Sodium: 230 mg

Cholesterol: 0 mg

## Sweet Potato Stew

*Serves six*

$^1/_2$ Tbs margarine

2 cups fresh sweet potatoes, cooked and sliced

8 oz can crushed pineapple in natural juice

$^1/_4$ tsp ground cinnamon

1/8 tsp salt

Heat margarine in a large frying pan. Add potato slices and pineapple. Sprinkle with cinnamon and salt. Simmer uncovered until most of the juice has evaporated (about 10 to 15 minutes), turning potato slices several times.

<u>Nutrition Analysis $^1/_2$ cup serving)</u>

Calories: 135

Total fat: 1.6 grams

Saturated fat: 0.3 grams

Dietary Fiber: 2.3 grams

Protein: 1.3 grams

Sodium: 78 mg

Cholesterol: 0 mg

## Papaya Sorbet

*Serves four*

1 ripe papaya (1$^1/_4$ pounds), diced

$^1/_4$ cup plain low-fat yogurt

$^1/_2$ cup light corn syrup

1 tsp fresh lime juice

Place papaya in a 9-inch square baking pan and freeze for about 1 hour. Place frozen papaya in food processor with yogurt, corn syrup, and lime juice. Process until smooth. Freeze for at least 1 hour. Makes 2 cups.

<u>Nutrition Analysis</u>

Calories: 160

Total fat: 0 grams

Saturated fat: 0 grams

Dietary Fiber: 0.3 grams

Protein: 1.4 grams

Sodium: 60 mg

Cholesterol: 1 mg

## Spicy Poached Pears

*Serves four*

1 cup apple juice

$^1/_2$ cup cranberry juice cocktail

1 Tbs orange juice

$^1/_3$ cup water

$^1/_4$ tsp ground cloves

$^1/_4$ tsp cinnamon

1/8 tsp ground ginger

4 ripe bosc pears, peeled

Pour juice, water, and spices into a deep saucepan; cover and bring to a boil. Trim the bottom off pears, if necessary, so they stand up straight. Remove core. Add pears and simmer uncovered until tender (15–25 minutes, depending on how ripe the pears are). Remove pears and set aside. Cook the remaining liquids over medium–high heat, stirring periodically, until mixture has reduced by half. Drizzle this juice-syrup over pears, and serve while warm, or chill and serve later.

Nutrition Analysis

Calories: 165

Total fat: 0.7 grams

Saturated fat: 0.1 grams

Dietary Fiber: 3.8 grams

Protein: 1 gram

Sodium: <5 mg

Cholesterol: 0 mg

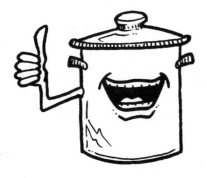

# Glossary

**ACE**   American Council on Exercise.

**ACSM**   American College of Sports Medicine.

**active lifestyle**   The lifestyle of folks who are constantly on the go. They do a lot of walking, taking the stairs, playing sports, or regularly working out.

**AFAA**   Aerobics and Fitness Association of America.

**anaphylactic shock**   A life-threatening whole-body allergic reaction to an offending substance. Symptoms include swelling of the mouth and throat, difficulty breathing, a drop in blood pressure, and a loss of consciousness. In other words, get help fast!

**anorexia nervosa**   A complex psychological disorder characterized by self-induced starvation. Meaning an "appetite loss of nervous origin," people who suffer from this disorder believe they are overweight, despite the fact that they are often skinny to an unhealthy degree.

**antibodies**   Large protein molecules that are produced by the body's immune system in response to foreign substances.

**bulimia**   Another psychological disorder personified through abnormal eating habits. Meaning "ox-like hunger," people suffering from bulimia are characterized by a vicious cycle of gorging massive amounts of food and inducing vomiting, taking laxatives, or excessively exercising in order to purge the food from their systems.

**calorically dense foods**   Foods that provide a lot of calories and fat in a relatively small portion size.

**calorie**   The amount of energy food provides. The number of calories a food provides is determined by burning it in a device called a calorimeter and measuring the amount of heat produced. One calorie is equal to the amount of energy needed to raise the temperature of one liter of water one degree Celsius. Carbohydrates and protein contain four calories per gram, fat contains nine calories per gram, and alcohol contains seven calories per gram.

**complementary proteins**   Two incomplete proteins in a food that compensate for one another's shortfalls when combined.

**complex carbohydrates (complex sugars)**   Compounds composed of long strands of many simple sugars linked together.

**cross conditioner/cross-country ski machines**   A great aerobic exercise that uses the entire body and burns tons of calories without any jarring impact. It's also good for quick warm-ups because it gets the whole body going. There is, however, one catch: Learning the movement can be a bit tricky for some people, and let's just say the term "poetry in motion" takes on a whole new meaning.

**diastolic pressure**   This number represents the pressure in your arteries while your heart is relaxing between beats. During this relaxation period, your heart is filling up with blood for the next squeeze. Although both systolic and diastolic numbers are critically important, your doctor might be more concerned with an elevated diastolic number because this indicates there is increased pressure on the artery walls even when your heart is resting.

**diverticulosis**   An illness or condition where tiny pouches (called diverticula) form in the wall of the colon. The condition is often without symptoms, but when the pouches become infected or inflamed, it can be painful. When this happens, the condition is known as diverticulitus, which can cause fever, abdominal pain, and diarrhea.

**empty calories**   Calories with no nutritional value.

**essential amino acids**   Amino acids that cannot be synthesized by the body. We must get these from outside food sources.

**fat-soluble nutrients**   Nutrients that dissolve in fat. Some essential nutrients such as the vitamins A, D, E, and K require fat for circulation and absorption.

**food allergy**   An over-reaction by the body's immune system, usually triggered by protein-containing foods (such as cow's milk, nuts, soybeans, shellfish, eggs, and wheat).

**food intolerance**   An adverse reactions to foods that generally do *not* involve the immune system (such as lactose intolerance).

**food poisoning**   An adverse reaction caused by contaminated food (microorganisms, parasites, or other toxins).

**food sensitivity**   A general term used to describe *any* abnormal response to food or a food additive.

**free radicals**   Unstable, hyperactive atoms that literally trek around your body damaging healthy cells and tissue.

**glucose (also called dextrose)**   A simple sugar found in fruits, honey, and vegetables. It is also the substance measured in blood. (Blood-sugar equals blood glucose.)

**hemorrhoid**   Painful swelling of a vein in the rectal area.

**homogenized milk**   Milk that has been processed to reduce the size of milkfat globules so the cream does not separate and the milk stays consistently smooth and uniform.

**hypertension**   The medical term for sustained high blood pressure. Contrary to how this term might sound, it does not refer to being tense, nervous, or hyperactive.

**hyponatremia**   Excessive loss of sodium and water due to persistent vomiting, diarrhea, or profuse sweating. Both water and salt must be replenished to maintain the correct balance for your body.

**incontinence**   The inability to control excretory functions.

**iron toxicity**   Although not very common, iron toxicity is a serious problem that occurs from either a genetic abnormality causing the body to store excessive amounts or the unnecessary over-supplementation of iron. The result can be liver and other organ damage.

**lacto-vegetarians**   This group of vegetarians eliminates meat and eggs from its diet but includes all dairy products.

**legumes**   Vegetables borne in pods of the bean and pea family that are especially rich in complex carbohydrates, protein, and fiber. They supply iron, zinc, magnesium, phosphorous, potassium, and several B-vitamins, including folic acid. Because foods that fall into this category provide ample amounts of both complex carbs and protein, they can fit in either the meat and beans group *or* the vegetable group. Legumes you might know by a more common name include black beans, pinto beans, kidney beans, lima beans, navy beans, soybeans (tofu), black-eyed peas, chickpeas (garbonzos), split peas, lentils, nuts, and seeds.

**NSCA**   National Strength and Conditioning Association.

**NASM**   National Academy of Sports Medicine.

**ovolacto-vegetarians**   This group of vegetarians eliminates all meat from its diet (red meat, poultry, fish, and seafood); however, it does include dairy products and eggs.

**pasteurized milk**   Milk that has been briefly heated to kill harmful bacteria and then rapidly chilled.

**proteins**   Compounds composed of carbon, hydrogen, oxygen, and nitrogen and arranged as strands of amino acids.

**pseudo vegetarians**   These people will not eat meat on the days they decide they're vegetarian but will, however, inhale hamburgers and steak sandwiches when they get a craving.

**rowing machines**   Another good "total-body" workout (and warm-up machine) without any impact. Be sure to get some pointers on technique; there is an easy way and the *right* way to do it. Obviously, the right way requires a lot more energy, concentration, and muscular effort.

**scurvy**   A disease resulting from a deficiency of vitamin C, characterized by bleeding and swollen gums, joint pain, muscle wasting, and bruises. Scurvy is now rare, except among alcoholics, and can be cured by as little as five to seven milligrams of vitamin C.

**sedentary lifestyle**   The lifestyle of folks who generally have desk jobs, watch a lot of TV, and tend to sit around most of the time.

**semi-vegetarians**   This group does not eat red meat but eats most chicken, turkey, and fish, along with all dairy and eggs.

**simple carbohydrates (simple sugars)**   Molecules of single sugar units or pairs of small sugar units bonded together.

**stairclimbers**   Cardiovascular equipment that provides a very challenging workout with some potential stress to your knees and lower back. (Listen carefully to your body.) This is a more advanced piece of machinery due to the importance of technique, and therefore, you need a base level of stamina and strength to use this machine even on lower levels.

**stationary bikes**   Now, they come in two flavors: the upright bike (like a regular outdoors bicycle) and the recumbent bike (legs out in front with high bucket seats lending more support for people with lower back pain). Both types of stationary bikes provide effective aerobic workouts that can give your joints a break because they are non—weight-bearing activities. Make sure that the tension is not too high and that the seat is not too low. If you are a beginning biker, ask a trainer to help you get into the proper position for an effective workout. When you are ready to pump up the intensity, play around with increasing your speed before increasing the tension.

**systolic pressure**   The top, larger number of a blood pressure measurement. This represents the amount of pressure in your arteries while your heart contracts (or beats). During this contraction, blood is ejected from the heart and into the blood vessels that travel throughout your body.

**tofu (firm)**   This tofu is stiff, dense, and perfect for stir-fry dishes, soups, or anywhere that you want tofu to maintain its shape. A 4-ounce serving of firm tofu supplies 13 grams of protein, 120 milligrams of calcium, and about 40 percent of your daily iron.

**tofu (silken)**   This tofu is creamy and custard-like and therefore also works well in pureed or blended recipes such as dips, soups, and pies. Silken tofu doesn't provide as much calcium as the more solid tofu varieties (only 40 milligrams), but it is the lowest in fat and is packed with $9^1/_2$ grams of protein per 4-ounce serving.

**tofu (soft)**   This tofu provides 9 grams of protein, 130 milligrams of calcium, and a little less than 40 percent of your daily iron from a 4-ounce serving. Soft tofu is good for dishes that require blended tofu (commonly used in soups).

**treadmills**   Cardiovascular equipment that presents light to moderate impact on your joints depending on whether you are running or walking. Walking on a flat grade is a good starting place for beginning exercisers. As your fitness and confidence levels build, you can experiment with increasing the incline and speed.

**vegetarians**   People who substitutes vegetables, nuts, and seeds for meat in a diet. They vary in strictness from avoiding all animal products to avoiding meat only. Vegetarian groups include ovolacto, pseudo, semi, and vegan.

**vegans**   These are the strictest types of vegetarians (sort of the Pope of all vegetarians). Vegans abstain from eating or using *all* animal products, from eating meat, dairy, and eggs to wearing wool, silk, or leather. If you're a vegan, you'll need to be extra responsible about getting adequate protein, iron, calcium, vitamin D, vitamin B-12, and zinc.

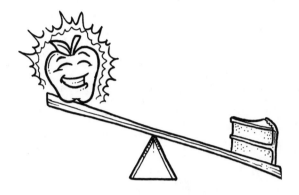

# Food Values

## A Closer Look at the Foods We Eat

This section provides a comprehensive nutrition profile for a wide variety of foods. It lists the nutrient values for calories, carbohydrate, protein, fat, saturated fat, dietary fiber, sugar, sodium, and cholesterol, plus seven other vitamins and minerals found in the foods and beverages we consume. Keep in mind that this chart provides you with the nutrient facts based on standard items—the nutritional content of packaged foods can vary from brand to brand. All information was derived from Nutritionist Five ©First Databank 1999.

The items for this table have been organized into several categories:

Breads and Grains

Fruits

Vegetables

Dairy: Cheese, Milk, Yogurt

Meats: Beef, Veal, Pork, Lamb

Poultry: Chicken, Turkey, Duck

Seafood

Eggs

Nuts and Seeds

Combination Foods

Fats: Oils, Salad Dressings, Spreads

Beverages

Sweets

Condiments

| GRAINS | Amount | Portion | Kcal | Protein | Carb | Fat | Chol | Sat Fat | Mono Fat | Poly Fat | Sodium | Potas |
|---|---|---|---|---|---|---|---|---|---|---|---|---|
| **BREADS:** | | | | | | | | | | | | |
| White Bread | 1 | SLICE | 66.75 | 2.05 | 12.38 | 0.90 | 0.25 | 0.20 | 0.40 | 0.19 | 134.50 | 29.75 |
| Wheat Bread | 1 | SLICE | 65.00 | 2.28 | 11.80 | 1.03 | 0.00 | 0.22 | 0.43 | 0.23 | 132.50 | 50.25 |
| Cracked Wheat Bread | 1 | SLICE | 65.00 | 2.18 | 12.38 | 0.98 | 0.00 | 0.23 | 0.48 | 0.17 | 134.50 | 44.25 |
| Mixed Grain Bread | 1 | SLICE | 65.00 | 2.60 | 12.06 | 0.99 | 0.00 | 0.21 | 0.40 | 0.24 | 126.62 | 53.04 |
| 100% Whole Wheat Bread | 1 | SLICE | 118.80 | 3.68 | 21.55 | 2.72 | 0.49 | 0.58 | 1.05 | 0.85 | 295.24 | 165.64 |
| Italian Bread | 1 | SLICE | 81.30 | 2.64 | 15.00 | 1.05 | 0.00 | 0.26 | 0.24 | 0.42 | 175.20 | 33.00 |
| Rye Bread | 1 | SLICE | 82.88 | 2.72 | 15.46 | 1.06 | 0.00 | 0.20 | 0.42 | 0.26 | 211.20 | 53.12 |
| Plain Hamburger Roll/Bun | 1 | ITEM | 122.98 | 3.66 | 21.63 | 2.19 | 0.00 | 0.52 | 0.36 | 1.08 | 240.80 | 60.63 |
| Hard Roll | 1 | ITEM | 167.01 | 5.64 | 30.04 | 2.45 | 0.00 | 0.35 | 0.65 | 0.98 | 310.08 | 61.56 |
| Submarine/Hoagie Roll | 1 | ITEM | 400.00 | 11.00 | 72.00 | 8.00 | 0.00 | 1.80 | 3.00 | 2.20 | 683.00 | 128.00 |
| Pita Bread | 1 | ITEM | 165.00 | 5.46 | 33.42 | 0.72 | 0.00 | 0.10 | 0.06 | 0.32 | 321.60 | 72.00 |
| English Muffin, Toasted | 1 | ITEM | 127.50 | 4.20 | 25.00 | 1.00 | 0.00 | 0.14 | 0.16 | 0.48 | 252.00 | 71.50 |
| Plain Bagel | 1 | ITEM | 195.25 | 7.46 | 37.91 | 1.14 | 0.00 | 0.16 | 0.09 | 0.49 | 379.14 | 71.71 |
| Plain Biscuit, Ready to Eat | 1 | ITEM | 127.40 | 2.17 | 16.98 | 5.78 | 0.35 | 0.87 | 2.42 | 2.17 | 368.20 | 78.40 |
| Plain Waffle, Prepared | 1 | ITEM | 218.25 | 5.93 | 24.68 | 10.58 | 51.75 | 2.15 | 2.64 | 5.09 | 383.25 | 119.25 |
| Plain Pancakes, Prepared | 3 | ITEM | 258.78 | 7.30 | 32.26 | 11.06 | 67.26 | 2.42 | 2.82 | 5.07 | 500.46 | 150.48 |
| Taco Shell | 1.00 | ITEM | 60.84 | 0.94 | 8.11 | 2.94 | 0.00 | 0.42 | 1.16 | 1.10 | 47.71 | 23.27 |
| Corn Tortilla | 1.00 | ITEM | 55.50 | 1.43 | 11.65 | 0.63 | 0.00 | 0.08 | 0.16 | 0.28 | 40.25 | 38.50 |
| Flour Tortilla | 1.00 | ITEM | 113.75 | 3.05 | 19.46 | 2.49 | 0.00 | 0.61 | 1.32 | 0.37 | 167.30 | 45.85 |
| **CRACKERS:** | | | | | | | | | | | | |
| Saltine Crackers | 10 | ITEM | 130.20 | 2.76 | 21.45 | 3.54 | 0.00 | 0.88 | 1.93 | 0.50 | 390.60 | 38.40 |
| Wheat Crackers | 10 | ITEM | 141.90 | 2.58 | 19.47 | 6.18 | 0.00 | 1.55 | 3.43 | 0.84 | 238.50 | 54.90 |
| Plain Rice Cakes (Brown Rice) | 3.00 | ITEM | 104.49 | 2.21 | 22.01 | 0.76 | 0.00 | 0.15 | 0.28 | 0.27 | 88.02 | 78.30 |
| Animal Cracker | 14 | ITEM | 124.88 | 1.93 | 20.75 | 3.86 | 0.00 | 0.97 | 2.17 | 0.51 | 110.04 | 28.00 |
| Plain Graham Crackers | 4 | ITEM | 118.44 | 1.93 | 21.50 | 2.83 | 0.00 | 0.43 | 1.14 | 1.07 | 169.40 | 37.80 |
| Cheese Crackers | 30 | ITEM | 150.90 | 3.03 | 17.46 | 7.59 | 3.90 | 2.81 | 3.63 | 0.74 | 298.50 | 43.50 |
| Plain Bread Sticks | 2 | ITEM | 49.44 | 1.44 | 8.21 | 1.14 | 0.00 | 0.17 | 0.43 | 0.44 | 78.84 | 14.88 |
| Seasoned Croutons, Ready to Eat | 1 | SERVING | 32.55 | 0.76 | 4.45 | 1.28 | 0.00 | 0.49 | 0.37 | 0.17 | 86.66 | 12.67 |
| **CEREALS:** | | | | | | | | | | | | |
| Oatmeal Cereal, Made with Milk | 1.00 | CUP | 237.78 | 12.34 | 32.76 | 6.51 | 17.34 | 3.03 | 1.96 | 0.95 | 350.08 | 434.00 |
| Shredded Wheat Cereal, Large Biscuit | 1.00 | ITEM | 84.96 | 2.57 | 19.19 | 0.39 | 0.00 | 0.07 | 0.06 | 0.21 | 0.47 | 77.17 |
| Shredded Wheat Cereal, Small Biscuit | 1.00 | CUP | 107.10 | 3.30 | 24.12 | 0.50 | 0.00 | 0.08 | 0.08 | 0.26 | 3.00 | 108.30 |
| Granola Cereal, Prepared | 1.00 | CUP | 569.74 | 17.93 | 64.66 | 30.01 | 0.00 | 5.80 | 9.60 | 12.90 | 29.28 | 656.36 |
| KELLOGG'S FROSTED FLAKES Cereal | 0.75 | CUP | 120.00 | 1.00 | 27.98 | 0.00 | 0.00 | 0.00 | 0.00 | 0.00 | 200.25 | 20.03 |
| KELLOGG'S ALL-BRAN Cereal | 0.50 | CUP | 80.00 | 4.00 | 22.00 | 1.00 | 0.00 | 0.00 | 0.00 | 0.50 | 280.00 | 340.00 |
| KELLOGG'S CORN FLAKES Cereal | 1.00 | CUP | 110.00 | 2.00 | 26.00 | 0.00 | 0.00 | 0.00 | 0.00 | 0.00 | 330.00 | 35.00 |
| KELLOGG'S FROOT LOOPS Cereal | 1.00 | CUP | 120.00 | 1.00 | 26.00 | 1.00 | 0.00 | 0.50 | 0.00 | 0.00 | 150.00 | 30.00 |
| KELLOGG'S Raisin Bran Cereal | 1.00 | CUP | 170.00 | 5.00 | 43.00 | 1.00 | 0.00 | 0.00 | 0.00 | 0.50 | 310.00 | 400.00 |
| KELLOGG'S RICE KRISPIES Cereal | 1.25 | CUP | 110.00 | 2.00 | 26.00 | 0.00 | 0.00 | 0.00 | 0.00 | 0.00 | 320.00 | 35.00 |
| KELLOGG'S SPECIAL K Cereal | 1.00 | CUP | 110.00 | 6.00 | 21.00 | 0.00 | 0.00 | 0.00 | 0.00 | 0.00 | 250.00 | 55.00 |
| KELLOGG'S FROSTED MINI-WHEATS Cereal | 1.00 | CUP | 190.00 | 5.00 | 45.00 | 1.00 | 0.00 | 0.00 | 0.00 | 0.50 | 0.00 | 160.00 |
| GENERAL MILLS MULTI-BRAN CHEX Cereal | 1.00 | CUP | 200.00 | 4.00 | 49.00 | 1.50 | 0.00 | 0.00 | 0.00 | 0.00 | 360.00 | 230.00 |
| GENERAL MILLS CORN CHEX Cereal | 1.00 | CUP | 110.00 | 2.00 | 26.00 | 0.00 | 0.00 | 0.00 | 0.00 | 0.00 | 300.00 | 30.00 |
| GENERAL MILLS CHEERIOS Cereal | 1.00 | CUP | 110.00 | 3.00 | 22.00 | 2.00 | 0.00 | 0.50 | 0.00 | 0.50 | 280.00 | 95.00 |
| GENERAL MILLS HONEY NUT CHEERIOS Cereal | 1.00 | CUP | 120.00 | 3.00 | 24.00 | 1.50 | 0.00 | 0.50 | 0.00 | 0.50 | 270.00 | 95.00 |
| GENERAL MILLS WHEATIES Cereal | 1.00 | CUP | 110.00 | 3.00 | 24.00 | 1.00 | 0.00 | 0.00 | 0.00 | 0.00 | 220.00 | 110.00 |
| GENERAL MILLS FIBER ONE Cereal | 0.50 | CUP | 60.00 | 2.00 | 24.00 | 1.00 | 0.00 | 0.00 | 0.00 | 0.00 | 140.00 | 250.00 |
| GENERAL MILLS TOTAL Raisin Bran Cereal | 1.00 | CUP | 180.00 | 4.00 | 43.00 | 1.00 | 0.00 | 0.00 | 0.00 | 0.00 | 240.00 | 280.00 |
| QUAKER OATS CAP'N CRUNCH Cereal | 0.75 | CUP | 110.00 | 1.00 | 23.00 | 1.50 | 0.00 | 0.00 | 0.32 | 0.39 | 210.00 | 35.00 |
| CREAM OF WHEAT Cereal, Regular, Prepared | 1.00 | CUP | 123.00 | 3.58 | 26.00 | 0.20 | 0.00 | 0.03 | 0.02 | 0.09 | 2.68 | 34.00 |
| POST GRAPE NUTS Cereal | 0.50 | CUP | 200.00 | 6.00 | 47.00 | 1.00 | 0.00 | 0.00 | 0.13 | 0.45 | 350.00 | 160.00 |
| POST Bran Flakes Cereal | 0.75 | CUP | 100.00 | 3.00 | 24.00 | 0.50 | 0.00 | 0.00 | 0.00 | 0.54 | 220.00 | 190.00 |
| POST Fruity PEBBLES Cereal | 0.75 | CUP | 110.00 | 0.50 | 24.00 | 1.00 | 0.00 | 0.00 | 0.25 | 0.25 | 160.00 | 30.00 |

| Vit A (IU) | Beta-C | Vit C | Calcium | Iron | Vit D (IU) | Vit E (IU) | Thiamin | Ribo | Niacin | Vit B6 | Folate | Vit B12 | Phosp | Magn | Zinc | Diet Fiber | Sugar |
|---|---|---|---|---|---|---|---|---|---|---|---|---|---|---|---|---|---|
| 0.00 | 0.00 | 0.00 | 27.00 | 0.76 | | | 0.12 | 0.09 | 0.99 | 0.02 | 23.75 | 0.01 | 23.50 | 6.00 | 0.16 | 0.58 | 0.98 |
| 0.00 | 0.00 | 0.00 | 26.25 | 0.83 | | | 0.11 | 0.07 | 1.03 | 0.02 | 19.25 | 0.00 | 37.50 | 11.50 | 0.26 | 1.08 | 1.12 |
| 0.00 | 0.00 | 0.00 | 10.75 | 0.70 | | | 0.09 | 0.06 | 0.92 | 0.08 | 15.25 | 0.01 | 38.25 | 13.00 | 0.31 | 1.38 | 1.00 |
| 0.00 | 0.00 | 0.08 | 23.66 | 0.90 | | | 0.11 | 0.09 | 1.14 | 0.09 | 20.80 | 0.02 | 45.76 | 13.78 | 0.33 | 1.66 | 1.01 |
| 9.95 | | 0.04 | 22.81 | 1.18 | | | 0.10 | 0.08 | 1.58 | 0.11 | 14.84 | 0.01 | 96.09 | 43.01 | 0.78 | 3.05 | |
| 0.00 | 0.00 | 0.00 | 23.40 | 0.88 | | | 0.14 | 0.09 | 1.31 | 0.01 | 28.50 | 0.00 | 30.90 | 8.10 | 0.26 | 0.81 | 0.98 |
| 2.24 | 0.00 | 0.13 | 23.36 | 0.91 | | | 0.14 | 0.11 | 1.22 | 0.02 | 27.52 | 0.00 | 40.00 | 12.80 | 0.37 | 1.86 | 3.07 |
| 0.00 | 0.00 | 0.04 | 59.77 | 1.36 | | | 0.21 | 0.13 | 1.69 | 0.02 | 40.85 | 0.03 | 37.84 | 8.60 | 0.27 | 1.16 | 3.18 |
| 0.00 | 0.00 | 0.00 | 54.15 | 1.87 | | | 0.27 | 0.19 | 2.42 | 0.02 | 54.15 | 0.00 | 57.00 | 15.39 | 0.54 | 1.31 | 2.22 |
| 0.00 | 0.00 | 0.00 | 100.00 | 3.80 | | | 0.54 | 0.33 | 4.50 | 0.05 | | | 115.00 | | | 3.75 | 10.00 |
| 0.00 | 0.00 | 0.00 | 51.60 | 1.57 | | | 0.36 | 0.20 | 2.78 | 0.02 | 57.00 | 0.00 | 58.20 | 15.60 | 0.50 | 1.32 | 3.24 |
| 0.00 | 0.00 | 0.05 | 94.50 | 1.36 | | | 0.19 | 0.14 | 1.90 | 0.02 | 14.50 | 0.02 | 72.50 | 11.00 | 0.38 | 1.45 | |
| 0.00 | 0.00 | 0.00 | 52.54 | 2.53 | | | 0.38 | 0.22 | 3.24 | 0.04 | 62.48 | 0.00 | 68.16 | 20.59 | 0.63 | 1.63 | 2.34 |
| 0.70 | | 0.00 | 17.15 | 1.16 | | | 0.15 | 0.10 | 1.17 | 0.02 | 20.65 | 0.05 | 150.50 | 5.95 | 0.17 | 0.46 | 1.54 |
| 171.00 | | 0.30 | 191.25 | 1.73 | | | 0.20 | 0.26 | 1.56 | 0.04 | 34.50 | 0.19 | 142.50 | 14.25 | 0.51 | 1.68 | 4.12 |
| 223.44 | | 0.34 | 249.66 | 2.05 | | | 0.23 | 0.32 | 1.79 | 0.05 | 43.32 | 0.25 | 181.26 | 18.24 | 0.64 | 1.13 | 5.46 |
| 0.00 | 0.00 | 0.00 | 20.80 | 0.33 | | | 0.03 | 0.01 | 0.18 | 0.04 | 13.65 | 0.00 | 32.24 | 13.65 | 0.18 | 0.98 | |
| 0.00 | 0.00 | 0.00 | 43.75 | 0.35 | | | 0.03 | 0.02 | 0.38 | 0.06 | 28.50 | 0.00 | 78.50 | 16.25 | 0.24 | 1.30 | |
| 0.00 | 0.00 | 0.00 | 43.75 | 1.16 | | | 0.19 | 0.10 | 1.25 | 0.02 | 43.05 | 0.00 | 43.40 | 9.10 | 0.25 | 1.16 | |
| 0.00 | 0.00 | 0.00 | 35.70 | 1.62 | | | 0.17 | 0.14 | 1.58 | 0.01 | 37.20 | 0.00 | 31.50 | 8.10 | 0.23 | 0.90 | 0.00 |
| 0.00 | 0.00 | 0.00 | 14.70 | 1.32 | | | 0.15 | 0.10 | 1.49 | 0.04 | 13.20 | 0.00 | 66.00 | 18.60 | 0.48 | 1.35 | |
| 12.42 | 0.00 | 0.00 | 2.97 | 0.40 | | | 0.02 | 0.05 | 2.11 | 0.04 | 5.67 | 0.00 | 97.20 | 35.37 | 0.81 | 1.13 | |
| 0.00 | 0.00 | 0.00 | 12.04 | 0.77 | | | 0.10 | 0.09 | 0.97 | 0.01 | 3.92 | 0.01 | 31.92 | 5.04 | 0.18 | 0.31 | |
| 0.00 | 0.00 | 0.00 | 6.72 | 1.04 | | | 0.06 | 0.09 | 1.15 | 0.02 | 16.80 | 0.00 | 29.12 | 8.40 | 0.23 | 0.78 | 5.18 |
| 48.60 | 0.00 | 0.00 | 45.30 | 1.43 | | | 0.17 | 0.13 | 1.40 | 0.17 | 24.00 | 0.14 | 65.40 | 10.80 | 0.34 | 0.72 | 0.48 |
| 0.00 | 0.00 | 0.00 | 2.64 | 0.51 | | | 0.07 | 0.07 | 0.63 | 0.01 | 14.64 | 0.00 | 14.52 | 3.84 | 0.11 | 0.36 | |
| 2.73 | | 0.00 | 6.72 | 0.20 | | | 0.04 | 0.03 | 0.33 | 0.01 | 6.16 | 0.01 | 9.80 | 2.94 | 0.07 | 0.35 | 0.00 |
| 392.89 | | 1.67 | 267.91 | 1.47 | | | 0.27 | 0.37 | 0.42 | 0.12 | 16.57 | 0.60 | 351.40 | 77.99 | 1.85 | 3.63 | |
| 0.00 | 0.00 | 0.00 | 9.68 | 0.74 | | | 0.07 | 0.07 | 1.08 | 0.06 | 11.80 | 0.00 | 85.67 | 40.12 | 0.59 | 2.31 | |
| 0.00 | 0.00 | 0.00 | 11.40 | 1.27 | | | 0.08 | 0.08 | 1.58 | 0.08 | 15.00 | 0.00 | 105.90 | 39.60 | 0.99 | 2.94 | |
| 45.14 | | 1.71 | 98.82 | 5.12 | 0.00 | | 0.90 | 0.34 | 2.50 | 0.39 | 104.92 | 0.00 | 563.64 | 217.16 | 4.95 | 12.81 | 33.40 |
| 750.00 | | 15.00 | 0.00 | 4.50 | 50.12 | | 0.38 | 0.43 | 5.00 | 0.50 | 99.75 | 0.00 | 0.00 | 0.00 | 0.00 | 0.00 | 12.98 |
| 750.00 | 0.00 | 15.00 | 100.00 | 4.50 | 50.00 | | 0.38 | 0.43 | 5.00 | 0.50 | 100.00 | 1.50 | 294.00 | 120.00 | 3.75 | 10.00 | 5.00 |
| 750.00 | 0.00 | 15.00 | 0.00 | 8.40 | 50.00 | | 0.38 | 0.43 | 5.00 | 0.50 | 100.00 | 0.00 | 0.00 | 0.00 | | 1.00 | 2.01 |
| 750.00 | | 15.00 | 0.00 | 4.50 | 50.00 | | 0.38 | 0.43 | 5.00 | 0.50 | 100.00 | 0.00 | 20.50 | 8.00 | 3.75 | 1.00 | 14.00 |
| 750.00 | | 0.00 | 40.00 | 4.50 | 50.00 | | 0.38 | 0.43 | 5.00 | 0.50 | 100.00 | 1.50 | 191.00 | 80.00 | 3.75 | 7.00 | 18.00 |
| 750.00 | | 15.00 | 0.00 | 1.80 | 50.00 | | 0.38 | 0.43 | 5.00 | 0.50 | 100.00 | 0.00 | 35.75 | 8.00 | 0.60 | 1.00 | 3.00 |
| 750.00 | | 15.00 | 0.00 | 8.40 | 50.00 | | 0.53 | 0.60 | 7.00 | 0.70 | 100.00 | 0.00 | 60.70 | 16.00 | 3.75 | 1.00 | 3.00 |
| 0.00 | 0.00 | 0.00 | 0.00 | 16.20 | 0.00 | | 0.38 | 0.43 | 5.00 | 0.50 | 100.00 | 1.50 | 160.00 | 60.00 | 1.50 | 6.00 | 12.00 |
| 0.00 | 0.00 | 6.00 | 0.00 | 16.20 | 0.00 | | 0.38 | 0.00 | 5.00 | 0.50 | 100.00 | 1.50 | 200.00 | 60.00 | 3.75 | 7.00 | 10.00 |
| 0.00 | 0.00 | 6.00 | 0.00 | 9.00 | 0.00 | | 0.38 | 0.07 | 5.00 | 0.50 | 100.00 | 1.50 | 11.70 | 4.20 | 0.11 | 0.54 | 3.00 |
| 500.00 | 0.00 | 6.00 | 40.00 | 8.10 | 40.00 | | 0.38 | 0.43 | 5.00 | 0.50 | 100.00 | 1.50 | 100.00 | 32.00 | 3.75 | 3.00 | 1.00 |
| 500.00 | 0.00 | 6.00 | 0.00 | 4.50 | 40.00 | | 0.38 | 0.43 | 5.00 | 0.50 | 100.00 | 1.50 | 100.00 | 24.00 | 3.75 | 2.00 | 11.00 |
| 500.00 | 0.00 | 6.00 | 0.00 | 8.10 | 40.00 | | 0.38 | 0.43 | 5.00 | 0.50 | 100.00 | 1.50 | 100.00 | 32.00 | 3.75 | 3.00 | 4.00 |
| 0.00 | 0.00 | 6.00 | 20.00 | 4.50 | 0.00 | | 0.38 | 0.43 | 5.00 | 0.50 | 100.00 | 1.50 | 150.00 | 60.00 | 1.20 | 13.00 | 10.00 |
| 500.00 | 0.00 | 0.00 | 200.00 | 18.00 | 40.00 | 30.00 | 1.50 | 1.70 | 20.00 | 2.00 | 400.00 | 6.00 | 100.00 | 40.00 | 15.00 | 5.00 | 19.00 |
| 0.00 | 0.00 | 0.00 | 4.38 | 4.50 | | | 0.38 | 0.43 | 5.00 | 0.50 | 174.00 | 1.71 | 34.30 | 10.90 | 2.93 | 1.00 | 12.00 |
| 0.00 | 0.00 | 0.00 | 55.60 | 10.80 | 0.00 | | 0.15 | 0.08 | 1.20 | 0.02 | 0.01 | 0.00 | 38.00 | 5.13 | 0.22 | 0.94 | 0.00 |
| 750.00 | 0.00 | 0.00 | 20.00 | 8.10 | 40.00 | | 0.38 | 0.43 | 5.00 | 0.50 | 100.00 | 1.50 | 150.00 | 60.00 | 1.20 | 5.00 | 7.00 |
| 750.00 | | 0.00 | 0.00 | 8.10 | 40.00 | | 0.38 | 0.43 | 5.00 | 0.50 | 100.00 | 1.50 | 150.00 | 60.00 | 1.50 | 5.00 | 6.00 |
| 750.00 | | 0.00 | 0.00 | 1.80 | 39.90 | | 0.38 | 0.43 | 5.00 | 0.50 | 99.75 | 1.50 | 0.00 | 0.00 | 1.50 | 0.00 | 12.00 |

*continues*

*continued*

| GRAINS | Amount | Portion | Kcal | Protein | Carb | Fat | Chol | Sat Fat | Mono Fat | Poly Fat | Sodium | Potas |
|---|---|---|---|---|---|---|---|---|---|---|---|---|
| **PASTA:** | | | | | | | | | | | | |
| Spaghetti, Enriched, Cooked | 0.50 | CUP | 98.70 | 3.34 | 19.84 | 0.47 | 0.00 | 0.07 | 0.06 | 0.19 | 0.70 | 21.70 |
| Egg Noodles, Enriched, Cooked | 0.50 | CUP | 106.40 | 3.80 | 19.87 | 1.18 | 26.40 | 0.25 | 0.34 | 0.33 | 5.60 | 22.40 |
| Ramen Noodles, Prepared | 0.50 | CUP | 103.50 | 2.95 | 15.35 | 4.30 | 17.75 | 0.19 | 0.22 | 0.21 | 414.50 | 34.45 |
| Japanese Somen Noodles, Wheat, Cooked | 0.50 | CUP | 115.28 | 3.52 | 24.24 | 0.16 | 0.00 | 0.02 | 0.02 | 0.06 | 141.68 | 25.52 |
| Chinese Cellophane Noodles (rice or mung bean), Dehydrated | 2.00 | OUNCE | 199.37 | 0.09 | 48.91 | 0.03 | 0.00 | 0.01 | 0.01 | 0.01 | 5.68 | 5.68 |
| Chow Fun Rice Noodles, Cooked, Fat Added | 0.50 | CUP | 69.54 | 1.13 | 15.23 | 0.27 | 0.00 | 0.07 | 0.08 | 0.07 | 1.71 | 14.44 |
| Cheese Gnocchi, Cooked | 0.50 | CUP | 63.89 | 3.38 | 2.99 | 4.23 | 24.29 | 1.64 | 1.65 | 0.67 | 102.88 | 25.49 |
| Potato Gnocchi, Cooked | 0.50 | CUP | 132.84 | 2.35 | 16.40 | 6.51 | 17.50 | 3.98 | 1.84 | 0.31 | 314.96 | 121.34 |
| **PURE GRAINS:** | | | | | | | | | | | | |
| Rice | 1.00 | SERVING | 99.34 | 1.94 | 21.76 | 0.18 | 0.00 | 0.05 | 0.06 | 0.05 | 92.06 | 31.32 |
| Brown Rice | 1.00 | SERVING | 257.94 | 5.34 | 54.28 | 1.91 | 0.00 | 0.38 | 0.69 | 0.68 | 8.18 | 190.97 |
| Short Grain White Rice, Cooked | 0.50 | CUP | 120.90 | 2.20 | 26.72 | 0.18 | 0.00 | 0.05 | 0.05 | 0.05 | 0.00 | 24.18 |
| Medium Grain White Rice, Cooked | 0.50 | CUP | 120.90 | 2.21 | 26.59 | 0.20 | 0.00 | 0.05 | 0.06 | 0.05 | 0.00 | 26.97 |
| Long Grain White Rice, Instant, Enriched, Boiled | 0.50 | CUP | 80.85 | 1.70 | 17.55 | 0.13 | 0.00 | 0.04 | 0.04 | 0.04 | 2.48 | 3.30 |
| Wild Brown Rice, Cooked | 0.50 | CUP | 82.82 | 3.27 | 17.50 | 0.28 | 0.00 | 0.04 | 0.04 | 0.18 | 2.46 | 82.82 |
| Medium Grain Brown Rice, Cooked | 0.50 | CUP | 109.20 | 2.26 | 22.92 | 0.81 | 0.00 | 0.16 | 0.29 | 0.29 | 0.98 | 77.03 |
| Long Grain Brown Rice, Cooked | 0.50 | CUP | 108.23 | 2.52 | 22.39 | 0.88 | 0.00 | 0.18 | 0.32 | 0.32 | 4.88 | 41.93 |
| Spanish Rice | 1.00 | CUP | 217.18 | 4.94 | 41.53 | 3.84 | 0.00 | 0.61 | 1.48 | 1.44 | 765.69 | 535.57 |
| Bulgur, Cooked | 0.50 | CUP | 75.53 | 2.80 | 16.91 | 0.22 | 0.00 | 0.04 | 0.03 | 0.09 | 4.55 | 61.88 |
| Barley | 2.00 | OUNCE | 200.72 | 7.08 | 41.66 | 1.30 | 0.00 | 0.27 | 0.17 | 0.63 | 6.80 | 256.28 |
| Buckwheat | 2.00 | OUNCE | 194.48 | 7.51 | 40.54 | 1.93 | 0.00 | 0.42 | 0.59 | 0.59 | 0.57 | 260.82 |
| Millet, Cooked | 0.50 | CUP | 142.80 | 4.21 | 28.40 | 1.20 | 0.00 | 0.21 | 0.22 | 0.61 | 2.40 | 74.40 |
| Oats | 2.00 | OUNCE | 220.56 | 9.58 | 37.58 | 3.91 | 0.00 | 0.69 | 1.24 | 1.44 | 1.13 | 243.24 |
| Quinoa | 2.00 | OUNCE | 212.06 | 7.43 | 39.07 | 3.29 | 0.00 | 0.34 | 0.87 | 1.33 | 11.91 | 419.58 |
| Rice Bran, Crude | 2.00 | OUNCE | 179.17 | 7.57 | 28.17 | 11.82 | 0.00 | 2.37 | 4.28 | 4.23 | 2.84 | 842.00 |
| Rye | 2.00 | OUNCE | 189.95 | 8.37 | 39.55 | 1.42 | 0.00 | 0.16 | 0.17 | 0.63 | 3.40 | 149.69 |
| Durum Wheat | 2.00 | OUNCE | 192.21 | 7.76 | 40.33 | 1.40 | 0.00 | 0.26 | 0.20 | 0.56 | 1.13 | 244.38 |
| Wheat Germ, Crude | 0.50 | CUP | 207.00 | 13.31 | 29.79 | 5.59 | 0.00 | 0.96 | 0.79 | 3.46 | 6.90 | 512.90 |
| Amaranth, Dry | 2.00 | OUNCE | 212.06 | 8.19 | 37.52 | 3.69 | 0.00 | 0.94 | 0.81 | 1.64 | 11.91 | 207.52 |
| **FLOUR:** | | | | | | | | | | | | |
| All Purpose Wheat Flour, White, Bleached, Enriched | 1.00 | CUP | 455.00 | 12.91 | 95.39 | 1.23 | 0.00 | 0.19 | 0.11 | 0.52 | 2.50 | 133.75 |
| Wheat Flour, White, Bread, Enriched | 1.00 | CUP | 494.57 | 16.41 | 99.37 | 2.27 | 0.00 | 0.33 | 0.19 | 1.00 | 2.74 | 137.00 |
| Whole Grain Wheat Flour | 1.00 | CUP | 406.80 | 16.44 | 87.08 | 2.24 | 0.00 | 0.39 | 0.28 | 0.94 | 6.00 | 486.00 |
| Barley Flour | 1.00 | CUP | 396.48 | 8.40 | 89.38 | 1.57 | 0.00 | 0.33 | 0.20 | 0.76 | 8.96 | 371.84 |
| White Rice Flour | 1.00 | CUP | 578.28 | 9.40 | 126.61 | 2.24 | 0.00 | 0.61 | 0.70 | 0.60 | 0.00 | 120.08 |
| Whole Grain Corn Flour | 1.00 | CUP | 422.37 | 8.11 | 89.91 | 4.52 | 0.00 | 0.64 | 1.19 | 2.06 | 5.85 | 368.55 |
| Brown Rice Flour | 1.00 | CUP | 573.54 | 11.42 | 120.84 | 4.39 | 0.00 | 0.88 | 1.59 | 1.57 | 12.64 | 456.62 |
| Dark Rye Flour | 1.00 | CUP | 414.72 | 17.96 | 87.99 | 3.44 | 0.00 | 0.40 | 0.42 | 1.54 | 1.28 | 934.40 |
| Semolina, Enriched | 1.00 | CUP | 601.20 | 21.18 | 121.63 | 1.75 | 0.00 | 0.25 | 0.21 | 0.72 | 1.67 | 310.62 |
| Oat Bran, Raw | 2.00 | OUNCE | 139.48 | 9.81 | 37.55 | 3.99 | 0.00 | 0.75 | 1.35 | 1.57 | 2.27 | 320.92 |
| Wheat Bran, Crude | 1.00 | CUP | 125.28 | 9.02 | 37.42 | 2.47 | 0.00 | 0.37 | 0.37 | 1.28 | 1.16 | 685.56 |
| White Bread Crumbs, Enriched | 1 | CUP | 93.45 | 2.87 | 17.33 | 1.26 | 0.35 | 0.28 | 0.56 | 0.26 | 188.30 | 41.65 |
| Plain Bread Crumbs | 1 | CUP | 426.60 | 13.50 | 78.30 | 5.83 | 0.00 | 1.31 | 2.58 | 1.20 | 930.96 | 238.68 |
| Seasoned Bread Crumbs | 1 | CUP | 440.40 | 17.04 | 84.48 | 3.12 | 1.20 | 0.87 | 1.16 | 0.79 | 3180.00 | 324.00 |
| **SNACKS:** | | | | | | | | | | | | |
| Plain Popcorn | 3.00 | CUP | 91.68 | 2.88 | 18.70 | 1.01 | 0.00 | 0.14 | 0.26 | 0.46 | 0.96 | 72.24 |
| Popcorn, with Oil and Salt, Popped | 3.00 | CUP | 165.00 | 2.97 | 18.88 | 9.27 | 0.00 | 1.61 | 2.70 | 4.43 | 291.72 | 74.25 |
| Popcorn, Buttered, Popped in Oil | 1.00 | CUP | 72.95 | 1.15 | 7.23 | 4.65 | 2.97 | 1.30 | 1.35 | 1.74 | 122.97 | 28.80 |
| Pretzels, Twisted, Thin | 5.00 | ITEM | 114.30 | 2.73 | 23.76 | 1.05 | 0.00 | 0.23 | 0.41 | 0.37 | 514.50 | 43.80 |
| Soft Pretzel | 1.00 | ITEM | 214.52 | 5.08 | 43.28 | 1.92 | 1.86 | 0.43 | 0.66 | 0.59 | 870.48 | 54.56 |
| Plain Corn Chips | 1.00 | OUNCE | 153.08 | 1.87 | 16.16 | 9.49 | 0.00 | 1.29 | 2.74 | 4.68 | 178.92 | 40.33 |
| Plain Tortilla Chip | 1.00 | OUNCE | 142.28 | 1.99 | 17.86 | 7.44 | 0.00 | 1.43 | 4.39 | 1.03 | 149.95 | 55.95 |

| Vit A (IU) | Beta-C | Vit C | Calcium | Iron | Vit D (IU) | Vit E (IU) | Thiamin | Ribo | Niacin | Vit B6 | Folate | Vit B12 | Phosp | Magn | Zinc | Diet Fiber | Sugar |
|---|---|---|---|---|---|---|---|---|---|---|---|---|---|---|---|---|---|
| 0.00 | 0.00 | 0.00 | 4.90 | 0.98 | | | 0.14 | 0.07 | 1.17 | 0.02 | 49.00 | 0.00 | 37.80 | 12.60 | 0.37 | 1.19 | 0.90 |
| 16.00 | | 0.00 | 9.60 | 1.27 | | | 0.15 | 0.07 | 1.19 | 0.03 | 51.20 | 0.07 | 55.20 | 15.20 | 0.50 | 0.88 | 1.03 |
| 552.50 | 98.50 | 0.09 | 8.75 | 0.89 | | | 0.08 | 0.05 | 0.71 | 0.03 | 4.00 | 0.01 | 35.00 | 8.50 | 0.31 | 1.02 | |
| 0.00 | 0.00 | 0.00 | 7.04 | 0.46 | | | 0.02 | 0.03 | 0.09 | 0.01 | 1.76 | 0.00 | 23.76 | 1.76 | 0.19 | | |
| 0.00 | 0.00 | 0.00 | 14.20 | 1.23 | | | 0.09 | 0.00 | 0.11 | 0.03 | 1.14 | 0.00 | 18.18 | 1.70 | 0.23 | 0.28 | |
| 0.00 | 0.00 | 0.00 | 3.04 | 0.07 | | | 0.02 | 0.00 | 0.44 | 0.07 | 0.53 | 0.00 | 18.62 | 7.22 | 0.17 | 0.46 | |
| 260.18 | | 0.01 | 75.87 | 0.28 | | | 0.02 | 0.07 | 0.18 | 0.01 | 3.60 | 0.11 | 56.30 | 4.43 | 0.31 | 0.08 | |
| 658.84 | | 1.72 | 21.76 | 0.73 | | | 0.11 | 0.09 | 1.08 | 0.09 | 5.14 | 0.05 | 39.22 | 10.27 | 0.22 | 0.88 | |
| 0.00 | 0.00 | 0.00 | 7.68 | 1.17 | 0.00 | | 0.16 | 0.01 | 1.14 | 0.05 | 62.87 | 0.00 | 31.30 | 6.81 | 0.30 | 0.35 | 0.15 |
| 0.00 | 0.00 | 0.00 | 27.08 | 1.30 | 0.00 | | 0.29 | 0.03 | 3.07 | 0.36 | 14.25 | 0.00 | 188.11 | 103.67 | 1.49 | 2.42 | 0.51 |
| 0.00 | 0.00 | 0.00 | 0.93 | 1.36 | | | 0.15 | 0.02 | 1.39 | 0.06 | 54.87 | 0.00 | 30.69 | 7.44 | 0.37 | 0.28 | 0.19 |
| 0.00 | 0.00 | 0.00 | 2.79 | 1.39 | | | 0.16 | 0.02 | 1.71 | 0.05 | 53.94 | 0.00 | 34.41 | 12.09 | 0.39 | 0.28 | 0.19 |
| 0.00 | 0.00 | 0.00 | 6.60 | 0.52 | | | 0.06 | 0.04 | 0.73 | 0.01 | 33.83 | 0.00 | 11.55 | 4.13 | 0.20 | 0.50 | 0.17 |
| 0.00 | 0.00 | 0.00 | 2.46 | 0.49 | | | 0.04 | 0.07 | 1.06 | 0.11 | 21.32 | 0.00 | 67.24 | 26.24 | 1.10 | 1.48 | 0.58 |
| 0.00 | 0.00 | 0.00 | 9.75 | 0.52 | | | 0.10 | 0.01 | 1.30 | 0.15 | 3.90 | 0.00 | 75.08 | 42.90 | 0.64 | 1.76 | 0.30 |
| 0.00 | 0.00 | 0.00 | 9.75 | 0.41 | | | 0.09 | 0.02 | 1.49 | 0.14 | 3.90 | 0.00 | 80.93 | 41.93 | 0.61 | 1.76 | 0.30 |
| 1145.12 | | 38.77 | 69.28 | 2.52 | | | 0.24 | 0.08 | 2.98 | 0.31 | 20.10 | 0.00 | 89.22 | 39.18 | 0.88 | 3.00 | 5.91 |
| 0.00 | 0.00 | 0.00 | 9.10 | 0.87 | | | 0.05 | 0.03 | 0.91 | 0.08 | 16.38 | 0.00 | 36.40 | 29.12 | 0.52 | 4.10 | |
| 12.47 | | 0.00 | 18.71 | 2.04 | | | 0.37 | 0.16 | 2.61 | 0.18 | 10.77 | 0.00 | 149.69 | 75.41 | 1.57 | 9.81 | |
| 0.00 | 0.00 | 0.00 | 10.21 | 1.25 | | | 0.06 | 0.24 | 3.98 | 0.12 | 17.01 | 0.00 | 196.75 | 130.98 | 1.36 | 5.67 | 1.47 |
| 0.00 | 0.00 | 0.00 | 3.60 | 0.76 | | | 0.13 | 0.10 | 1.60 | 0.13 | 22.80 | 0.00 | 120.00 | 52.80 | 1.09 | 1.56 | 0.35 |
| 0.00 | 0.00 | 0.00 | 30.62 | 2.68 | | | 0.43 | 0.08 | 0.55 | 0.07 | 31.75 | 0.00 | 296.54 | 100.36 | 2.25 | 6.01 | 1.02 |
| 0.00 | 0.00 | 0.00 | 34.02 | 5.25 | | | 0.11 | 0.23 | 1.66 | 0.13 | 27.78 | 0.00 | 232.47 | 119.07 | 1.87 | 3.35 | |
| 0.00 | 0.00 | 0.00 | 32.32 | 10.51 | | | 1.56 | 0.16 | 19.28 | 2.31 | 35.72 | 0.00 | 950.86 | 442.83 | 3.43 | 11.91 | 0.51 |
| 0.00 | 0.00 | 0.00 | 18.71 | 1.51 | | | 0.18 | 0.14 | 2.42 | 0.17 | 34.02 | 0.00 | 212.06 | 68.61 | 2.12 | 8.28 | |
| 0.00 | 0.00 | 0.00 | 19.28 | 2.00 | | | 0.24 | 0.07 | 3.82 | 0.24 | 24.55 | 0.00 | 288.04 | 81.65 | 2.36 | 6.91 | 1.04 |
| 0.00 | 0.00 | 0.00 | 22.43 | 3.60 | | | 1.08 | 0.29 | 3.92 | 0.75 | 161.58 | 0.00 | 484.15 | 137.43 | 7.07 | 7.59 | 7.00 |
| 0.00 | 0.00 | 2.38 | 86.75 | 4.30 | | | 0.05 | 0.12 | 0.73 | 0.13 | 27.78 | 0.00 | 257.99 | 150.82 | 1.80 | 8.62 | 1.11 |
| 0.00 | 0.00 | 0.00 | 18.75 | 5.80 | 0.98 | 0.62 | 7.38 | 0.06 | 32.50 | 0.00 | 135.00 | 27.50 | 0.88 | | 3.38 | 2.13 | |
| 0.00 | 0.00 | 0.00 | 20.55 | 6.04 | | | 1.11 | 0.70 | 10.35 | 0.05 | 210.98 | 0.00 | 132.89 | 34.25 | 1.16 | 3.29 | 2.33 |
| 0.00 | 0.00 | 0.00 | 40.80 | 4.66 | | | 0.54 | 0.26 | 7.64 | 0.41 | 52.80 | 0.00 | 415.20 | 165.60 | 3.52 | 14.64 | 2.40 |
| 0.00 | 0.00 | 0.00 | 32.48 | 1.41 | | | 0.13 | 0.06 | 5.14 | 0.31 | 25.76 | 0.00 | 252.00 | 90.72 | 2.09 | 4.26 | |
| 0.00 | 0.00 | 0.00 | 15.80 | 0.55 | | | 0.22 | 0.03 | 4.09 | 0.69 | 6.32 | 0.00 | 154.84 | 55.30 | 1.26 | 3.79 | 1.58 |
| 548.73 | | 0.00 | 8.19 | 2.79 | | | 0.29 | 0.09 | 2.22 | 0.43 | 29.25 | 0.00 | 318.24 | 108.81 | 2.02 | 15.68 | |
| 0.00 | 0.00 | 0.00 | 17.38 | 3.13 | | | 0.70 | 0.13 | 10.02 | 1.16 | 25.28 | 0.00 | 532.46 | 176.96 | 3.87 | 7.27 | 1.60 |
| 0.00 | 0.00 | 0.00 | 71.68 | 8.26 | | | 0.40 | 0.32 | 5.47 | 0.57 | 76.80 | 0.00 | 808.96 | 317.44 | 7.19 | 28.93 | 5.92 |
| 0.00 | 0.00 | 0.00 | 28.39 | 7.28 | | | 1.35 | 0.95 | 10.00 | 0.17 | 257.18 | 0.00 | 227.12 | 78.49 | 1.75 | 6.51 | 3.07 |
| 0.00 | 0.00 | 0.00 | 32.89 | 3.07 | | | 0.66 | 0.13 | 0.53 | 0.09 | 29.48 | 0.00 | 416.18 | 133.25 | 1.76 | 8.73 | 1.47 |
| 0.00 | 0.00 | 0.00 | 42.34 | 6.13 | | | 0.30 | 0.34 | 7.88 | 0.76 | 45.82 | 0.00 | 587.54 | 354.38 | 4.22 | 24.82 | 2.50 |
| 0.00 | 0.00 | 0.00 | 37.80 | 1.06 | | | 0.17 | 0.12 | 1.39 | 0.02 | 11.90 | 0.01 | 32.90 | 8.40 | 0.22 | 0.81 | 1.37 |
| 0.00 | 0.00 | 0.00 | 245.16 | 6.61 | | | 0.83 | 0.47 | 7.40 | 0.11 | 117.72 | 0.02 | 158.76 | 49.68 | 1.32 | 2.59 | 4.10 |
| 15.60 | | 0.48 | 118.80 | 3.82 | | | 0.19 | 0.20 | 3.28 | 0.18 | 130.80 | 0.05 | 159.60 | 45.60 | 1.09 | 5.04 | 4.44 |
| 47.04 | | 0.00 | 2.40 | 0.64 | | | 0.05 | 0.07 | 0.47 | 0.06 | 5.52 | 0.00 | 72.00 | 31.44 | 0.83 | 3.62 | 0.10 |
| 50.82 | | 0.10 | 3.30 | 0.92 | | | 0.04 | 0.05 | 0.51 | 0.07 | 5.61 | 0.00 | 82.50 | 35.64 | 0.87 | 3.30 | 0.33 |
| 61.01 | | 0.04 | 1.59 | 0.35 | | | 0.02 | 0.02 | 0.20 | 0.03 | 2.19 | 0.00 | 31.92 | 13.68 | 0.33 | 1.26 | |
| 0.00 | 0.00 | 0.00 | 10.80 | 1.30 | | | 0.14 | 0.19 | 1.58 | 0.04 | 24.90 | 0.00 | 33.90 | 10.50 | 0.26 | 0.96 | |
| 0.00 | 0.00 | 0.00 | 14.26 | 2.43 | | | 0.26 | 0.18 | 2.65 | 0.01 | 8.68 | 0.00 | 48.98 | 13.02 | 0.58 | 1.05 | |
| 26.70 | 12.20 | 0.00 | 36.07 | 0.38 | | | 0.01 | 0.04 | 0.34 | 0.07 | 5.68 | 0.00 | 52.54 | 21.58 | 0.36 | 1.39 | |
| 55.66 | 12.20 | 0.00 | 43.74 | 0.43 | | | 0.02 | 0.05 | 0.36 | 0.08 | 2.84 | 0.00 | 58.22 | 24.99 | 0.44 | 1.85 | |

| FRUITS | Amount | Portion | Kcal | Protein | Carb | Fat | Chol | Sat Fat |
|---|---|---|---|---|---|---|---|---|
| Apple | 1.00 | ITEM | 81.42 | 0.26 | 21.05 | 0.50 | 0.00 | 0.08 |
| Applesauce | 1.00 | SERVING | 102.90 | 0.29 | 26.43 | 0.47 | 0.00 | 0.08 |
| Avocado, California | 0.25 | ITEM | 76.55 | 0.91 | 2.99 | 7.50 | 0.00 | 1.12 |
| Banana, Peeled | 1.00 | ITEM | 108.56 | 1.22 | 27.65 | 0.57 | 0.00 | 0.22 |
| Grapes, European Type (Adherent Skin) | 1.00 | CUP | 113.60 | 1.06 | 28.43 | 0.93 | 0.00 | 0.30 |
| Lemon | 1.00 | ITEM | 21.60 | 1.30 | 11.56 | 0.32 | 0.00 | 0.04 |
| Cantaloupe | 1.00 | CUP | 56.00 | 1.41 | 13.38 | 0.45 | 0.00 | 0.11 |
| Honeydew | 1.00 | CUP | 61.95 | 0.81 | 16.25 | 0.18 | 0.00 | 0.04 |
| Watermelon | 1.00 | CUP | 48.64 | 0.94 | 10.91 | 0.65 | 0.00 | 0.07 |
| Casaba Melon | 0.75 | CUP | 33.15 | 1.15 | 7.91 | 0.13 | 0.00 | 0.03 |
| Orange | 1.00 | ITEM | 61.57 | 1.23 | 15.39 | 0.16 | 0.00 | 0.02 |
| Tangerine | 2.00 | ITEM | 73.92 | 1.06 | 18.80 | 0.32 | 0.00 | 0.04 |
| Grapefruit | 0.50 | CUP | 36.80 | 0.73 | 9.29 | 0.12 | 0.00 | 0.02 |
| Peach | 1.00 | ITEM | 42.14 | 0.69 | 10.88 | 0.09 | 0.00 | 0.01 |
| Pear | 1.00 | CUP | 97.35 | 0.64 | 24.93 | 0.66 | 0.00 | 0.04 |
| Nectarine | 1.00 | CUP | 67.62 | 1.30 | 16.26 | 0.64 | 0.00 | 0.07 |
| Apricots | 4.00 | ITEM | 67.20 | 1.96 | 15.57 | 0.55 | 0.00 | 0.04 |
| Papaya | 0.50 | CUP | 27.30 | 0.43 | 6.87 | 0.10 | 0.00 | 0.03 |
| Pineapple | 0.50 | CUP | 37.98 | 0.30 | 9.60 | 0.33 | 0.00 | 0.03 |
| Cherries | 24.00 | ITEM | 85.44 | 1.58 | 19.01 | 0.38 | 0.00 | 0.00 |
| Raspberries | 0.50 | CUP | 30.14 | 0.56 | 7.12 | 0.34 | 0.00 | 0.01 |
| Strawberries | 0.50 | CUP | 21.60 | 0.44 | 5.05 | 0.27 | 0.00 | 0.01 |
| Blackberries | 0.50 | CUP | 37.44 | 0.52 | 9.19 | 0.28 | 0.00 | 0.01 |
| Blueberries | 0.50 | CUP | 35.23 | 0.51 | 7.79 | 0.24 | 0.00 | 0.00 |
| Cranberries, Chopped | 0.50 | CUP | 26.95 | 0.21 | 6.97 | 0.11 | 0.00 | 0.01 |
| Figs | 3.00 | ITEM | 111.00 | 1.13 | 28.77 | 0.45 | 0.00 | 0.09 |
| Fruit Cocktail, Canned in Light Syrup | 0.50 | CUP | 68.97 | 0.48 | 18.07 | 0.09 | 0.00 | 0.01 |
| Fruit Cocktail, Canned in Heavy Syrup | 0.50 | CUP | 90.52 | 0.48 | 23.45 | 0.09 | 0.00 | 0.01 |
| Guava | 1.00 | ITEM | 45.90 | 0.74 | 10.69 | 0.54 | 0.00 | 0.16 |
| Kiwi Fruit | 1.00 | ITEM | 46.36 | 0.75 | 11.31 | 0.33 | 0.00 | 0.02 |
| Kumquats | 3.00 | ITEM | 35.91 | 0.51 | 9.37 | 0.06 | 0.00 | 0.01 |
| Lychee | 0.75 | CUP | 94.05 | 1.18 | 23.56 | 0.63 | 0.00 | 0.14 |
| Mango | 0.50 | ITEM | 67.28 | 0.53 | 17.60 | 0.28 | 0.00 | 0.07 |
| Passion Fruit (Granadilla) | 0.50 | CUP | 114.46 | 2.60 | 27.59 | 0.83 | 0.00 | 0.07 |
| Persimmon | 5.00 | ITEM | 158.75 | 1.00 | 41.88 | 0.50 | 0.00 | 0.05 |
| Pomegranate | 1.00 | ITEM | 104.72 | 1.46 | 26.44 | 0.46 | 0.00 | 0.06 |
| *DRIED FRUITS:* | | | | | | | | |
| Dried Apples, Sulfured | 0.25 | CUP | 52.25 | 0.20 | 14.17 | 0.07 | 0.00 | 0.01 |
| Raisins, Seedless | 0.25 | CUP | 108.75 | 1.17 | 28.69 | 0.17 | 0.00 | 0.05 |
| Dried Apricot Halves, Sulfured | 0.25 | CUP | 77.35 | 1.19 | 20.07 | 0.15 | 0.00 | 0.01 |
| Dates | 1.00 | OUNCE | 71.75 | 0.66 | 19.13 | 0.07 | 0.00 | 0.00 |
| Prunes, Dried | 0.25 | CUP | 101.58 | 1.11 | 26.66 | 0.22 | 0.00 | 0.02 |
| Dried Figs | 0.25 | CUP | 126.86 | 1.52 | 32.51 | 0.58 | 0.00 | 0.12 |

**338**

| Sodium | Potas | Beta-C | Vit C | Calcium | Iron | Vit E (IU) | Zinc | Diet Fiber | Sugar |
|---|---|---|---|---|---|---|---|---|---|
| 0.00 | 158.70 | | 7.87 | 9.66 | 0.25 | | 0.06 | 3.73 | 18.40 |
| 5.80 | 224.84 | 6.40 | 5.57 | 13.06 | 0.36 | | 0.09 | 2.66 | 16.00 |
| 5.19 | 274.21 | | 3.42 | 4.76 | 0.51 | | 0.18 | 2.12 | 0.39 |
| 1.18 | 467.28 | 50.93 | 10.74 | 7.08 | 0.37 | | 0.19 | 2.83 | 18.43 |
| 3.20 | 296.00 | | 17.28 | 17.60 | 0.42 | | 0.08 | 1.60 | 29.00 |
| 3.24 | 156.60 | 3.24 | 83.16 | 65.88 | 0.76 | | 0.11 | 5.08 | 2.70 |
| 14.40 | 494.40 | 3100.00 | 67.52 | 17.60 | 0.34 | | 0.26 | 1.28 | 13.90 |
| 17.70 | 479.67 | | 43.90 | 10.62 | 0.12 | | 0.12 | 1.06 | 14.58 |
| 3.04 | 176.32 | | 14.59 | 12.16 | 0.26 | | 0.11 | 0.76 | 13.68 |
| 15.30 | 267.75 | 3.83 | 20.40 | 6.38 | 0.51 | | 0.20 | 1.02 | 6.00 |
| 0.00 | 237.11 | | 69.69 | 52.40 | 0.13 | | 0.09 | 3.14 | 12.10 |
| 1.68 | 263.76 | | 51.74 | 23.52 | 0.17 | | 0.40 | 3.86 | 12.90 |
| 0.00 | 159.85 | 13.80 | 39.56 | 13.80 | 0.10 | | 0.08 | 1.27 | 7.10 |
| 0.00 | 193.06 | | 6.47 | 4.90 | 0.11 | | 0.14 | 1.96 | 8.56 |
| 0.00 | 206.25 | | 6.60 | 18.15 | 0.41 | | 0.20 | 3.96 | 17.40 |
| 0.00 | 292.56 | 102.49 | 7.45 | 6.90 | 0.21 | | 0.12 | 2.21 | 11.77 |
| 1.40 | 414.40 | | 14.00 | 19.60 | 0.76 | | 0.36 | 3.36 | 13.01 |
| 2.10 | 179.90 | 69.50 | 43.26 | 16.80 | 0.07 | | 0.05 | 1.26 | 4.15 |
| 0.78 | 87.58 | | 11.94 | 5.43 | 0.29 | | 0.06 | 0.93 | 9.20 |
| 1.22 | 295.20 | 0.05 | 11.18 | 16.68 | 0.72 | | 0.10 | 3.19 | 20.26 |
| 0.00 | 93.48 | | 15.38 | 13.53 | 0.35 | | 0.28 | 4.18 | 5.85 |
| 0.72 | 119.52 | | 40.82 | 10.08 | 0.27 | | 0.09 | 1.66 | 4.16 |
| 0.00 | 141.12 | | 15.12 | 23.04 | 0.41 | | 0.19 | 3.82 | 5.85 |
| 0.78 | 59.99 | 0.03 | 7.02 | 6.13 | 0.20 | | 0.10 | 3.29 | 5.23 |
| 0.55 | 39.05 | 2.75 | 7.43 | 3.85 | 0.11 | | 0.07 | 2.31 | |
| 1.50 | 348.00 | 21.00 | 3.00 | 52.50 | 0.56 | | 0.23 | 4.95 | 10.35 |
| 7.26 | 107.69 | 25.40 | 2.30 | 7.26 | 0.35 | | 0.11 | 1.21 | |
| 7.44 | 109.12 | | 2.36 | 7.44 | 0.36 | | 0.10 | 1.24 | |
| 2.70 | 255.60 | 71.10 | 165.15 | 18.00 | 0.28 | | 0.21 | 4.86 | 5.40 |
| 3.80 | 252.32 | 13.70 | 74.48 | 19.76 | 0.31 | | 0.13 | 2.58 | 7.98 |
| 3.42 | 111.15 | 17.10 | 21.32 | 25.08 | 0.22 | | 0.05 | 3.76 | 5.70 |
| 1.43 | 243.68 | 0.00 | 101.89 | 7.13 | 0.44 | | 0.10 | 1.85 | |
| 2.07 | 161.46 | 402.50 | 28.67 | 10.35 | 0.14 | | 0.04 | 1.86 | 15.30 |
| 33.04 | 410.64 | 82.60 | 35.40 | 14.16 | 1.89 | | 0.12 | 12.27 | 13.24 |
| 1.25 | 387.50 | | 82.50 | 33.75 | 3.13 | | | | |
| 4.62 | 398.86 | 0.00 | 9.39 | 4.62 | 0.46 | | 0.19 | 0.92 | 15.50 |
| | | | | | | | | | |
| 18.71 | 96.75 | 0.00 | 0.84 | 3.01 | 0.30 | | 0.04 | 1.87 | |
| 4.35 | 272.24 | | 1.20 | 17.76 | 0.75 | | 0.10 | 1.45 | 23.55 |
| 3.25 | 447.85 | | 0.78 | 14.63 | 1.53 | | 0.24 | 2.93 | 12.65 |
| 0.25 | 186.54 | | | 11.75 | 0.28 | | 0.10 | 2.11 | 18.24 |
| 1.70 | 316.63 | | 1.40 | 21.68 | 1.05 | | 0.23 | 3.02 | 18.69 |
| 5.47 | 354.22 | 6.48 | 0.40 | 71.64 | 1.11 | | 0.25 | 6.07 | 31.00 |

| VEGGIES | Amount | Portion | Kcal | Protein | Carb | Fat | Chol | Sat Fat |
|---|---|---|---|---|---|---|---|---|
| **LEGUMES:** | | | | | | | | |
| Black Beans, Boiled | 0.50 | CUP | 113.52 | 7.62 | 20.39 | 0.46 | 0.00 | 0.12 |
| Split Peas, Boiled | 0.50 | CUP | 115.64 | 8.17 | 20.69 | 0.38 | 0.00 | 0.05 |
| Pinto Beans, Boiled | 0.50 | CUP | 117.14 | 7.02 | 21.93 | 0.45 | 0.00 | 0.09 |
| White Beans, Boiled | 0.50 | CUP | 124.41 | 8.71 | 22.47 | 0.31 | 0.00 | 0.08 |
| Lima Beans, Boiled, Drained | 0.50 | CUP | 104.55 | 5.79 | 20.09 | 0.27 | 0.00 | 0.06 |
| Kidney Beans, Boiled | 0.50 | CUP | 112.40 | 7.67 | 20.19 | 0.44 | 0.00 | 0.06 |
| Red Kidney Beans, Canned with Liquid | 0.50 | CUP | 108.80 | 6.72 | 19.97 | 0.44 | 0.00 | 0.06 |
| Lentils, Boiled | 0.50 | CUP | 114.84 | 8.93 | 19.94 | 0.38 | 0.00 | 0.05 |
| Garbanzo Beans, Boiled | 0.50 | CUP | 134.48 | 7.27 | 22.48 | 2.12 | 0.00 | 0.22 |
| Boston Baked Beans | 0.50 | CUP | 193.45 | 7.70 | 27.33 | 6.42 | 6.41 | 2.27 |
| Navy Beans, Boiled | 0.50 | CUP | 129.22 | 7.92 | 23.94 | 0.52 | 0.00 | 0.14 |
| Refried Beans, Canned | 0.50 | CUP | 118.91 | 6.95 | 19.65 | 1.59 | 10.12 | 0.60 |
| Hummus | 0.50 | CUP | 210.33 | 6.03 | 24.81 | 10.39 | 0.00 | 1.56 |
| **SOY:** | | | | | | | | |
| Soybeans, Boiled | 0.50 | CUP | 148.78 | 14.31 | 8.53 | 7.71 | 0.00 | 1.12 |
| Tofu, Raw, Soft, with Calcium Sulfate | 1.00 | PIECE | 73.20 | 7.86 | 2.16 | 4.43 | 0.00 | 0.64 |
| Tofu, Raw, Firm, with Calcium Sulfate | 0.50 | CUP | 182.70 | 19.88 | 5.39 | 10.99 | 0.00 | 1.59 |
| Miso (Fermented Soybeans), Paste | 1.00 | TBSP | 35.41 | 2.03 | 4.81 | 1.04 | 0.00 | 0.15 |
| Tempeh | 0.50 | CUP | 165.17 | 15.73 | 14.14 | 6.37 | 0.00 | 0.92 |
| **STARCHY VEGETABLES:** | | | | | | | | |
| Sweet Corn, Frozen, Boiled, Drained | 0.50 | CUP | 65.60 | 2.26 | 16.04 | 0.35 | 0.00 | 0.05 |
| Sweet Corn, Cream Style, Canned | 0.50 | CUP | 92.16 | 2.23 | 23.21 | 0.54 | 0.00 | 0.08 |
| Green Peas, Boiled, Drained | 0.50 | CUP | 67.20 | 4.29 | 12.51 | 0.18 | 0.00 | 0.03 |
| Blackeye Peas | 1.00 | SERVING | 102.39 | 6.82 | 18.33 | 0.47 | 0.00 | 0.12 |
| Cowpeas (Black-Eyed, Croweder, Southern), Common, Boiled | 0.50 | CUP | 99.18 | 6.61 | 17.76 | 0.45 | 0.00 | 0.12 |
| Potatoes, Baked | 1.00 | ITEM | 220.18 | 4.65 | 50.97 | 0.20 | 0.00 | 0.05 |
| Potatoes, Mashed, Dehydrated Granules, Dry | 1.00 | CUP | 744.00 | 16.44 | 171.02 | 1.08 | 0.00 | 0.28 |
| Baked Sweet Potatoes | 1.00 | SERVING | 60.96 | 0.58 | 12.18 | 1.36 | 0.00 | 0.24 |
| Sweet Potato, Candied | 1.00 | PIECE | 143.85 | 0.91 | 29.25 | 3.41 | 8.40 | 1.42 |
| **ALL OTHERS:** | | | | | | | | |
| Broccoli | 1.00 | CUP | 24.64 | 2.62 | 4.61 | 0.31 | 0.00 | 0.05 |
| Cabbage, Shredded | 1.00 | CUP | 17.50 | 1.01 | 3.80 | 0.19 | 0.00 | 0.02 |
| Carrots | 1.00 | CUP | 52.46 | 1.26 | 12.37 | 0.23 | 0.00 | 0.04 |
| Peas and Carrots, Frozen, Boiled, Drained | 0.50 | CUP | 38.40 | 2.47 | 8.10 | 0.34 | 0.00 | 0.06 |
| Cauliflower, Boiled, Drained | 0.50 | CUP | 14.26 | 1.14 | 2.55 | 0.28 | 0.00 | 0.04 |
| Celery, Stalk | 1.00 | ITEM | 6.40 | 0.30 | 1.46 | 0.06 | 0.00 | 0.02 |
| Collards, Boiled, Drained | 0.50 | CUP | 24.70 | 2.00 | 4.66 | 0.34 | 0.00 | 0.05 |
| Cucumber | 1.00 | ITEM | 39.13 | 2.08 | 8.31 | 0.39 | 0.00 | 0.10 |
| Green Beans, Frozen, Boiled, Drained | 0.50 | CUP | 18.90 | 1.01 | 4.35 | 0.12 | 0.00 | 0.03 |
| Iceberg Lettuce | 1.00 | CUP | 6.60 | 0.56 | 1.15 | 0.11 | 0.00 | 0.01 |
| Onions, Red, Sliced | 1.00 | CUP | 43.70 | 1.33 | 9.92 | 0.18 | 0.00 | 0.03 |
| Sweet (Bell) Pepper | 1.00 | CUP | 21.56 | 1.36 | 4.72 | 0.18 | 0.00 | 0.00 |
| Hot Chili Peppers, Green | 1.00 | ITEM | 18.00 | 0.90 | 4.26 | 0.09 | 0.00 | 0.01 |
| Pumpkin, Canned | 0.50 | CUP | 41.65 | 1.35 | 9.90 | 0.34 | 0.00 | 0.18 |
| Spinach, Trimmed Leaves | 1.00 | CUP | 3.16 | 0.90 | 0.05 | 0.10 | 0.00 | 0.00 |
| Tomato, Red | 1.00 | ITEM | 25.83 | 1.05 | 5.71 | 0.41 | 0.00 | 0.06 |
| Romaine Lettuce, Shredded | 1.00 | CUP | 7.84 | 0.91 | 1.33 | 0.11 | 0.00 | 0.02 |
| Mushrooms | 1.00 | CUP | 26.60 | 3.12 | 2.65 | 1.77 | 0.00 | 0.24 |
| Summer Squash, All Varieties | 0.50 | CUP | 18.00 | 0.82 | 3.88 | 0.28 | 0.00 | 0.06 |
| Winter Squash, All Varieties | 1.00 | CUP | 42.92 | 1.68 | 10.21 | 0.27 | 0.00 | 0.05 |
| Vegetable Combinations (Broccoli, Carrots, Corn, Cauliflower, etc.), Cooked | 0.50 | CUP | 27.65 | 1.57 | 6.18 | 0.14 | 0.00 | 0.02 |
| Mixed Vegetables, Frozen, Boiled, Drained | 0.50 | CUP | 53.69 | 2.60 | 11.91 | 0.14 | 0.00 | 0.03 |

| Sodium | Potas | Beta-C | Vit C | Calcium | Iron | Vit E (IU) | Zinc | Diet Fiber | Sugar |
|---|---|---|---|---|---|---|---|---|---|
| 0.86 | 305.30 | | 0.00 | 23.22 | 1.81 | | 0.96 | 7.48 | 0.95 |
| 1.96 | 354.76 | 0.96 | 0.39 | 13.72 | 1.26 | | 0.98 | 8.13 | 2.83 |
| 1.71 | 400.14 | 0.00 | 1.80 | 41.04 | 2.23 | | 0.92 | 7.35 | 1.88 |
| 5.37 | 502.10 | 0.00 | 0.00 | 80.55 | 3.31 | | 1.24 | 5.64 | 1.97 |
| 14.45 | 484.50 | 25.50 | 8.59 | 27.20 | 2.08 | | 0.67 | 4.51 | 2.50 |
| 1.77 | 356.66 | 0.00 | 1.06 | 24.78 | 2.60 | | 0.95 | 5.66 | 1.95 |
| 436.48 | 328.96 | 0.00 | 1.41 | 30.72 | 1.61 | | 0.70 | 8.19 | 2.82 |
| 1.98 | 365.31 | 0.99 | 1.49 | 18.81 | 3.30 | | 1.26 | 7.82 | 1.80 |
| 5.74 | 238.62 | | 1.07 | 40.18 | 2.37 | | 1.26 | 6.23 | 3.94 |
| 575.19 | 536.78 | | 1.06 | 87.61 | 3.12 | | 1.16 | 4.99 | |
| 0.91 | 334.88 | 0.00 | 0.82 | 63.70 | 2.26 | | 0.97 | 5.82 | 2.00 |
| 378.24 | 337.76 | 0.00 | 7.59 | 44.28 | 2.10 | | 1.48 | 6.71 | |
| 300.12 | 214.02 | 2.46 | 9.72 | 61.50 | 1.93 | | 1.35 | 6.27 | |
| | | | | | | | | | |
| 0.86 | 442.90 | 0.86 | 1.46 | 87.72 | 4.42 | | 0.99 | 5.16 | 2.60 |
| 9.60 | 144.00 | 9.62 | 0.24 | 133.20 | 1.33 | | 0.77 | 0.24 | 0.84 |
| 17.64 | 298.62 | | 0.25 | 860.58 | 13.19 | | 1.98 | 2.90 | 0.17 |
| 626.85 | 28.19 | | 0.00 | 11.34 | 0.47 | | 0.57 | 0.93 | |
| 4.98 | 304.61 | | 0.00 | 77.19 | 1.88 | | 1.50 | | |
| | | | | | | | | | |
| 4.10 | 120.54 | | 2.54 | 3.28 | 0.29 | | 0.33 | 1.97 | 1.48 |
| 364.80 | 171.52 | 12.80 | 5.89 | 3.84 | 0.49 | | 0.68 | 1.54 | |
| 2.40 | 216.80 | 51.00 | 11.36 | 21.60 | 1.23 | | 0.95 | 4.40 | 4.64 |
| 3.53 | 245.39 | 1.62 | 0.35 | 21.19 | 2.22 | | 1.14 | 5.74 | 2.92 |
| | | | | | | | | | |
| 3.42 | 237.69 | 1.57 | 0.34 | 20.52 | 2.15 | | 1.10 | 5.56 | 2.83 |
| 16.16 | 844.36 | 0.00 | 26.06 | 20.20 | 2.75 | | 0.65 | 4.85 | 3.23 |
| 134.00 | 1406.00 | | 74.00 | 82.00 | 2.18 | | 1.82 | 14.20 | |
| 32.24 | 122.36 | 240.78 | 8.04 | 11.65 | 0.39 | | 0.07 | 0.98 | 7.60 |
| 73.50 | 198.45 | 592.00 | 7.04 | 27.30 | 1.19 | | 0.16 | 2.52 | |
| | | | | | | | | | |
| 23.76 | 286.00 | 136.00 | 82.02 | 42.24 | 0.77 | | 0.35 | 2.64 | 1.75 |
| 12.60 | 172.20 | 9.10 | 22.54 | 32.90 | 0.41 | | 0.13 | 1.61 | 2.52 |
| 42.70 | 394.06 | 3431.25 | 11.35 | 32.94 | 0.61 | | 0.24 | 3.66 | 8.05 |
| 54.40 | 126.40 | 617.00 | 6.48 | 18.40 | 0.75 | | 0.36 | 2.48 | 4.00 |
| 9.30 | 88.04 | | 27.47 | 9.92 | 0.21 | | 0.11 | 1.67 | 2.36 |
| 34.80 | 114.80 | 5.20 | 2.80 | 16.00 | 0.16 | | 0.05 | 0.68 | 0.44 |
| 8.55 | 247.00 | 316.17 | 17.29 | 113.05 | 0.44 | | 0.40 | 2.66 | |
| 6.02 | 433.44 | | 15.95 | 42.14 | 0.78 | | 0.60 | 2.41 | 6.92 |
| 6.08 | 85.05 | | 2.77 | 33.08 | 0.59 | | 0.32 | 2.03 | 1.76 |
| 4.95 | 86.90 | 18.16 | 2.15 | 10.45 | 0.28 | | 0.12 | 0.77 | 0.99 |
| 3.45 | 180.55 | 0.00 | 7.36 | 23.00 | 0.26 | | 0.22 | 2.07 | 7.13 |
| 2.07 | 269.08 | 0.24 | 113.07 | 12.45 | 0.52 | | 0.15 | 2.43 | 3.58 |
| 3.15 | 153.00 | 483.60 | 109.13 | 8.10 | 0.54 | | 0.14 | 0.68 | 1.13 |
| 6.13 | 252.35 | 175.50 | 5.15 | 31.85 | 1.70 | | 0.21 | 3.55 | 4.05 |
| 37.97 | 134.09 | 1.01 | 7.50 | 25.01 | 2.13 | | 0.18 | 2.77 | 0.00 |
| 11.07 | 273.06 | 139.00 | 23.49 | 6.15 | 0.55 | | 0.11 | 1.35 | 3.40 |
| 4.48 | 162.40 | 18.50 | 13.44 | 20.16 | 0.62 | | 0.14 | 0.95 | 1.12 |
| 4.06 | 341.41 | 0.00 | 0.00 | 2.69 | 0.55 | | | 0.68 | 1.89 |
| 0.90 | 172.80 | 25.95 | 4.95 | 24.30 | 0.32 | | 0.35 | 1.26 | 1.89 |
| 4.64 | 406.00 | | 14.27 | 35.96 | 0.67 | | 0.15 | 1.74 | 2.55 |
| | | | | | | | | | |
| 183.85 | 112.62 | | 14.15 | 20.85 | 0.34 | | 0.19 | 2.09 | |
| 31.85 | 153.79 | | 2.91 | 22.75 | 0.75 | | 0.45 | 4.00 | 3.93 |

| DAIRY | Amount | Portion | Kcal | Protein | Carb | Fat | Chol | Sat Fat | Sodium |
|---|---|---|---|---|---|---|---|---|---|
| **CHEESE:** | | | | | | | | | |
| American Cheese | 1.00 | OUNCE | 106.44 | 6.28 | 0.45 | 8.86 | 26.76 | 5.58 | 405.52 |
| Cheddar Cheese, Shredded | 0.25 | CUP | 113.73 | 7.03 | 0.36 | 9.36 | 29.63 | 5.96 | 175.29 |
| Cottage Cheese, 1% Fat | 0.50 | CUP | 81.81 | 14.00 | 3.07 | 1.15 | 4.97 | 0.73 | 458.78 |
| Cottage Cheese, 4% Fat, Creamed | 0.50 | CUP | 108.51 | 13.12 | 2.81 | 4.74 | 15.65 | 3.00 | 425.04 |
| Fat Free Cream Cheese | 2.00 | TBSP | 28.80 | 4.32 | 1.74 | 0.41 | 2.40 | 0.27 | 163.50 |
| Lowfat Cream Cheese | 2.00 | TBSP | 69.30 | 3.18 | 2.10 | 5.28 | 16.80 | 3.33 | 88.80 |
| Cream Cheese | 2.00 | TBSP | 101.22 | 2.19 | 0.77 | 10.11 | 31.81 | 6.37 | 85.70 |
| Mozzarella Cheese, Part Skim Milk | 1.00 | OUNCE | 71.19 | 6.79 | 0.78 | 4.46 | 16.18 | 2.83 | 130.48 |
| Mozzarella Cheese, Whole Milk | 1.00 | OUNCE | 78.79 | 5.44 | 0.62 | 6.05 | 21.95 | 3.68 | 104.47 |
| Monterey Jack Cheese | 1.00 | OUNCE | 104.53 | 6.85 | 0.19 | 8.48 | 24.92 | 5.34 | 150.16 |
| Parmesan Cheese, Grated | 1.00 | TBSP | 22.79 | 2.08 | 0.19 | 1.50 | 3.94 | 0.95 | 93.08 |
| Provolone Cheese | 1.00 | OUNCE | 98.42 | 7.16 | 0.60 | 7.45 | 19.29 | 4.78 | 245.14 |
| Ricotta Cheese, Whole Milk | 0.50 | CUP | 213.95 | 13.85 | 3.74 | 15.97 | 62.24 | 10.20 | 103.44 |
| Ricotta Cheese, Part Skim Milk | 0.50 | CUP | 169.81 | 14.01 | 6.32 | 9.73 | 37.88 | 6.06 | 153.38 |
| Swiss Cheese | 1.00 | OUNCE | 105.21 | 7.96 | 0.95 | 7.69 | 25.68 | 4.98 | 72.80 |
| Romano Cheese | 1.00 | OUNCE | 108.26 | 8.90 | 1.02 | 7.54 | 29.12 | 4.79 | 336.00 |
| Brie Cheese | 1.00 | OUNCE | 93.42 | 5.81 | 0.13 | 7.75 | 28.00 | 4.88 | 176.23 |
| Muenster Cheese | 1.00 | OUNCE | 103.14 | 6.56 | 0.31 | 8.41 | 26.77 | 5.35 | 175.76 |
| Blue Cheese, Crumbled | 0.50 | CUP | 238.31 | 14.45 | 1.58 | 19.40 | 50.76 | 12.60 | 941.83 |
| Goat Cheese, Hard | 1.00 | OUNCE | 128.37 | 8.67 | 0.62 | 10.11 | 29.82 | 6.99 | 98.26 |
| Goat Cheese, Soft | 1.00 | OUNCE | 76.11 | 5.26 | 0.25 | 5.99 | 13.06 | 4.14 | 104.51 |
| **MILK:** | | | | | | | | | |
| Whole Milk, 3.3% | 8.00 | FL OZ | 149.92 | 8.03 | 11.37 | 8.15 | 33.18 | 5.07 | 119.56 |
| Reduced Fat Milk, 2% | 8.00 | FL OZ | 121.20 | 8.13 | 11.71 | 4.69 | 18.30 | 2.92 | 121.76 |
| Lowfat Milk, 1% | 8.00 | FL OZ | 102.15 | 8.03 | 11.66 | 2.59 | 9.76 | 1.61 | 123.22 |
| Nonfat/Skim/Fat Free Milk | 8.00 | FL OZ | 85.53 | 8.35 | 11.88 | 0.44 | 4.41 | 0.29 | 126.18 |
| Chocolate Milk, Whole | 8 | FL OZ | 208.38 | 7.93 | 25.85 | 8.48 | 30.50 | 5.26 | 149.00 |
| Reduced Fat Chocolate Milk, 2% | 8 | FL OZ | 178.84 | 8.03 | 26.00 | 5.00 | 17.00 | 3.10 | 150.50 |
| Chocolate Flavored Milk, Powder | 2.5 | TSP | 75.38 | 0.71 | 19.51 | 0.67 | 0.00 | 0.40 | 45.36 |
| **YOGURT:** | | | | | | | | | |
| Lowfat Fruit Yogurt, with Nonfat Milk Solids | 1.00 | CUP | 257.56 | 11.91 | 45.57 | 3.45 | 13.48 | 2.23 | 159.01 |
| Lowfat Plain Yogurt, with Nonfat Milk Solids | 1.00 | CUP | 155.05 | 12.86 | 17.25 | 3.80 | 14.95 | 2.45 | 171.99 |
| Nonfat Plain Yogurt, with Nonfat Milk Solids | 1.00 | CUP | 136.64 | 14.04 | 18.82 | 0.44 | 4.41 | 0.28 | 187.43 |
| Nonfat Fruit Yogurt, Sweetened with Low-Calorie Sweetener | 1.00 | CUP | 121.89 | 10.62 | 19.38 | 0.39 | 3.25 | 0.21 | 139.48 |
| **CREAM:** | | | | | | | | | |
| Half and Half Cream | 2.00 | TBSP | 39.11 | 0.89 | 1.29 | 3.45 | 11.07 | 2.15 | 12.21 |
| Heavy Whipping Cream, Liquid | 2.00 | TBSP | 103.43 | 0.62 | 0.84 | 11.10 | 41.13 | 6.91 | 11.28 |
| Sour Cream | 2.00 | TBSP | 51.42 | 0.76 | 1.03 | 5.03 | 10.66 | 3.13 | 12.79 |
| Cream Substitute, Liquid | 1.00 | TBSP | 20.35 | 0.15 | 1.71 | 1.50 | 0.00 | 0.29 | 11.88 |
| Cream Substitute, Powder | 1.00 | TSP | 10.93 | 0.10 | 1.10 | 0.71 | 0.00 | 0.65 | 3.62 |

| Potas | Beta-C | Vit C | Calcium | Iron | Vit E (IU) | Zinc | Diet Fiber | Sugar |
|---|---|---|---|---|---|---|---|---|
| 45.93 | | 0.00 | 174.49 | 0.11 | | 0.85 | 0.00 | 0.45 |
| 27.80 | | 0.00 | 203.77 | 0.19 | | 0.88 | 0.00 | 0.51 |
| 96.62 | | 0.00 | 68.82 | 0.16 | | 0.43 | 0.00 | 3.08 |
| 88.52 | | 0.00 | 63.00 | 0.15 | | 0.39 | 0.00 | 0.63 |
| 48.90 | | 0.00 | 55.50 | 0.05 | | 0.26 | 0.00 | |
| 50.10 | | 0.00 | 33.60 | 0.50 | | 0.23 | 0.00 | |
| 34.63 | | 0.00 | 23.17 | 0.35 | | 0.16 | 0.00 | 0.50 |
| 23.44 | | 0.00 | 180.80 | 0.06 | | 0.77 | 0.00 | 0.11 |
| 18.79 | | 0.00 | 144.76 | 0.05 | | 0.62 | 0.00 | 0.11 |
| 22.60 | 6.86 | 0.00 | 208.99 | 0.20 | | 0.84 | 0.00 | 0.00 |
| 5.36 | | 0.00 | 68.79 | 0.05 | | 0.16 | 0.00 | |
| 38.72 | | 0.00 | 211.65 | 0.15 | | 0.90 | 0.00 | |
| 128.66 | | 0.00 | 254.61 | 0.47 | | 1.43 | 0.00 | 1.85 |
| 153.75 | | 0.00 | 334.56 | 0.54 | | 1.65 | 0.00 | 1.72 |
| 31.00 | | 0.00 | 269.05 | 0.05 | | 1.09 | 0.00 | 0.19 |
| 24.16 | | 0.00 | 297.86 | 0.22 | | 0.72 | 0.00 | |
| 42.56 | 2.52 | 0.00 | 51.52 | 0.14 | | 0.67 | 0.00 | |
| 37.63 | 3.64 | 0.00 | 200.84 | 0.12 | | 0.79 | 0.00 | |
| 173.00 | 5.40 | 0.00 | 356.13 | 0.21 | | 1.80 | 0.00 | |
| 13.63 | | 0.00 | 254.18 | 0.53 | | 0.45 | 0.00 | |
| 7.38 | | 0.00 | 39.76 | 0.54 | | 0.26 | 0.00 | |
| 369.66 | | 2.29 | 291.34 | 0.12 | | 0.93 | 0.00 | 12.00 |
| 376.74 | | 2.32 | 296.70 | 0.12 | | 0.95 | 0.00 | 11.20 |
| 380.88 | | 2.37 | 300.12 | 0.12 | | 0.95 | 0.00 | 11.20 |
| 405.72 | | 2.40 | 302.33 | 0.10 | | 0.98 | 0.00 | 10.80 |
| 417.25 | | 2.28 | 280.25 | 0.60 | | 1.03 | 2.00 | |
| 422.00 | | 2.30 | 284.00 | 0.60 | | 1.03 | 1.25 | |
| 127.66 | 0.43 | 0.15 | 7.99 | 0.68 | | 0.34 | 1.25 | 8.67 |
| 529.94 | | 1.81 | 413.81 | 0.17 | | 2.01 | 0.00 | 37.78 |
| 572.81 | | 1.96 | 447.37 | 0.20 | | 2.18 | 0.00 | 12.52 |
| 624.51 | | 2.13 | 487.80 | 0.22 | | 2.38 | 0.00 | 12.52 |
| 549.90 | | 26.40 | 369.51 | 0.62 | | 1.83 | 1.27 | |
| 38.88 | | 0.26 | 31.47 | 0.02 | | 0.15 | 0.00 | |
| 22.62 | 0.00 | 0.17 | 19.38 | 0.01 | | 0.07 | 0.00 | 0.84 |
| 34.56 | | 0.21 | 27.94 | 0.01 | | 0.07 | 0.00 | |
| 28.58 | | 0.00 | 1.40 | 0.00 | | 0.00 | 0.00 | |
| 16.24 | | 0.00 | 0.45 | 0.02 | | 0.01 | 0.00 | |

**343**

| MEATS | Amount | Portion | Kcal | Protein | Carb | Fat | Chol | Sat Fat |
|---|---|---|---|---|---|---|---|---|
| **BEEF:** | | | | | | | | |
| Ground Beef, Extra Lean, Broiled Medium | 3.00 | OUNCE | 217.60 | 21.59 | 0.00 | 13.88 | 71.40 | 5.46 |
| Ground Beef, Regular, Broiled-Medium | 3.00 | OUNCE | 245.65 | 20.46 | 0.00 | 17.59 | 76.50 | 6.91 |
| Beef Chuck Arm Pot Roast, Separable Lean, 1/4in. Fat, Braised | 3.00 | OUNCE | 183.60 | 28.07 | 0.00 | 7.06 | 85.85 | 2.56 |
| Beef Short Ribs, Choice, Separable Lean, Braised | 3.00 | OUNCE | 250.75 | 26.15 | 0.00 | 15.41 | 79.05 | 6.58 |
| Beef Round, Full Cut, Choice, Separable Lean, 1/4in. Fat, Broiled | 3.00 | OUNCE | 162.35 | 24.83 | 0.00 | 6.21 | 66.30 | 2.18 |
| Beef Eye of Round, Separable Lean, 1/4in. Fat, Roasted | 3.00 | OUNCE | 142.80 | 24.64 | 0.00 | 4.17 | 58.65 | 1.51 |
| Beef Round Tip, Separable Lean and Fat, 1/4in. Fat, Roasted | 3.00 | OUNCE | 198.90 | 22.87 | 0.00 | 11.25 | 69.70 | 4.27 |
| Beef Short Loin, T-Bone Steak, Choice, Separable Lean, 1/4in. Fat, Broiled | 3.00 | OUNCE | 174.25 | 22.76 | 0.00 | 8.54 | 50.15 | 3.06 |
| Beef Top Sirloin, All Grades, Separable Lean, 0in. Fat, Broiled | 3.00 | OUNCE | 162.35 | 25.82 | 0.00 | 5.78 | 75.65 | 2.25 |
| Corned Beef Brisket, Cooked | 3.00 | OUNCE | 213.35 | 15.44 | 0.40 | 16.13 | 83.30 | 5.39 |
| **PORK:** | | | | | | | | |
| Ham, Whole, Lean, Cured | 3.00 | OUNCE | 124.95 | 18.97 | 0.04 | 4.85 | 44.20 | 1.63 |
| Ham, Boneless, 11% Fat, Roasted | 3.00 | OUNCE | 151.30 | 19.23 | 0.00 | 7.67 | 50.15 | 2.65 |
| Pork, Center Loin (Chops), Separable Lean, Bone-In, Broiled | 3.00 | OUNCE | 171.70 | 25.66 | 0.00 | 6.86 | 69.70 | 2.51 |
| Pork, Center Loin (Roasts), Separable Lean and Fat, Bone-In, Roasted | 3.00 | OUNCE | 198.90 | 22.36 | 0.00 | 11.44 | 68.00 | 4.30 |
| Pork Spareribs, Separable Lean and Fat, Braised | 3.00 | OUNCE | 337.45 | 24.70 | 0.00 | 25.76 | 102.85 | 9.45 |
| Bacon, Pork | 2.00 | SLICE | 72.58 | 3.84 | 0.07 | 6.20 | 10.71 | 2.20 |
| **VEAL:** | | | | | | | | |
| Ground Veal, Broiled | 3.00 | OUNCE | 146.20 | 20.72 | 0.00 | 6.43 | 87.55 | 2.58 |
| Braised Veal Chops | 1.00 | SERVING | 215.61 | 37.49 | 0.00 | 6.21 | 148.69 | 1.88 |
| Veal Loin, Separable Lean and Fat, Roasted | 3.00 | OUNCE | 184.45 | 21.08 | 0.00 | 10.47 | 87.55 | 4.47 |
| **LAMB:** | | | | | | | | |
| Roasted Lamb Leg | 1.00 | SERVING | 178.43 | 28.66 | 0.00 | 6.29 | 89.22 | 2.24 |
| Roasted Lamb Shoulder | 1.00 | SERVING | 218.69 | 29.69 | 0.00 | 10.27 | 100.23 | 3.68 |
| Braised Lamb Chops | 1.00 | SERVING | 267.65 | 36.34 | 0.00 | 12.57 | 122.67 | 4.50 |
| Lamb Foreshank, Choice, Separable Lean and Fat, 1/4in. Fat, Braised | 3.00 | OUNCE | 206.55 | 24.12 | 0.00 | 11.44 | 90.10 | 4.79 |
| **DEER:** | | | | | | | | |
| Deer, Raw | 3.00 | OUNCE | 102.00 | 19.52 | 0.00 | 2.06 | 72.25 | 0.81 |
| **PROCESSED MEATS:** | | | | | | | | |
| Pork Sausage, Patty, Cooked | 2.00 | ITEM | 199.26 | 10.61 | 0.56 | 16.83 | 44.82 | 5.84 |
| Pork Sausage, Link, Cooked | 2.00 | ITEM | 95.94 | 5.11 | 0.27 | 8.10 | 21.58 | 2.81 |
| Beef Frankfurter | 1.00 | ITEM | 141.75 | 5.40 | 0.81 | 12.83 | 27.45 | 5.42 |
| Chicken Frankfurter | 1.00 | ITEM | 115.65 | 5.82 | 3.06 | 8.77 | 45.45 | 2.49 |
| Turkey Frankfurter | 1.00 | ITEM | 101.70 | 6.43 | 0.67 | 7.97 | 48.15 | 2.65 |
| Ham Luncheon Meat, Sliced, Prepackaged or Deli | 1.00 | SLICE | 34.02 | 3.84 | 0.48 | 1.76 | 11.13 | 0.57 |
| Turkey or Chicken Breast Luncheon Meat, Prepackaged or Deli | 2.00 | OUNCE | 61.60 | 12.60 | 0.00 | 0.88 | 22.96 | 0.27 |
| Turkey Loaf, Breast Meat | 2.00 | SLICE | 46.75 | 9.56 | 0.00 | 0.67 | 17.43 | 0.20 |
| Pepperoni with Beef and Pork | 10.00 | SLICE | 273.35 | 11.53 | 1.56 | 24.18 | 43.45 | 8.87 |
| Bologna, Beef and Pork, Sliced | 1.00 | SLICE | 89.59 | 3.31 | 0.79 | 8.01 | 15.59 | 3.03 |
| Pork and Beef Salami, Dry | 6.00 | SLICE | 250.80 | 13.72 | 1.55 | 20.63 | 47.40 | 7.32 |

**344**

| Sodium | Potas | Beta-C | Vit C | Calcium | Iron | Vit E (IU) | Zinc | Diet Fiber | Sugar |
|---|---|---|---|---|---|---|---|---|---|
| 59.50 | 266.05 | 0.00 | 0.00 | 5.95 | 2.00 | | 4.63 | 0.00 | 0.00 |
| 70.55 | 248.20 | 0.00 | 0.00 | 9.35 | 2.07 | | 4.40 | 0.00 | 0.00 |
| 56.10 | 245.65 | 0.00 | 0.00 | 7.65 | 3.22 | | 7.36 | 0.00 | 0.00 |
| 49.30 | 266.05 | 0.00 | 0.00 | 9.35 | 2.86 | | 6.63 | 0.00 | 0.00 |
| 54.40 | 358.70 | 0.00 | 0.00 | 4.25 | 2.30 | | 3.94 | 0.00 | 0.00 |
| 52.70 | 335.75 | 0.00 | 0.00 | 4.25 | 1.66 | | 4.03 | 0.00 | 0.00 |
| 53.55 | 305.15 | 0.00 | 0.00 | 5.10 | 2.34 | | 5.53 | 0.00 | 0.00 |
| 60.35 | 321.30 | 0.00 | 0.00 | 5.10 | 2.69 | | 4.51 | 0.00 | 0.00 |
| 56.10 | 342.55 | 0.00 | 0.00 | 9.35 | 2.86 | | 5.54 | 0.00 | 0.00 |
| 963.90 | 123.25 | 0.00 | 0.00 | 6.80 | 1.58 | | 3.89 | 0.00 | 0.60 |
| 1288.60 | 315.35 | 0.00 | 0.00 | 5.95 | 0.69 | | 1.73 | 0.00 | 0.00 |
| 1275.00 | 347.65 | 0.00 | 0.00 | 6.80 | 1.14 | | 2.10 | 0.00 | 0.00 |
| 51.00 | 318.75 | 0.00 | 0.34 | 26.35 | 0.72 | | 2.02 | 0.00 | 0.00 |
| 53.55 | 299.20 | 0.00 | 0.77 | 22.95 | 0.84 | | 1.72 | 0.00 | 0.00 |
| 79.05 | 272.00 | 0.00 | 0.00 | 39.95 | 1.57 | | 3.91 | 0.00 | 0.00 |
| 201.10 | 61.24 | 0.00 | 0.00 | 1.51 | 0.20 | | 0.41 | 0.00 | 0.00 |
| 70.55 | 286.45 | 0.00 | 0.00 | 14.45 | 0.84 | | 3.29 | 0.00 | 0.00 |
| 169.14 | 602.21 | 0.00 | 0.00 | 31.60 | 1.39 | | 4.63 | 0.00 | 0.00 |
| 79.05 | 276.25 | 0.00 | 0.00 | 16.15 | 0.74 | | 2.58 | 0.00 | 0.00 |
| 86.43 | 402.87 | 0.00 | 0.00 | 8.36 | 2.54 | | 5.35 | 0.00 | 0.00 |
| 106.31 | 416.12 | 0.00 | 0.00 | 22.78 | 2.52 | | 7.24 | 0.00 | 0.00 |
| 130.11 | 509.28 | 0.00 | 0.00 | 27.88 | 3.09 | | 8.87 | 0.00 | 0.00 |
| 61.20 | 218.45 | 0.00 | 0.00 | 17.00 | 1.82 | | 6.54 | 0.00 | 0.00 |
| 43.35 | 270.30 | 0.00 | 0.00 | 4.25 | 2.89 | | 1.78 | 0.00 | 0.00 |
| 698.76 | 194.94 | 0.00 | 0.00 | 1.08 | 17.28 | | 0.93 | | 0.39 |
| 336.44 | 93.86 | 0.00 | 0.00 | 0.52 | 8.32 | | 0.45 | | 0.19 |
| 461.70 | 74.70 | 0.00 | 0.00 | 0.00 | 9.00 | | 0.69 | | 0.13 |
| 616.50 | 37.80 | 58.50 | 0.00 | 0.00 | 42.75 | 0.00 | 0.11 | | 0.37 |
| 641.70 | 80.55 | 0.00 | 0.00 | 0.00 | 47.70 | 0.00 | 0.13 | | 0.32 |
| 268.38 | 62.37 | 0.00 | 0.00 | 0.00 | 1.47 | | 0.17 | | |
| 801.36 | 155.68 | 0.00 | 0.00 | 0.00 | 3.92 | | 1.13 | | |
| 608.18 | 118.15 | 0.00 | 0.00 | 0.00 | 2.98 | 0.20 | 0.86 | | 0.25 |
| 1122.00 | 190.85 | 0.00 | 0.00 | 0.00 | 5.50 | | 1.38 | | 1.03 |
| 288.89 | 51.03 | 0.00 | 0.00 | 0.00 | 3.40 | | 0.38 | | 0.08 |
| 1116.00 | 226.80 | 0.00 | 0.00 | 0.00 | 4.80 | | 1.14 | | 0.64 |

**345**

| POULTRY **CHICKEN:** | Amount | Portion | Kcal | Protein | Carb | Fat | Chol | Sat Fat |
|---|---|---|---|---|---|---|---|---|
| Chicken Breast, Meat Only, Roasted | 3.00 | OUNCE | 140.25 | 26.37 | 0.00 | 3.03 | 72.25 | 0.86 |
| Chicken Breast, Meat and Skin, Roasted | 3.00 | OUNCE | 167.45 | 25.33 | 0.00 | 6.61 | 71.40 | 1.86 |
| Chicken Breast, Meat Only, Fried | 3.00 | OUNCE | 158.95 | 28.42 | 0.43 | 4.00 | 77.35 | 1.10 |
| Chicken Leg and Thigh, Meat and Skin, Roasted | 3.00 | OUNCE | 197.20 | 22.07 | 0.00 | 11.44 | 78.20 | 3.16 |
| Chicken Wing, Meat and Skin, Roasted | 3.00 | OUNCE | 246.50 | 22.83 | 0.00 | 16.54 | 71.40 | 4.63 |
| Chicken Drumstick, Meat and Skin, Roasted | 3.00 | OUNCE | 183.60 | 22.98 | 0.00 | 9.48 | 77.35 | 2.59 |
| Chicken, Boneless Pieces, Breaded and Fried **TURKEY:** | 6 | PIECE | 287.26 | 18.02 | 15.158 | 17.172 | 61.48 | 3.636 |
| Turkey, Light Meat, Meat Only, Roasted | 3.00 | OUNCE | 133.45 | 25.42 | 0.00 | 2.74 | 58.65 | 0.88 |
| Turkey Light Meat, Meat and Skin, Roasted | 3.00 | OUNCE | 167.45 | 24.29 | 0.00 | 7.08 | 64.60 | 1.99 |
| Turkey Leg and Thigh, Meat and Skin, Roasted **DUCK:** | 3.00 | OUNCE | 176.80 | 23.69 | 0.00 | 8.35 | 72.25 | 2.60 |
| Duck, Domesticated, Meat and Skin, Roasted | 3.00 | OUNCE | 286.45 | 16.14 | 0.00 | 24.10 | 71.40 | 8.22 |
| Duck, Domesticated, Meat Only, Roasted | 3.00 | OUNCE | 170.85 | 19.96 | 0.00 | 9.52 | 75.65 | 3.55 |

| Sodium | Potas | Beta-C | Vit C | Calcium | Iron | Vit E (IU) | Zinc | Diet Fiber | Sugar |
|---|---|---|---|---|---|---|---|---|---|
| 62.90 | 217.60 | 0.00 | 0.00 | 12.75 | 0.88 | | 0.85 | 0.00 | 0.00 |
| 60.35 | 208.25 | 0.00 | 0.00 | 11.90 | 0.91 | | 0.87 | 0.00 | 0.00 |
| 67.15 | 234.60 | 0.00 | 0.00 | 13.60 | 0.97 | | 0.92 | 0.00 | 0.00 |
| 73.95 | 191.25 | 0.00 | 0.00 | 10.20 | 1.13 | | 2.21 | 0.00 | 0.00 |
| 69.70 | 156.40 | 0.00 | 0.00 | 12.75 | 1.08 | | 1.55 | 0.00 | 0.00 |
| 76.50 | 194.65 | 0.00 | 0.00 | 10.20 | 1.13 | | 2.44 | 0.00 | 0.00 |
| 513.04 | 305.28 | 0 | 0 | 13.78 | 0.943 | | 0.996 | 0 | 0 |
| | | | | | | | | | |
| 54.40 | 259.25 | 0.00 | 0.00 | 16.15 | 1.15 | | 1.73 | 0.00 | 0.00 |
| 53.55 | 242.25 | 0.00 | 0.00 | 17.85 | 1.20 | | 1.73 | 0.00 | 0.00 |
| 65.45 | 238.00 | 0.00 | 0.00 | 27.20 | 1.96 | | 3.63 | 0.00 | 0.00 |
| | | | | | | | | | |
| 50.15 | 173.40 | 0.00 | 0.00 | 9.35 | 2.30 | | 1.58 | 0.00 | 0.00 |
| 55.25 | 214.20 | 0.00 | 0.00 | 10.20 | 2.30 | | 2.21 | 0.00 | 0.00 |

| SEAFOOD | Amount | Portion | Kcal | Protein | Carb | Fat | Chol | Sat Fat | Sodium |
|---|---|---|---|---|---|---|---|---|---|
| **SHELLFISH:** | | | | | | | | | |
| Clams, Mixed Species, Cooked, Moist Heat | 3.00 | OUNCE | 125.80 | 21.72 | 4.36 | 1.66 | 56.95 | 0.16 | 0.47 |
| Shrimp, Mixed Species, Cooked, Moist Heat | 3.00 | OUNCE | 84.15 | 17.77 | 0.00 | 0.92 | 165.75 | 0.25 | 0.37 |
| Bay and Sea Scallops, Steamed | 3.00 | OUNCE | 90.39 | 13.77 | 1.95 | 2.67 | 27.03 | | |
| Alaska King Crab, Cooked, Moist Heat | 3.00 | OUNCE | 82.45 | 16.45 | 0.00 | 1.31 | 45.05 | 0.11 | 0.46 |
| Imperial Crab | 3.00 | OUNCE | 127.30 | 13.17 | 2.78 | 6.78 | 106.38 | 1.60 | 1.69 |
| Northern Lobster, Cooked, Moist Heat | 3.00 | OUNCE | 83.30 | 17.43 | 1.09 | 0.50 | 61.20 | 0.09 | 0.08 |
| **ALL OTHERS:** | | | | | | | | | |
| Tuna, White, Canned in Water, Drained | 3.00 | OUNCE | 108.80 | 20.08 | 0.00 | 2.52 | 35.70 | 0.67 | 320.45 |
| Tuna, White, Canned in Oil, Drained | 3.00 | OUNCE | 158.10 | 22.55 | 0.00 | 6.87 | 26.35 | 1.40 | 2.87 |
| Light Tuna, Canned in Oil, Drained | 1.00 | OUNCE | 168.30 | 24.76 | 0.00 | 6.98 | 15.30 | 1.30 | 300.90 |
| Bluefin Tuna, Cooked, Dry Heat | 3.00 | OUNCE | 156.40 | 25.42 | 0.00 | 5.34 | 41.65 | 1.37 | 1.57 |
| Yellowtail, Mixed Species, Cooked, Dry Heat | 3.00 | OUNCE | 158.95 | 25.22 | 0.00 | 5.71 | 60.35 | 1.45 | 1.53 |
| Atlantic Cod, Cooked, Dry Heat | 3.00 | OUNCE | 89.25 | 19.41 | 0.00 | 0.73 | 46.75 | 0.14 | 0.25 |
| Haddock, Cooked, Dry Heat | 3.00 | OUNCE | 95.20 | 20.60 | 0.00 | 0.79 | 62.90 | 0.14 | 0.26 |
| Sea Trout, Mixed Species, Cooked, Dry Heat | 3.00 | OUNCE | 113.05 | 18.24 | 0.00 | 3.94 | 90.10 | 1.10 | 0.79 |
| Rainbow Trout, Farmed, Cooked, Dry Heat | 3.00 | OUNCE | 143.65 | 20.63 | 0.00 | 6.12 | 57.80 | 1.79 | 1.98 |
| Striped Bass, Cooked, Dry Heat | 3.00 | OUNCE | 105.40 | 19.32 | 0.00 | 2.54 | 87.55 | 0.55 | 0.85 |
| Sea Bass, Mixed Species, Cooked, Dry Heat | 3.00 | OUNCE | 105.40 | 20.09 | 0.00 | 2.18 | 45.05 | 0.56 | 0.81 |
| Bluefish, Cooked, Dry Heat | 3.00 | OUNCE | 135.15 | 21.84 | 0.00 | 4.62 | 64.60 | 1.00 | 1.15 |
| Halibut, Cooked, Dry Heat | 3.00 | OUNCE | 119.00 | 22.69 | 0.00 | 2.50 | 34.85 | 0.35 | 0.80 |
| Atlantic Herring, Pickled | 1.00 | PIECE | 39.30 | 2.13 | 1.45 | 2.70 | 1.95 | 0.36 | 0.25 |
| Atlantic Mackerel, Cooked, Dry Heat | 3.00 | OUNCE | 222.70 | 20.27 | 0.00 | 15.14 | 63.75 | 3.55 | 3.66 |
| Pacific/Jack Mackerel, Mixed Species, Cooked, Dry Heat | 3.00 | OUNCE | 170.85 | 21.87 | 0.00 | 8.60 | 51.00 | 2.45 | 2.12 |
| Snapper, Mixed Species, Cooked, Dry Heat | 3.00 | OUNCE | 108.80 | 22.36 | 0.00 | 1.46 | 39.95 | 0.31 | 0.50 |
| Atlantic Salmon, Wild, Cooked, Dry Heat | 3.00 | OUNCE | 154.70 | 21.62 | 0.00 | 6.91 | 60.35 | 1.07 | 2.77 |
| Atlantic Salmon, Farmed, Cooked, Dry Heat | 3.00 | OUNCE | 175.10 | 18.79 | 0.00 | 10.50 | 53.55 | 2.13 | 3.76 |
| Pink Salmon, Cooked, Dry Heat | 3.00 | OUNCE | 126.65 | 21.73 | 0.00 | 3.76 | 56.95 | 0.61 | 1.47 |
| Sturgeon, Steamed | 3.00 | OUNCE | 110.63 | 17.01 | 0.00 | 4.26 | 63.22 | 0.97 | 0.73 |
| Sturgeon, Mixed Species, Cooked, Dry Heat | 3.00 | OUNCE | 114.75 | 17.60 | 0.00 | 4.40 | 65.45 | 1.00 | 0.75 |
| Swordfish, Cooked, Dry Heat | 3.00 | OUNCE | 131.75 | 21.58 | 0.00 | 4.37 | 42.50 | 1.20 | 1.01 |
| Swordfish, Broiled, with Margarine | 3.00 | OUNCE | 151.03 | 20.26 | 0.38 | 7.06 | 39.81 | 1.69 | 1.77 |
| Gelfilte Fish, Sweet Recipe | 2.00 | PIECE | 70.56 | 7.62 | 6.22 | 1.45 | 25.20 | 0.35 | 0.24 |
| Sablefish, Cooked, Dry Heat | 3.00 | OUNCE | 212.50 | 14.61 | 0.00 | 16.68 | 53.55 | 3.48 | 2.23 |
| Sablefish, Smoked | 3.00 | OUNCE | 218.45 | 15.00 | 0.00 | 17.12 | 54.40 | 3.58 | 2.29 |
| Whitefish, Mixed Species, Cooked, Dry Heat | 3.00 | OUNCE | 146.20 | 20.80 | 0.00 | 6.38 | 65.45 | 0.99 | 2.34 |
| Perch, Mixed Species, Cooked, Dry Heat | 3.00 | OUNCE | 99.45 | 21.13 | 0.00 | 1.00 | 97.75 | 0.20 | 0.40 |
| Atlantic Sardine, Solids with Bone, Canned in | 2.00 | ITEM | 49.92 | 5.91 | 0.00 | 2.75 | 34.08 | 0.37 | 1.24 |
| Anchovy, Canned in Oil, Drained | 14.00 | ITEM | 117.60 | 16.18 | 0.00 | 5.44 | 47.60 | 1.23 | 1.44 |
| Octopus, Common, Cooked, Moist Heat | 3.00 | OUNCE | 139.40 | 25.35 | 3.74 | 1.77 | 81.60 | 0.39 | 0.41 |
| Atlantic Smelt, Canned | 3.00 | OUNCE | 170.00 | 15.64 | 0.00 | 11.48 | | | |
| Rainbow Smelt, Cooked, Dry Heat | 3.00 | OUNCE | 105.40 | 19.21 | 0.00 | 2.64 | 76.50 | 0.49 | 0.97 |
| Caviar, Red and Black, Granular | 1.00 | TBSP | 40.32 | 3.94 | 0.64 | 2.86 | 94.08 | 0.65 | 1.19 |
| Eel, Steamed or Poached | 3.00 | OUNCE | 197.97 | 19.84 | 0.00 | 12.55 | 135.57 | 2.54 | 1.02 |

| Potas | Beta-C | Vit C | Calcium | Iron | Vit E (IU) | Zinc | Diet Fiber | Sugar |
|---|---|---|---|---|---|---|---|---|
| 95.20 | 484.50 | 0.05 | 18.79 | 78.20 | 0.00 | 15.30 | 2.32 | 0.00 |
| 190.40 | 186.15 | 0.00 | 1.87 | 33.15 | 0.00 | 28.90 | 1.33 | 0.00 |
| 365.86 | 128.59 | | 1.97 | 20.55 | | | | 0.00 |
| 911.20 | 24.65 | 0.00 | 6.46 | 50.15 | 0.00 | 53.55 | 6.48 | 0.00 |
| 358.37 | 271.10 | | 4.58 | 82.07 | | 22.08 | 2.48 | 0.14 |
| 323.00 | 73.95 | 0.00 | 0.00 | 51.85 | 0.00 | 29.75 | 2.48 | 0.00 |
| | | | | | | | | |
| 201.45 | | 0.00 | 11.90 | 0.83 | | 0.41 | 0.00 | 0.00 |
| 336.60 | 68.00 | 0.00 | 0.00 | 3.40 | 0.00 | 28.90 | 0.40 | 0.00 |
| 175.95 | | 0.00 | 11.05 | 1.18 | | 0.77 | 0.00 | 0.00 |
| 42.50 | 2142.00 | 2.83 | 0.00 | 8.50 | 0.00 | 54.40 | 0.66 | 0.00 |
| 42.50 | 88.40 | | 2.47 | 24.65 | | 32.30 | 0.57 | 0.00 |
| 66.30 | 39.10 | 36.60 | 0.85 | 11.90 | 0.00 | 35.70 | 0.49 | 0.00 |
| 73.95 | 53.55 | 9.45 | 0.00 | 35.70 | 0.00 | 42.50 | 0.41 | 0.00 |
| 62.90 | 97.75 | | 0.00 | 18.70 | | 34.00 | 0.49 | 0.00 |
| 35.70 | 243.95 | | 2.81 | 73.10 | | 27.20 | 0.42 | 0.00 |
| 74.80 | 88.40 | | 0.00 | 16.15 | | 43.35 | 0.43 | 0.00 |
| 73.95 | 181.05 | 3.39 | 0.00 | 11.05 | 0.84 | 45.05 | 0.44 | 0.00 |
| 65.45 | 390.15 | | 0.00 | 7.65 | | 35.70 | 0.88 | 0.00 |
| 58.65 | 152.15 | | 0.00 | 51.00 | 0.00 | 90.95 | 0.45 | 0.00 |
| 130.50 | 129.15 | 0.00 | 0.00 | 11.55 | 0.00 | 1.20 | 0.08 | 0.00 |
| 70.55 | 153.00 | 2.83 | 0.34 | 12.75 | 0.00 | 82.45 | 0.80 | 0.00 |
| | | | | | | | | |
| 93.50 | 39.95 | | 1.79 | 24.65 | | 30.60 | 0.73 | 0.00 |
| 48.45 | 97.75 | | 1.36 | 34.00 | 0.00 | 31.45 | 0.37 | 0.00 |
| 47.60 | 37.40 | | 0.00 | 12.75 | | 31.45 | 0.70 | 0.00 |
| 51.85 | 42.50 | | 3.15 | 12.75 | | 25.50 | 0.37 | 0.00 |
| 73.10 | 115.60 | | 0.00 | 14.45 | | 28.05 | 0.60 | 0.00 |
| 388.55 | 663.73 | | 0.00 | 11.17 | | 29.51 | 0.36 | 0.00 |
| 58.65 | 686.80 | 0.00 | 0.00 | 14.45 | 0.00 | 38.25 | 0.46 | 0.00 |
| 97.75 | 116.45 | 3.39 | 0.94 | 5.10 | 0.00 | 28.90 | 1.25 | 0.00 |
| 430.92 | 365.16 | | 2.74 | 5.66 | | 27.92 | 1.18 | 0.02 |
| 440.16 | 74.76 | 0.00 | 0.67 | 19.32 | 0.00 | 7.56 | 0.69 | 0.00 |
| 61.20 | 287.30 | | 0.00 | 38.25 | | 60.35 | 0.35 | 0.00 |
| 626.45 | 346.80 | | 0.00 | 42.50 | | 62.90 | 0.37 | 0.00 |
| 55.25 | 111.35 | | 0.00 | 28.05 | | 35.70 | 1.08 | 0.00 |
| 67.15 | 27.20 | 0.07 | 1.45 | 86.70 | 0.00 | 32.30 | 1.22 | 0.00 |
| 121.20 | 53.76 | | 0.00 | 91.68 | 0.00 | 9.36 | 0.31 | 0.00 |
| 2054.08 | 39.20 | 0.00 | 0.00 | 129.92 | 168.00 | 38.64 | 1.37 | 0.00 |
| 391.00 | 229.50 | | 6.80 | 90.10 | | 51.00 | 2.86 | 0.00 |
| | 81.59 | | 0.00 | 304.30 | 255.00 | | | 0.00 |
| 65.45 | 49.30 | 0.06 | 0.00 | 65.45 | 0.00 | 32.30 | 1.80 | 0.00 |
| 240.00 | 298.88 | 0.00 | 0.00 | 44.00 | 0.00 | 48.00 | 0.15 | 0.00 |
| 49.39 | 3179.29 | | 1.45 | 21.52 | | 19.37 | 1.74 | 0.00 |

**349**

| EGGS | Amount | Portion | Kcal | Protein | Carb | Fat | Chol | Sat Fat | Sodium | Potas |
|---|---|---|---|---|---|---|---|---|---|---|
| Egg, Raw | 1.00 | ITEM | 74.50 | 6.25 | 0.61 | 5.01 | 212.50 | 1.55 | 63.00 | 60.50 |
| Egg Yolk, Raw | 1.00 | ITEM | 59.43 | 2.78 | 0.30 | 5.12 | 212.65 | 1.59 | 7.14 | 15.60 |
| Egg White, Raw | 1.00 | ITEM | 16.70 | 3.51 | 0.34 | 0.00 | 0.00 | 0.00 | 54.78 | 47.76 |
| Egg Substitute, Liquid | 0.50 | CUP | 105.58 | 15.07 | 0.80 | 4.16 | 1.26 | 0.83 | 222.31 | 414.48 |
| **PREPARED:** | | | | | | | | | | |
| Hard Boiled Egg | 1.00 | ITEM | 77.50 | 6.29 | 0.56 | 5.31 | 212.00 | 1.63 | 62.00 | 63.00 |
| Fried Egg | 1.00 | ITEM | 91.54 | 6.23 | 0.63 | 6.90 | 211.14 | 1.92 | 162.38 | 60.72 |
| Scrambled Eggs | 1.00 | SERVING | 81.12 | 6.50 | 0.97 | 5.48 | 212.63 | 1.63 | 211.64 | 72.94 |
| Scrambled Egg or Omelet, Fat Added in Cooking | 1.00 | SERVING | 189.94 | 12.94 | 2.98 | 13.69 | 399.49 | 4.07 | 466.76 | 173.44 |
| Poached Egg | 1.00 | ITEM | 74.50 | 6.22 | 0.61 | 4.99 | 211.50 | 1.54 | 140.00 | 60.00 |

| NUTS & SEEDS | Amount | Portion | Kcal | Protein | Carb | Fat | Chol | Sat Fat | Sodium | Potas |
|---|---|---|---|---|---|---|---|---|---|---|
| **NUTS:** | | | | | | | | | | |
| Peanuts, All Types, Oil Roasted, with Salt | 0.50 | CUP | 418.32 | 18.97 | 13.63 | 35.50 | 0.00 | 4.93 | 311.76 | 491.04 |
| Peanut Butter, Smooth, with Salt | 2 | TBSP | 189.76 | 8.07 | 6.17 | 16.33 | 0.00 | 3.31 | 149.44 | 214.08 |
| Black Walnut, Chopped, Dried | 0.50 | CUP | 379.38 | 15.22 | 7.56 | 35.36 | 0.00 | 2.27 | 0.63 | 327.50 |
| Almonds, Dry Roasted, Unblanched, Salted | 0.25 | CUP | 202.52 | 5.63 | 8.34 | 17.80 | 0.00 | 1.69 | 269.10 | 265.65 |
| Almonds, Oil Roasted, Unblanched, Salted | 0.25 | CUP | 242.57 | 8.00 | 6.23 | 22.64 | 0.00 | 2.15 | 305.76 | 268.08 |
| Brazil Nuts, Whole, Unblanched, Dried | 0.50 | CUP | 459.20 | 10.04 | 8.96 | 46.35 | 0.00 | 11.31 | 1.40 | 420.00 |
| Cashew Nut, Oil Roasted | 0.50 | CUP | 374.40 | 10.50 | 18.54 | 31.34 | 0.00 | 6.19 | 11.05 | 344.50 |
| Coconut, Shredded | 2.00 | TBSP | 35.40 | 0.33 | 1.52 | 3.35 | 0.00 | 2.97 | 2.00 | 35.60 |
| Pecan Halves, Dried | 0.50 | CUP | 360.18 | 4.19 | 9.85 | 36.53 | 0.00 | 2.93 | 0.54 | 211.68 |
| Cashews, Dry Roasted | 0.50 | CUP | 393.19 | 10.49 | 22.39 | 31.75 | 0.00 | 6.27 | 10.96 | 387.03 |
| Macadamia Nut, Oil Roasted | 0.50 | CUP | 481.06 | 4.86 | 8.64 | 51.27 | 0.00 | 7.68 | 4.69 | 220.43 |
| Mixed Nuts with Peanuts, Dry Roasted | 0.50 | CUP | 406.89 | 11.85 | 17.37 | 35.24 | 0.00 | 4.73 | 8.22 | 408.95 |
| Pistachio Nuts, Dry Roasted | 0.50 | CUP | 387.84 | 9.56 | 17.62 | 33.81 | 0.00 | 4.28 | 3.84 | 620.80 |
| Pine Nut (Pingolia), Dried | 1.00 | TBSP | 48.68 | 2.06 | 1.22 | 4.36 | 0.00 | 0.67 | 0.34 | 51.51 |
| **SEEDS:** | | | | | | | | | | |
| Pumpkin Seed | 0.25 | CUP | 187.08 | 8.81 | 4.56 | 18.95 | 0.00 | 2.99 | 6.21 | 278.19 |
| Sesame Seeds, Dried | 1.00 | TBSP | 51.57 | 1.60 | 2.11 | 4.47 | 0.00 | 0.63 | 0.99 | 42.12 |
| Sesame Seeds, Roasted, Toasted | 1.00 | TBSP | 50.85 | 1.53 | 2.32 | 4.32 | 0.00 | 0.61 | 0.99 | 42.75 |
| Psyllium Seed, Ground | 1.00 | TBSP | 4.19 | 0.24 | 6.77 | 0.04 | 0.00 | 0.00 | 2.93 | 14.99 |
| Sunflower Seed Kernels, Dry Roasted | 0.25 | CUP | 186.24 | 6.19 | 7.70 | 15.94 | 0.00 | 1.67 | 0.96 | 272.00 |
| Sunflower Seed Kernels, Oil Roasted | 0.25 | CUP | 207.56 | 7.21 | 4.97 | 19.39 | 0.00 | 2.03 | 1.01 | 163.01 |

| Beta-C | Vit C | Calcium | Iron | Vit E (IU) | Zinc | Diet Fiber | Sugar |
|---|---|---|---|---|---|---|---|
| 0.00 | 0.00 | 24.50 | 0.72 | | 0.55 | 0.00 | 0.00 |
| 0.00 | 0.00 | 22.74 | 0.59 | | 0.52 | 0.00 | 0.00 |
| 0.00 | 0.00 | 2.00 | 0.01 | | 0.00 | 0.00 | 0.00 |
| 308.25 | 0.00 | 66.57 | 2.64 | | 1.63 | 0.00 | 0.00 |
| | | | | | | | |
| 0.00 | 0.00 | 25.00 | 0.60 | | 0.53 | 0.00 | 0.00 |
| | 0.00 | 25.30 | 0.72 | | 0.55 | 0.00 | 0.00 |
| 0.00 | 0.07 | 33.83 | 0.72 | | 0.58 | 0.00 | 0.32 |
| | | | | | | | |
| | 0.32 | 93.14 | 1.37 | | 1.17 | 0.00 | |
| 0.00 | 0.00 | 24.50 | 0.72 | | 0.55 | 0.00 | 0.00 |

| Beta-C | Vit C | Calcium | Iron | Vit E (IU) | Zinc | Diet Fiber | Sugar |
|---|---|---|---|---|---|---|---|
| 0.00 | 0.00 | 63.36 | 1.32 | | 4.77 | 6.62 | 2.67 |
| 0.00 | 0.00 | 12.16 | 0.59 | | 0.93 | 1.89 | 2.67 |
| 7.50 | 2.00 | 36.25 | 1.92 | | 2.14 | 3.13 | 1.32 |
| | | | | | | | |
| 0.00 | 0.24 | 97.29 | 1.31 | | 1.69 | 4.73 | |
| | | | | | | | |
| 0.00 | 0.28 | 91.85 | 1.50 | | 1.92 | 4.40 | |
| | | | | | | | |
| 0.00 | 0.49 | 123.20 | 2.38 | | 3.21 | 3.78 | 1.82 |
| 0.00 | 0.00 | 26.65 | 2.67 | | 3.09 | 2.47 | 4.03 |
| 0.00 | 0.33 | 1.40 | 0.24 | | 0.11 | 0.90 | 0.35 |
| | 1.08 | 19.44 | 1.15 | | 2.95 | 4.10 | 2.32 |
| 0.00 | 0.00 | 30.83 | 4.11 | | 3.84 | 2.06 | 4.25 |
| 0.67 | 0.00 | 30.15 | 1.21 | | 0.74 | 6.23 | 4.15 |
| | | | | | | | |
| 0.69 | 0.27 | 47.95 | 2.53 | | 2.60 | 6.17 | 2.74 |
| 15.35 | 4.67 | 44.80 | 2.03 | | 0.87 | 6.91 | 4.23 |
| | 0.16 | 2.24 | 0.79 | | 0.37 | 0.39 | |
| | | | | | | | |
| 13.12 | 0.66 | 15.55 | 3.40 | | 2.58 | 0.58 | 0.35 |
| 0.09 | 0.00 | 87.75 | 1.31 | | 0.70 | 1.06 | 0.10 |
| | | | | | | | |
| 0.09 | 0.00 | 89.01 | 1.33 | | 0.64 | 1.26 | 0.10 |
| | 0.03 | 17.00 | 0.29 | | 0.22 | 6.03 | |
| | | | | | | | |
| 0.00 | 0.45 | 22.40 | 1.22 | | 1.69 | 3.55 | |
| | | | | | | | |
| 1.69 | 0.47 | 18.90 | 2.26 | | 1.76 | 2.30 | 1.96 |

| COMBINATION FOODS | Amount | Portion | Kcal | Protein | Carb | Fat | Chol | Sat Fat |
|---|---|---|---|---|---|---|---|---|
| **BREAKFAST ITEMS:** | | | | | | | | |
| Grilled Cheese Sandwich | 1 | ITEM | 291.51 | 9.79 | 27.07 | 15.94 | 19.45 | 6.22 |
| Scrambled Egg, No Added Fat | 2 | ITEM | 158.41 | 12.9 | 2.94 | 10.16 | 399.51 | 3.4 |
| Cheese Omelet | 1 | ITEM | 425.13 | 27.8 | 7.1 | 31.24 | 638.09 | 12.7 |
| Egg, Ham and Cheese Sandwich on English Muffin | 1 | ITEM | 299.31 | 19.33 | 24.66 | 13.15 | 212.46 | 5.28 |
| French Toast, Prepared with 2% Lowfat Milk | 1 | SLICE | 148.85 | 5.01 | 16.25 | 7.02 | 75.4 | 1.77 |
| **SOUPS:** | | | | | | | | |
| Chili con Carne | 0.5 | CUP | 160.36 | 11.20 | 13.56 | 7.05 | 29.80 | 2.50 |
| Vegetable Soup | 1 | CUP | 100.25 | 4.30 | 12.29 | 4.51 | 0.00 | 0.89 |
| Tomato Soup, Condensed, Prepared with Water | 1 | CUP | 85.40 | 2.05 | 16.59 | 1.93 | 0.00 | 0.37 |
| Chicken Broth, Condensed, Prepared with Water | 1 | CUP | 39.04 | 4.93 | 0.93 | 1.39 | 0.00 | 0.39 |
| Chicken Noodle Soup | 1 | CUP | 127.11 | 17.83 | 6.97 | 2.71 | 60.13 | 0.68 |
| Chunky Beef Soup, Canned, Ready to Eat | 1 | CUP | 170.40 | 11.74 | 19.56 | 5.14 | 14.40 | 2.54 |
| Chunky Chicken Soup, Canned, Ready to Eat | 1 | CUP | 178.21 | 12.70 | 17.27 | 6.63 | 30.12 | 1.98 |
| Green Pea Soup, Condensed, Prepared with Water | 1 | CUP | 165.00 | 8.60 | 26.50 | 2.93 | 0.00 | 1.40 |
| Cream of Mushroom Soup, Condensed, Canned | 0.5 | CUP | 129.27 | 2.02 | 9.29 | 9.50 | 1.26 | 2.57 |
| **PIZZA, PASTA & RICE:** | | | | | | | | |
| Fried Rice, with Meat and/or Poultry | 1 | CUP | 329.49 | 11.91 | 41.34 | 12.44 | 102.44 | 2.27 |
| Ravioli, Canned, Meat-Filled with Tomato or Meat Sauce | 1 | CUP | 219.76 | 8.75 | 37.90 | 4.10 | 16.56 | 1.58 |
| Macaroni and Cheese Mix with Prepared Cheese Sauce, Prepared | 0.5 | CUP | 178.96 | 6.76 | 25.01 | 5.57 | 13.76 | 3.19 |
| Spaghetti with Tomato Sauce, Meatless | 1 | CUP | 229.41 | 7.03 | 41.48 | 3.65 | 0.00 | 0.52 |
| Lasagna with Meat and/or Poultry | 1 | PIECE | 369.89 | 21.74 | 37.63 | 14.67 | 54.94 | 7.56 |
| Cheese Pizza, Thick Crust | 1 | SLICE | 202.02 | 7.49 | 27.54 | 6.69 | 7.29 | 2.49 |
| **SALADS:** | | | | | | | | |
| Tuna Salad | 0.5 | CUP | 191.68 | 16.44 | 9.65 | 9.49 | 13.33 | 1.58 |
| Potato Salad | 0.5 | CUP | 178.75 | 3.35 | 13.96 | 10.25 | 85.00 | 1.79 |
| Coleslaw | 0.5 | CUP | 41.40 | 0.77 | 7.45 | 1.57 | 4.80 | 0.23 |
| Chicken Salad | 0.5 | CUP | 208.62 | 14.75 | 1.25 | 15.93 | 53.01 | 2.82 |
| Macaroni Salad | 0.5 | CUP | 134.43 | 2.76 | 21.32 | 4.42 | 3.12 | 0.65 |
| **ENTREES:** | | | | | | | | |
| Hot Dog on Bun | 1 | ITEM | 259.57 | 8.57 | 19.62 | 15.99 | 24.23 | 5.65 |
| Hamburger, Single Patty with Condiments | 1 | ITEM | 272.42 | 12.32 | 34.25 | 9.77 | 29.68 | 3.56 |
| Cheeseburger, Single Patty with Condiments | 1 | ITEM | 294.93 | 15.96 | 26.53 | 14.15 | 37.29 | 6.31 |
| Fish Sticks, Frozen, Heated | 3 | ITEM | 228.48 | 13.15 | 19.95 | 10.27 | 94.08 | 2.65 |
| Taco, Prepared | 1 | ITEM | 369.36 | 20.66 | 26.73 | 20.55 | 56.43 | 11.37 |
| Bean and Cheese Burrito | 1 | ITEM | 188.79 | 7.53 | 27.48 | 5.85 | 13.95 | 3.42 |
| **SIDES:** | | | | | | | | |
| Bread Stuffing, Prepared from Mix | 0.5 | CUP | 178.00 | 3.20 | 21.70 | 8.60 | 0.00 | 1.73 |
| Hashed Brown Potatoes | 0.5 | CUP | 163.02 | 1.89 | 16.63 | 10.85 | 0.00 | 4.24 |
| Mashed Potatoes with Whole Milk | 0.5 | CUP | 80.85 | 2.04 | 18.43 | 0.62 | 2.10 | 0.35 |
| Potato Chips, Salted | 1 | OUNCE | 152.22 | 1.99 | 15.02 | 9.83 | 0.00 | 3.11 |
| Potatoes, Scalloped | 0.5 | CUP | 105.35 | 3.52 | 13.21 | 4.51 | 14.70 | 2.76 |
| Potato Puffs, Frozen, Heated | 0.5 | CUP | 142.08 | 2.14 | 19.51 | 6.87 | 0.00 | 3.26 |
| French Fried Potatoes, Frozen, Heated | 10 | ITEM | 100 | 1.585 | 15.595 | 3.78 | 0 | 0.631 |
| Onion Rings, Frozen, Heated | 7 | ITEM | 284.90 | 3.74 | 26.71 | 18.69 | 0.00 | 6.01 |
| | 3.00 | OUNCE | 117.57 | 1.41 | 14.78 | 6.15 | 0.00 | 0.78 |

| Sodium | Potas | Beta-C | Vit C | Calcium | Iron | Vit E (IU) | Zinc | Diet Fiber | Sugar |
|---|---|---|---|---|---|---|---|---|---|
| 695.65 | 137.02 | | 0.01 | 218.58 | 1.76 | | 1.15 | 1.17 | |
| 425.39 | 171.58 | | 0.3 | 91.76 | 1.36 | | 1.17 | 0 | |
| 1207.35 | 368.8 | | 0.47 | 374.87 | 2.4 | | 2.99 | 0 | |
| 934.29 | 246.97 | | 0.04 | 219.21 | 2.25 | | 2.03 | 1.33 | |
| 311.35 | 87.1 | | 0.19 | 65 | 1.08 | | 0.44 | 1.92 | |
| | | | | | | | | | |
| 655.97 | 381.05 | | 10.59 | 29.86 | 1.90 | | 2.06 | 3.72 | |
| 607.96 | 532.76 | | 11.61 | 43.91 | 1.05 | | 0.54 | 2.12 | |
| 695.40 | 263.52 | 68.30 | 66.37 | 12.20 | 1.76 | | 0.24 | 0.49 | 0.00 |
| 775.92 | 209.84 | 0.00 | 0.00 | 9.76 | 0.51 | | 0.25 | 0.00 | |
| 792.74 | 287.60 | | 3.66 | 23.80 | 1.12 | | 1.39 | 0.99 | |
| 866.40 | 336.00 | | 6.96 | 31.20 | 2.33 | | 2.64 | 1.44 | 2.37 |
| 888.54 | 175.70 | 75.30 | 1.26 | 25.10 | 1.73 | | 1.00 | 1.51 | |
| 917.50 | 190.00 | 20.00 | 1.75 | 27.50 | 1.95 | | 1.71 | 2.75 | 3.29 |
| 868.46 | 84.09 | 0.00 | 1.13 | 32.63 | 0.53 | | 0.59 | 0.38 | |
| | | | | | | | | | |
| 820.98 | 181.66 | | 3.38 | 36.40 | 2.66 | | 1.42 | 1.28 | |
| | | | | | | | | | |
| 1354.15 | 336.54 | | 21.53 | 27.54 | 2.04 | | 1.19 | 1.55 | |
| | | | | | | | | | |
| 392.64 | 54.27 | | 0.02 | 58.38 | 1.25 | | 0.67 | 1.11 | |
| 590.93 | 454.86 | | 11.46 | 38.84 | 2.50 | | 0.80 | 4.07 | |
| 741.32 | 433.88 | | 13.65 | 255.39 | 2.91 | | 3.15 | 2.60 | |
| 423.57 | 123.54 | | 2.60 | 117.58 | 1.79 | | 0.73 | 1.29 | |
| | | | | | | | | | |
| 412.05 | 182.45 | | 2.26 | 17.43 | 1.03 | | 0.57 | 0.00 | |
| 661.25 | 317.50 | | 12.50 | 23.75 | 0.81 | | 0.39 | 1.63 | |
| 13.80 | 108.60 | 132.00 | 19.62 | 27.00 | 0.35 | | 0.12 | 0.90 | |
| 145.10 | 165.30 | | 1.59 | 19.25 | 0.79 | | 1.11 | 0.39 | |
| 480.53 | 58.89 | | 1.12 | 11.24 | 0.89 | | 0.33 | 1.03 | |
| | | | | | | | | | |
| 747.32 | 132.45 | 0.00 | 0.00 | 56.13 | 1.72 | | 1.12 | 0.99 | |
| 534.24 | 251.22 | | 2.23 | 126.14 | 2.71 | | 2.25 | 2.33 | |
| 615.85 | 222.61 | | 1.92 | 110.74 | 2.43 | | 2.09 | | |
| 488.88 | 219.24 | | 0.00 | 16.80 | 0.62 | | 0.55 | 0.00 | 6.70 |
| 801.99 | 473.67 | 62.80 | 2.22 | 220.59 | 2.41 | | 3.93 | | 10.50 |
| 583.11 | 248.31 | 3.16 | 0.84 | 106.95 | 1.14 | | 0.82 | | |
| | | | | | | | | | |
| 543.00 | 74.00 | | 0.00 | 32.00 | 1.09 | | 0.28 | 2.90 | 0.87 |
| 18.72 | 250.38 | 0.00 | 4.45 | 6.24 | 0.63 | | 0.23 | 1.56 | |
| 318.15 | 313.95 | 0.00 | 7.04 | 27.30 | 0.28 | | 0.31 | 2.10 | 0.16 |
| 168.70 | 362.10 | 0.00 | 8.83 | 6.82 | 0.46 | | 0.31 | 1.28 | 4.10 |
| 410.38 | 463.05 | 4.50 | 12.99 | 69.83 | 0.70 | | 0.49 | 2.33 | 0.28 |
| 477.44 | 243.20 | 4.42 | 4.42 | 19.20 | 1.00 | | 0.19 | 2.05 | |
| 15 | 209 | 0 | 5.05 | 4 | 0.62 | | 0.2 | 1.6 | 0.25 |
| 262.50 | 90.30 | 0.32 | 0.98 | 21.70 | 1.18 | | 0.29 | 0.91 | |
| 197.29 | 277.77 | | 8.11 | 5.51 | 0.25 | | 0.23 | 1.42 | |

| FATS | Amount | Portion | Kcal | Protein | Carb | Fat | Chol | Sat Fat | Sodium | Potas |
|---|---|---|---|---|---|---|---|---|---|---|
| Butter | 1 | TBSP | 107.55 | 0.13 | 0.01 | 12.17 | 32.84 | 7.57 | 123.90 | 3.90 |
| Butter, Whipped | 1 | TBSP | 81.72 | 0.10 | 0.01 | 9.25 | 24.96 | 5.76 | 94.22 | 2.96 |
| Margarine, with Unspecified Oils | 1 | TBSP | 101.34 | 0.13 | 0.13 | 11.35 | 0.00 | 2.23 | 133.02 | 5.98 |
| Whipped Margarine | 1 | TBSP | 64.44 | 0.07 | 0.05 | 7.24 | 0.00 | 1.17 | 97.11 | 3.42 |
| Fat Free Margarine-Like Spread, Salted | 1 | TBSP | 4.90 | 0.20 | 0.20 | 0.21 | 0.00 | 0.03 | 90.02 | 0.00 |
| Mayonnaise, with Soybean Oil | 1 | TBSP | 98.91 | 0.15 | 0.37 | 10.96 | 8.14 | 1.63 | 78.44 | 4.69 |
| Low Calorie Mayonnaise | 1 | TBSP | 37.05 | 0.04 | 2.56 | 3.07 | 3.84 | 0.53 | 79.52 | 1.60 |
| Sour Cream Dip | 2 | TBSP | 66.97 | 1.16 | 2.47 | 6.01 | 12.55 | 3.69 | 227.56 | 56.16 |
| *OILS:* | | | | | | | | | | |
| Corn Oil | 1 | TBSP | 120.22 | 0.00 | 0.00 | 13.60 | 0.00 | 1.73 | 0.00 | 0.00 |
| Olive Oil | 1 | TBSP | 119.34 | 0.00 | 0.00 | 13.50 | 0.00 | 1.82 | 0.01 | 0.00 |
| Coconut Oil | 1 | TBSP | 117.23 | 0.00 | 0.00 | 13.60 | 0.00 | 11.76 | 0.00 | 0.00 |
| Peanut Oil | 1.00 | TBSP | 119.34 | 0.00 | 0.00 | 13.50 | 0.00 | 2.28 | 0.02 | 0.00 |
| Soybean Oil, with Soybean and Cottonseed Oil | 1.00 | TBSP | 120.22 | 0.00 | 0.00 | 13.60 | 0.00 | 2.45 | 0.00 | 0.00 |
| Sesame Vegetable Oil | 1.00 | TBSP | 120.22 | 0.00 | 0.00 | 13.60 | 0.00 | 1.93 | 0.00 | 0.00 |
| Canola Oil | 1.00 | TBSP | 120.22 | 0.00 | 0.00 | 13.60 | 0.00 | 0.97 | 0.00 | 0.00 |
| Cottonseed Oil | 1.00 | TBSP | 120.22 | 0.00 | 0.00 | 13.60 | 0.00 | 3.52 | 0.00 | 0.00 |
| Grapeseed Oil | 1.00 | TBSP | 120.22 | 0.00 | 0.00 | 13.60 | 0.00 | 1.31 | 0.00 | 0.00 |
| Soybean Oil | 1.00 | TBSP | 120.22 | 0.00 | 0.00 | 13.60 | 0.00 | 1.96 | 0.00 | 0.00 |
| Flaxseed Oil | 1.00 | TBSP | 114.92 | 0.00 | 0.00 | 13.00 | 0.00 | 1.22 | 0.00 | 0.00 |
| *DRESSING:* | | | | | | | | | | |
| Blue Cheese Salad Dressing | 1 | TBSP | 77.11 | 0.73 | 1.13 | 8.00 | 2.60 | 1.52 | 167.38 | 5.66 |
| French Salad Dressing | 1 | TBSP | 67.03 | 0.09 | 2.73 | 6.40 | 0.00 | 1.48 | 213.72 | 12.32 |
| Italian Salad Dressing | 1 | TBSP | 68.69 | 0.10 | 1.50 | 7.10 | 0.00 | 1.03 | 115.69 | 2.21 |
| Mayonnaise-Type Salad Dressing | 1 | TBSP | 57.28 | 0.13 | 3.51 | 4.91 | 3.82 | 0.72 | 104.49 | 1.32 |
| Thousand Island Salad Dressing | 1 | TBSP | 58.85 | 0.14 | 2.37 | 5.57 | 4.06 | 0.94 | 109.20 | 17.63 |
| Low Calorie Thousand Island Salad Dressing | 2 | TBSP | 48.53 | 0.24 | 4.96 | 3.27 | 4.59 | 0.49 | 306.00 | 34.58 |

| Beta-C | Vit C | Calcium | Iron | Vit E (IU) | Zinc | Diet Fiber | Sugar |
|--------|-------|---------|------|------------|------|------------|-------|
| 12.42 | 0.00 | 3.60 | 0.02 | | 0.01 | 0.00 | 0.00 |
| 9.45 | 0.00 | 2.68 | 0.02 | | 0.01 | 0.00 | 0.00 |
| 12.60 | 0.02 | 4.22 | 0.01 | | 0.00 | 0.00 | 0.00 |
| | 0.01 | 2.34 | 0.00 | | 0.00 | 0.00 | 0.00 |
| | 0.00 | 0.00 | 0.00 | | 0.00 | 0.00 | |
| | 0.00 | 2.48 | 0.07 | | 0.02 | 0.00 | 0.00 |
| 0.00 | 0.00 | 0.00 | 0.00 | | 0.02 | 0.00 | |
| | 0.30 | 35.94 | 0.05 | | 0.09 | 0.25 | |
| | | | | | | | |
| 0.00 | 0.00 | 0.00 | 0.00 | | 0.00 | 0.00 | 0.00 |
| 0.00 | 0.00 | 0.02 | 0.05 | | 0.01 | 0.00 | 0.00 |
| 0.00 | 0.00 | 0.00 | 0.01 | | 0.00 | 0.00 | 0.00 |
| 0.00 | 0.00 | 0.01 | 0.00 | | 0.00 | 0.00 | 0.00 |
| | | | | | | | |
| 0.00 | 0.00 | 0.00 | 0.00 | | 0.00 | 0.00 | 0.00 |
| 0.00 | 0.00 | 0.00 | 0.00 | | 0.00 | 0.00 | 0.00 |
| 0.00 | 0.00 | 0.00 | 0.00 | | 0.00 | 0.00 | 0.00 |
| 0.00 | 0.00 | 0.00 | 0.00 | | 0.00 | 0.00 | 0.00 |
| 0.00 | 0.00 | 0.00 | 0.00 | | 0.00 | 0.00 | 0.00 |
| 0.00 | 0.00 | 0.01 | 0.00 | | 0.00 | 0.00 | 0.00 |
| 0.00 | 0.00 | 0.00 | 0.00 | | 0.00 | 0.00 | 0.00 |
| | | | | | | | |
| | 0.31 | 12.39 | 0.03 | | 0.04 | 0.00 | |
| | 0.00 | 1.72 | 0.06 | | 0.01 | 0.00 | 2.21 |
| | 0.00 | 1.47 | 0.03 | | 0.02 | 0.00 | 0.37 |
| | 0.00 | 2.06 | 0.03 | | 0.03 | 0.00 | |
| | 0.00 | 1.72 | 0.09 | | 0.02 | 0.00 | |
| | | | | | | | |
| | 0.00 | 3.37 | 0.18 | | 0.05 | 0.37 | |

| BEVERAGES | Amount | Portion | Kcal | Protein | Carb | Fat | Chol | Sat Fat |
|---|---|---|---|---|---|---|---|---|
| **JUICE:** | | | | | | | | |
| Apple Juice, Canned | 8 | FL OZ | 116.56 | 0.15 | 28.97 | 0.27 | 0.00 | 0.05 |
| Grapefruit Juice | 8 | FL OZ | 96.33 | 1.24 | 22.72 | 0.25 | 0.00 | 0.04 |
| Orange Juice | 8 | FL OZ | 111.60 | 1.74 | 25.79 | 0.50 | 0.00 | 0.06 |
| Pineapple Juice, Canned | 8 | FL OZ | 140.00 | 0.80 | 34.45 | 0.20 | 0.00 | 0.01 |
| Lemonade, Frozen Concentrate, Prepared with Water | 8 | FL OZ | 99.20 | 0.25 | 26.04 | 0.00 | 0.00 | 0.00 |
| Grape Juice, Unsweetened | 1 | CUP | 154.33 | 1.42 | 37.85 | 0.20 | 0.00 | 0.06 |
| Cranberry Juice Drink with Vitamin C Added | 1 | CUP | 144.21 | 0.00 | 36.43 | 0.25 | 0.00 | 0.02 |
| Fruit Punch Drink Mix, Prepared with Water | 8 | FL OZ | 96.94 | 0.00 | 24.89 | 0.00 | 0.00 | 0.00 |
| Tomato Juice, Canned | 8 | FL OZ | 41.48 | 1.85 | 10.32 | 0.15 | 0.00 | 0.02 |
| Carrot Juice, Canned | 8 | FL OZ | 98.40 | 2.34 | 22.85 | 0.37 | 0.00 | 0.07 |
| Vegetable Juice, Canned | 8 | FL OZ | 45.98 | 1.53 | 11.01 | 0.22 | 0.00 | 0.03 |
| **ALCOHOL:** | | | | | | | | |
| Beer | 12 | FL OZ | 146.12 | 1.07 | 13.19 | 0.00 | 0.00 | 0.00 |
| Light Beer | 12 | FL OZ | 99.12 | 0.71 | 4.60 | 0.00 | 0.00 | 0.00 |
| Distilled Alcohol, 80 Proof | 1 | FL OZ | 64.22 | 0.00 | 0.00 | 0.00 | 0.00 | 0.00 |
| Distilled Alcohol, 86 Proof | 1 | FL OZ | 69.50 | 0.00 | 0.03 | 0.00 | 0.00 | 0.00 |
| Table Wine | 4 | FL OZ | 82.6 | 0.236 | 1.652 | 0 | 0 | 0 |
| **SOFT DRINKS:** | | | | | | | | |
| Club Soda | 12 | FL OZ | 0.00 | 0.00 | 0.00 | 0.00 | 0.00 | 0.00 |
| Cola | 12 | FL OZ | 151.53 | 0.00 | 38.43 | 0.00 | 0.00 | 0.00 |
| Low Calorie Cola | 12 | FL OZ | 3.55 | 0.36 | 0.36 | 0.00 | 0.00 | 0.00 |
| Ginger Ale | 12 | FL OZ | 124.44 | 0.00 | 31.84 | 0.00 | 0.00 | 0.00 |
| Root Beer | 12 | FL OZ | 151.54 | 0.00 | 39.18 | 0.00 | 0.00 | 0.00 |
| **COFFEE/TEA:** | | | | | | | | |
| Coffee, Brewed | 8 | FL OZ | 4.74 | 0.24 | 0.95 | 0.00 | 0.00 | 0.00 |
| Tea, Brewed | 8 | FL OZ | 2.37 | 0.00 | 0.71 | 0.00 | 0.00 | 0.00 |
| Herbal Tea, Prepared with Water | 8 | FL OZ | 2.37 | 0.00 | 0.47 | 0.00 | 0.00 | 0.00 |
| Coffee, Brewed, Decaffeinated | 8 | FL OZ | 4.74 | 0.24 | 0.94 | 0.00 | 0.00 | 0.00 |
| Decaffeinated Tea, Leaf, Unsweetened | 8 | FL OZ | 2.37 | 0.00 | 0.71 | 0.00 | 0.00 | 0.00 |
| **MISC:** | | | | | | | | |
| Tap Water | 8 | FL OZ | 0.00 | 0.00 | 0.00 | 0.00 | 0.00 | 0.00 |
| Soy Milk | 8.00 | FL OZ | 79.20 | 6.60 | 4.34 | 4.58 | 0.00 | 0.51 |

| Sodium | Potas | Beta-C | Vit C | Calcium | Iron | Vit E (IU) | Zinc | Diet Fiber | Sugar |
|---|---|---|---|---|---|---|---|---|---|
| 7.44 | 295.12 | 0.00 | 2.23 | 17.36 | 0.92 | | 0.07 | 0.25 | 27.00 |
| 2.47 | 400.14 | | 93.86 | 22.23 | 0.49 | | 0.12 | 0.25 | 15.50 |
| 2.48 | 496.00 | | 124.00 | 27.28 | 0.50 | | 0.12 | 0.50 | 25.30 |
| 2.50 | 335.00 | 0.00 | 26.75 | 42.50 | 0.65 | | 0.28 | 0.50 | 31.30 |
| 7.44 | 37.20 | | 9.67 | 7.44 | 0.40 | | 0.10 | 0.25 | 22.80 |
| 7.59 | 333.96 | | 0.25 | 22.77 | 0.61 | | 0.13 | 0.25 | |
| 5.06 | 45.54 | 0.00 | 89.56 | 7.59 | 0.38 | | 0.18 | 0.25 | |
| 36.68 | 2.62 | 0.00 | 30.92 | 41.92 | 0.13 | | 0.08 | 0.00 | 9.51 |
| 880.84 | 536.80 | 137.00 | 44.65 | 21.96 | 1.42 | | 0.34 | 0.98 | 8.00 |
| 71.34 | 718.32 | 6334.00 | 20.91 | 59.04 | 1.13 | | 0.44 | 1.97 | |
| 653.40 | 467.06 | 283.00 | 67.03 | 26.62 | 1.02 | | 0.48 | 1.94 | 8.20 |
| | | | | | | | | | |
| 17.82 | 89.10 | 0.00 | 0.00 | 17.82 | 0.11 | | 0.07 | 0.71 | 1.49 |
| 10.62 | 63.72 | 0.00 | 0.00 | 17.70 | 0.14 | | 0.11 | 0.00 | 2.50 |
| 0.28 | 0.56 | 0.00 | 0.00 | 0.00 | 0.01 | | 0.01 | 0.00 | 0.00 |
| 0.28 | 0.56 | 0.00 | 0.00 | 0.00 | 0.01 | | 0.01 | 0.00 | 0.00 |
| 9.44 | 105.02 | 0 | 0 | 9.44 | 0.484 | | 0.083 | 0 | 1.652 |
| | | | | | | | | | |
| 74.59 | 7.10 | 0.00 | 0.00 | 17.76 | 0.04 | | 0.36 | 0.00 | 0.00 |
| 14.78 | 3.69 | 0.00 | 0.00 | 11.08 | 0.11 | | 0.03 | 0.00 | 38.40 |
| 21.31 | 0.00 | 0.00 | 0.00 | 14.21 | 0.11 | | 0.28 | 0.00 | 0.00 |
| 25.62 | 3.66 | 0.00 | 0.00 | 10.98 | 0.66 | | 0.18 | 0.00 | 31.80 |
| 48.05 | 3.70 | 0.00 | 0.00 | 18.48 | 0.19 | | 0.26 | 0.00 | 39.24 |
| | | | | | | | | | |
| 4.74 | 127.98 | 0.00 | 0.00 | 4.74 | 0.12 | | 0.05 | 0.00 | 0.00 |
| 7.10 | 87.62 | 0.00 | 0.00 | 0.00 | 0.05 | | 0.05 | 0.00 | 0.00 |
| 2.37 | 21.31 | 0.00 | 0.00 | 4.74 | 0.19 | | 0.10 | 0.00 | 0.00 |
| 4.74 | 128.00 | 0.00 | 0.00 | 4.74 | 0.12 | | 0.05 | 0.00 | 0.00 |
| 7.11 | 87.69 | 0.00 | 0.00 | 0.00 | 0.05 | | 0.05 | 0.00 | |
| | | | | | | | | | |
| 7.11 | 0.00 | 0.00 | 0.00 | 4.74 | 0.02 | | 0.07 | 0.00 | 0.00 |
| 28.80 | 338.40 | 7.20 | 0.00 | 9.60 | 1.39 | | 0.55 | 3.12 | |

| SWEETS | Amount | Portion | Kcal | Protein | Carb | Fat | Chol | Sat Fat | Sodium | Potas |
|---|---|---|---|---|---|---|---|---|---|---|
| **CAKES & PIES:** | | | | | | | | | | |
| Devil's Food Cake with Chocolate Frosting, Prepared from Mix | 1.00 | SLICE | 235.00 | 3.00 | 40.00 | 8.00 | 37.00 | 3.50 | 181.00 | 90.00 |
| Devil's Food Cupcake with Chocolate Frosting | 1.00 | ITEM | 120.00 | 2.00 | 20.00 | 4.00 | 19.00 | 1.80 | 92.00 | 46.00 |
| White Cake with Frosting | 1.00 | SLICE | 251.92 | 2.84 | 38.76 | 10.23 | 2.79 | 2.79 | 185.92 | 71.30 |
| Carrot Cake with Cream Cheese Frosting, Prepared | 1.00 | SLICE | 484.00 | 5.11 | 52.40 | 29.30 | 59.90 | 5.43 | 273.00 | 124.00 |
| Butter Pound Cake, Ready to Eat | 1.00 | SLICE | 116.40 | 1.65 | 14.64 | 5.97 | 66.30 | 3.47 | 119.40 | 35.70 |
| Yellow Cake, Ready to Eat, with Chocolate Frosting | 1.00 | SLICE | 242.56 | 2.43 | 35.46 | 11.14 | 35.20 | 2.98 | 215.68 | 113.92 |
| Apple Pie, Prepared | 1.00 | SLICE | 410.75 | 3.72 | 57.51 | 19.38 | 0.00 | 4.73 | 327.05 | 122.45 |
| Pumpkin Pie, Prepared | 1.00 | SLICE | 316.20 | 6.98 | 40.92 | 14.42 | 65.10 | 4.92 | 348.75 | 288.30 |
| Chocolate Creme Pie, Ready to Eat | 1.00 | SLICE | 343.52 | 2.94 | 37.97 | 21.92 | 5.65 | 5.61 | 153.68 | 143.51 |
| **BAKED GOODS:** | | | | | | | | | | |
| Fig Bar | 2.00 | ITEM | 111.36 | 1.18 | 22.69 | 2.34 | 0.00 | 0.36 | 112.00 | 66.24 |
| Cinnamon Bun, Frosted | 1.00 | ITEM | 208.56 | 2.77 | 31.12 | 8.40 | 29.12 | 2.09 | 193.80 | 50.91 |
| Brownie, Prepared | 1.00 | ITEM | 111.84 | 1.49 | 12.05 | 6.98 | 17.52 | 1.76 | 82.32 | 42.24 |
| Corn Muffin, Prepared with 2% Lowfat Milk | 1.00 | ITEM | 180.12 | 4.05 | 25.19 | 7.01 | 23.94 | 1.32 | 333.45 | 82.65 |
| Oat Bran Muffin | 1.00 | ITEM | 153.90 | 3.99 | 27.53 | 4.22 | 0.00 | 0.62 | 224.01 | 288.99 |
| Plain Cake Doughnut, Glazed | 1.00 | ITEM | 191.70 | 2.34 | 22.86 | 10.31 | 14.40 | 2.67 | 180.90 | 45.90 |
| **COOKIES:** | | | | | | | | | | |
| Vanilla Sandwich Cookie with Creme Filling | 3.00 | ITEM | 144.90 | 1.35 | 21.63 | 6.00 | 0.00 | 0.89 | 104.70 | 27.30 |
| Chocolate Sandwich Cookie, with Creme Filling | 3.00 | ITEM | 141.60 | 1.41 | 21.09 | 6.18 | 0.00 | 1.10 | 181.20 | 52.50 |
| Butter Cookie, Ready to Eat | 6.00 | ITEM | 140.10 | 1.83 | 20.67 | 5.64 | 35.10 | 3.32 | 105.30 | 33.30 |
| Chocolate Chip Cookie, Prepared with Butter | 2.00 | ITEM | 156.16 | 1.82 | 18.62 | 9.09 | 22.40 | 4.50 | 109.12 | 70.72 |
| Oatmeal Cookie with Raisins, Prepared | 2.00 | ITEM | 130.50 | 1.95 | 20.52 | 4.86 | 9.90 | 0.97 | 161.40 | 71.70 |
| Peanut Butter Cookie, Ready to Eat | 2.00 | ITEM | 143.10 | 2.88 | 17.67 | 7.08 | 0.30 | 1.35 | 124.50 | 50.10 |
| Shortbread Cookie, Ready to Eat | 3.00 | ITEM | 120.48 | 1.46 | 15.48 | 5.78 | 4.80 | 1.47 | 109.20 | 24.00 |
| Granola Bar, with Oats, Sugar, Raisins, Coconut | 1.00 | ITEM | 195.22 | 4.21 | 28.68 | 7.57 | 0.00 | 5.46 | 119.54 | 140.18 |
| Sugar Cookie, Ready to Eat | 2.00 | ITEM | 143.40 | 1.53 | 20.37 | 6.33 | 15.30 | 1.63 | 107.10 | 18.90 |
| **FROZEN DESSERTS:** | | | | | | | | | | |
| Vanilla Ice Cream, Rich | 0.50 | CUP | 178.34 | 2.59 | 16.58 | 11.99 | 45.14 | 7.38 | 41.44 | 117.66 |
| Ice Cream with Cone, Flavor Other Than Chocolate | 1.00 | ITEM | 166.41 | 2.94 | 20.88 | 8.40 | 32.36 | 5.04 | 65.21 | 151.34 |
| Ice Cream Bar, Chocolate Covered | 1.00 | ITEM | 169.33 | 1.66 | 14.36 | 12.51 | 19.47 | 9.59 | 35.55 | 103.57 |
| Ice Cream Sandwich | 1.00 | ITEM | 143.63 | 2.62 | 21.75 | 5.61 | 19.78 | 3.24 | 36.37 | 122.39 |
| Ice Pop (Popsicle), Ready to Eat | 1.00 | ITEM | 42.48 | 0.00 | 11.15 | 0.00 | 0.00 | 0.00 | 7.08 | 2.36 |
| Sherbet, All Flavors | 0.50 | CUP | 133.17 | 1.06 | 29.34 | 1.93 | 4.83 | 1.12 | 44.39 | 92.64 |
| Frozen Yogurt, Fruit Varieties | 0.50 | CUP | 143.51 | 3.39 | 24.41 | 4.07 | 14.69 | 2.63 | 71.19 | 176.28 |
| Vanilla Frozen Yogurt, Soft Serve | 0.50 | CUP | 114.48 | 2.88 | 17.42 | 4.03 | 1.44 | 2.46 | 62.64 | 151.92 |
| **CANDIES:** | | | | | | | | | | |
| Gumdrops | 10.00 | ITEM | 138.96 | 0.00 | 35.60 | 0.00 | 0.00 | 0.00 | 15.84 | 1.80 |
| Hard Candy | 2.00 | PIECE | 47.28 | 0.00 | 11.76 | 0.02 | 0.00 | 0.00 | 4.56 | 0.60 |
| Marshmallows | 4.00 | ITEM | 91.58 | 0.52 | 23.41 | 0.06 | 0.00 | 0.02 | 13.54 | 1.44 |
| Taffy | 3.00 | PIECE | 169.20 | 0.05 | 41.10 | 1.49 | 4.05 | 0.92 | 39.90 | 1.80 |
| Fruit Leather Roll | 1.00 | ITEM | 73.50 | 0.21 | 17.70 | 0.63 | 0.00 | 0.14 | 12.81 | 61.74 |
| Licorice | 1.00 | ITEM | 69.73 | 0.00 | 17.69 | 0.10 | 0.00 | 0.03 | 4.75 | 7.03 |
| Chocolate Pudding, Canned | 0.50 | CUP | 173.57 | 3.52 | 29.75 | 5.22 | 3.92 | 0.93 | 168.35 | 234.90 |
| Milk Chocolate Bar | 1.00 | ITEM | 503.23 | 6.55 | 52.73 | 29.85 | 20.02 | | 83.72 | 413.00 |

| Beta-C | Vit C | Calcium | Iron | Vit E (IU) | Zinc | Diet Fiber | Sugar |
|---|---|---|---|---|---|---|---|
| | 0.00 | 41.00 | 1.40 | | | 1.52 | |
| | 0.00 | 21.00 | 0.70 | | | 0.70 | |
| | 0.00 | 65.07 | 0.63 | | 0.24 | 0.78 | |
| | 1.22 | 27.80 | 1.39 | | 0.54 | 1.33 | |
| | 0.00 | 10.50 | 0.41 | | 0.14 | 0.15 | |
| | 0.00 | 23.68 | 1.33 | | 0.40 | 1.15 | |
| | 2.64 | 10.85 | 1.74 | | 0.29 | | 47.90 |
| | 2.64 | 145.70 | 1.97 | | 0.71 | | |
| 0.00 | 0.00 | 40.68 | 1.21 | | 0.26 | 2.26 | |
| | 0.10 | 20.48 | 0.93 | | 0.13 | 1.47 | |
| | 0.89 | 33.12 | 0.71 | | 0.27 | 1.06 | |
| | 0.07 | 13.68 | 0.44 | | 0.23 | | |
| | 0.17 | 147.63 | 1.49 | | 0.35 | 1.14 | |
| 0.00 | 0.00 | 35.91 | 2.39 | | 1.05 | 2.62 | 2.11 |
| | 0.05 | 27.00 | 0.48 | | 0.20 | 0.68 | 7.61 |
| 0.00 | 0.00 | 8.10 | 0.66 | | 0.12 | 0.45 | |
| 0.00 | 0.00 | 7.80 | 1.16 | | 0.24 | 0.96 | 12.30 |
| | 0.00 | 8.70 | 0.09 | | 0.11 | 0.24 | |
| | 0.06 | 12.16 | 0.79 | | 0.30 | | 8.00 |
| | 0.15 | 30.00 | 0.80 | | 0.26 | | |
| | 0.00 | 10.50 | 0.75 | | 0.16 | 0.54 | |
| | 0.00 | 8.40 | 0.66 | | 0.13 | 0.43 | |
| | 0.43 | 25.80 | 1.37 | | 0.69 | 1.33 | |
| | 0.03 | 6.30 | 0.64 | | 0.13 | 0.23 | |
| | 0.52 | 86.58 | 0.04 | | 0.30 | 0.00 | 13.02 |
| | 0.44 | 95.25 | 0.23 | | 0.54 | 0.13 | |
| | 0.27 | 57.35 | 0.14 | | 0.35 | 0.18 | |
| | 0.27 | 60.02 | 0.28 | | 0.44 | 0.55 | |
| 0.00 | 0.00 | 0.00 | 0.00 | | 0.01 | 0.00 | |
| | 4.15 | 52.11 | 0.14 | | 0.46 | 0.48 | |
| 0.00 | 0.79 | 113.00 | 0.52 | | 0.32 | 0.00 | |
| | 0.58 | 102.96 | 0.22 | | 0.30 | 0.00 | |
| 0.00 | 0.00 | 1.08 | 0.14 | | 0.00 | 0.00 | 23.76 |
| 0.00 | 0.00 | 0.36 | 0.04 | | 0.00 | 0.00 | 7.55 |
| 0.00 | 0.00 | 0.86 | 0.07 | | 0.01 | 0.03 | 16.13 |
| | 0.00 | 1.35 | 0.03 | | 0.02 | 0.00 | 30.00 |
| 0.21 | 1.28 | 6.72 | 0.21 | | 0.04 | 0.76 | |
| 0.00 | 0.00 | 0.57 | 0.21 | | 0.01 | 0.00 | |
| | 2.35 | 117.45 | 0.67 | | 0.55 | 1.31 | |
| 0.00 | 0.82 | 195.65 | 1.09 | | 1.00 | 1.73 | |

| CONDIMENTS | Amount | Portion | Kcal | Protein | Carb | Fat | Chol | Sat Fat | Sodium | Potas |
|---|---|---|---|---|---|---|---|---|---|---|
| **SAUCE/GRAVY:** | | | | | | | | | | |
| Tomato Sauce, Canned | 0.25 | CUP | 18.37 | 0.81 | 4.40 | 0.10 | 0.00 | 0.02 | 370.56 | 227.24 |
| Tomato Paste, Canned | 2 | TBSP | 26.90 | 1.20 | 6.33 | 0.18 | 0.00 | 0.03 | 28.86 | 307.34 |
| Barbecue Sauce | 2 | TBSP | 23.43 | 0.56 | 4.00 | 0.56 | 0.00 | 0.08 | 254.69 | 54.38 |
| Sweet and Sour Sauce | 0.25 | CUP | 73.75 | 0.18 | 18.18 | 0.02 | 0.00 | 0.00 | 195.00 | 16.45 |
| Beef Gravy, Canned | 0.25 | CUP | 30.74 | 2.17 | 2.79 | 1.37 | 1.74 | 0.67 | 324.80 | 46.98 |
| Turkey Gravy, Canned | 0.25 | CUP | 30.60 | 1.56 | 3.06 | 1.26 | 1.20 | 0.37 | 346.20 | 65.40 |
| Steak Sauce, Tomato-Base | 1 | TBSP | 9.67 | 0.25 | 2.45 | 0.04 | 0.00 | 0.01 | 232.63 | 64.26 |
| Pepper Sauce (Tabasco) | 1 | TSP | 0.60 | 0.06 | 0.04 | 0.04 | 0.00 | 0.01 | 31.65 | 6.40 |
| Soy Sauce (Shoyu) | 1 | TBSP | 9.54 | 0.93 | 1.53 | 0.01 | 0.00 | 0.00 | 1028.70 | 32.40 |
| Spaghetti Sauce with Beef/Meat (not Lamb or Mutton) | 0.5 | CUP | 143.82 | 8.12 | 10.60 | 8.37 | 23.28 | 2.26 | 588.69 | 549.98 |
| Cocktail Sauce | 0.25 | CUP | 59.47 | 0.92 | 15.15 | 0.44 | 0.00 | 0.06 | 626.85 | 275.51 |
| Tartar Sauce | 1 | TBSP | 72.07 | 0.14 | 1.98 | 7.25 | 5.42 | 1.07 | 99.75 | 5.11 |
| Cranberry Sauce, Sweetened with Sugar, Canned | 0.25 | CUP | 104.56 | 0.13 | 26.94 | 0.10 | 0.00 | 0.01 | 20.08 | 18.01 |
| **TOPPINGS/ACCOMPANIMENTS:** | | | | | | | | | | |
| Salsa | 2 | TBSP | 4.48 | 0.20 | 1.00 | 0.04 | 0.00 | 0.01 | 69.44 | 34.08 |
| Catsup | 1 | TBSP | 15.60 | 0.22 | 4.09 | 0.05 | 0.00 | 0.01 | 177.90 | 72.15 |
| Yellow Mustard | 1 | TSP | 5.00 | 0.10 | 0.10 | 0.20 | 0.00 | 0.00 | 63.00 | 7.00 |
| Dill Pickle | 1 | ITEM | 11.70 | 0.40 | 2.68 | 0.12 | 0.00 | 0.03 | 833.30 | 75.40 |
| Sweet (Gherkin) Pickle, Small | 1 | ITEM | 17.55 | 0.05 | 4.77 | 0.04 | 0.00 | 0.01 | 140.85 | 4.80 |
| Black Olives, Ripe, Canned | 3 | ITEM | 15.18 | 0.11 | 0.83 | 1.41 | 0.00 | 0.19 | 115.10 | 1.06 |
| Bacon Bits, Meatless | 1 | TBSP | 31.08 | 2.24 | 2.00 | 1.81 | 0.00 | 0.28 | 123.90 | 10.15 |
| Honey | 1 | TSP | 21.28 | 0.02 | 5.77 | 0.00 | 0.00 | 0.00 | 0.28 | 3.64 |
| Jam (Preserves) | 1.00 | TBSP | 48.40 | 0.14 | 12.88 | 0.04 | 0.00 | 0.00 | 8.00 | 15.40 |
| Jelly | 1.00 | TBSP | 51.49 | 0.08 | 13.45 | 0.02 | 0.00 | 0.00 | 6.84 | 12.16 |
| Light Corn Syrup | 1 | TBSP | 56.40 | 0.00 | 15.32 | 0.00 | 0.00 | 0.00 | 24.20 | 0.80 |
| Maple Syrup | 0.25 | CUP | 209.60 | 0.00 | 53.76 | 0.16 | 0.00 | 0.03 | 7.20 | 163.20 |
| Reduced Calorie Pancake Syrup | 0.25 | CUP | 98.40 | 0.00 | 26.58 | 0.00 | 0.00 | 0.00 | 120.00 | 1.80 |
| Chocolate Syrup, Thin | 2 | TBSP | 81.75 | 0.71 | 22.09 | 0.34 | 0.00 | 0.19 | 36.00 | 84.00 |
| Whipped Cream Topping, Pressurized | 2 | TBSP | 19.29 | 0.24 | 0.94 | 1.67 | 5.70 | 1.04 | 9.75 | 11.05 |
| Non-Dairy Dessert Topping, Semi Solid, Frozen | 1 | TBSP | 38.19 | 0.15 | 2.77 | 3.04 | 0.00 | 2.61 | 3.04 | 2.18 |
| White Granulated Sugar | 1 | TSP | 15.48 | 0.00 | 4.00 | 0.00 | 0.00 | 0.00 | 0.04 | 0.08 |
| Brown Sugar | 1 | TSP | 11.28 | 0.00 | 2.92 | 0.00 | 0.00 | 0.00 | 1.17 | 10.38 |
| Powdered Sugar, Sifted | 1 | CUP | 389.00 | 0.00 | 99.50 | 0.10 | 0.00 | 0.02 | 1.00 | 2.00 |

| Beta-C | Vit C | Calcium | Iron | Vit E (IU) | Zinc | Diet Fiber | Sugar |
|---|---|---|---|---|---|---|---|
|  | 8.02 | 8.58 | 0.47 |  | 0.15 | 0.86 | 2.33 |
|  | 13.91 | 11.48 | 0.64 |  | 0.26 | 1.35 | 0.79 |
| 27.25 | 2.19 | 5.94 | 0.28 |  | 0.06 | 0.38 | 3.65 |
| 0.00 | 0.00 | 10.18 | 0.41 |  | 0.02 | 0.16 |  |
| 0.00 | 0.00 | 3.48 | 0.41 |  | 0.58 | 0.23 |  |
| 0.00 | 0.00 | 2.40 | 0.42 |  | 0.48 | 0.24 |  |
|  | 2.58 | 2.80 | 0.14 |  | 0.06 | 0.28 |  |
| 3.05 | 0.23 | 0.60 | 0.06 |  | 0.01 | 0.03 | 0.00 |
| 0.00 | 0.00 | 3.06 | 0.36 |  | 0.07 | 0.14 | 1.53 |
|  | 18.72 | 29.49 | 1.76 |  | 1.72 | 2.10 |  |
|  | 9.64 | 17.03 | 0.41 |  | 0.22 | 1.90 |  |
|  | 0.07 | 3.12 | 0.11 |  | 0.03 | 0.03 |  |
|  | 1.39 | 2.77 | 0.15 |  | 0.04 | 0.69 |  |
|  | 2.22 | 4.80 | 0.16 |  | 0.04 | 0.26 |  |
| 14.40 | 2.27 | 2.85 | 0.11 |  | 0.03 | 0.20 | 1.67 |
| 0.00 | 0.00 | 4.00 | 0.10 |  |  | 0.06 | 0.00 |
| 6.50 | 1.24 | 5.85 | 0.35 |  | 0.09 | 0.78 |  |
| 1.35 | 0.18 | 0.60 | 0.09 |  | 0.01 | 0.17 |  |
| 0.79 | 0.12 | 11.62 | 0.44 |  | 0.03 | 0.42 |  |
| 0.00 | 0.13 | 7.07 | 0.05 |  | 0.13 | 0.71 |  |
| 0.00 | 0.04 | 0.42 | 0.03 |  | 0.02 | 0.01 | 5.73 |
| 0.10 | 1.76 | 4.00 | 0.10 |  | 0.01 | 0.22 | 9.70 |
| 0.19 | 0.17 | 1.52 | 0.04 |  | 0.01 | 0.19 | 7.89 |
| 0.00 | 0.00 | 0.60 | 0.01 |  | 0.00 | 0.00 | 10.20 |
| 0.00 | 0.00 | 53.60 | 0.96 |  | 3.33 | 0.00 | 50.96 |
| 0.00 | 0.00 | 0.60 | 0.01 |  | 0.01 | 0.00 | 23.03 |
|  | 0.08 | 5.25 | 0.79 |  | 0.27 | 0.68 | 22.01 |
|  | 0.00 | 7.58 | 0.00 |  | 0.03 | 0.00 |  |
|  | 0.00 | 0.76 | 0.01 |  | 0.00 | 0.00 |  |
| 0.00 | 0.00 | 0.04 | 0.00 |  | 0.00 | 0.00 | 3.88 |
| 0.00 | 0.00 | 2.55 | 0.06 |  | 0.01 | 0.00 | 2.69 |
| 0.00 | 0.00 | 1.00 | 0.06 |  | 0.03 | 0.00 | 93.00 |

# Index